THYROID AND PARATHYROID DISEASES – NEW INSIGHTS INTO SOME OLD AND SOME NEW ISSUES

Edited by **Laura Sterian Ward**

Thyroid and Parathyroid Diseases – New Insights into Some Old and Some New Issues
Edited by Laura Sterian Ward

Published by InTech
Janeza Trdine 9, 51000 Rijeka, Croatia

Publishing Process Manager Ana Skalamera

Technical Editor Teodora Smiljanic

Cover Designer InTech Design Team

Additional hard copies can be obtained from orders@intechopen.com

Thyroid and Parathyroid Diseases – New Insights into Some Old and Some New Issues,
Edited by Laura Sterian Ward
p. cm.
ISBN 978-953-51-0221-2

For EU product safety concerns:
IN TECH d.o.o., Prolaz Marije Krucifikse Kozulić 3, 51000 Rijeka, Croatia,
info@intechopen.com or visit our website at intechopen.com.

Meet the editor

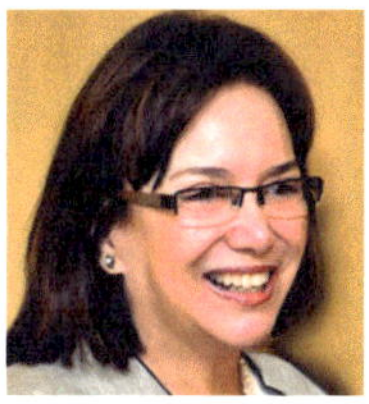

Laura Sterian Ward was born in Bucarest, Romenia, but emigrated to Brasil where she graduated from the Federal University of São Paulo (UNIFESP)) - Escola Paulista de Medicina in 1979. She completed her residency in Clinical Endocrinology in the Hospital São Paulo, in 1981; received her master degree in 1985, and her PhD from the same UNIFESP in 1992. She further specialized in thyroidology. During the years 1995-1997, Prof Ward developed a Post-Doctoral Fellowship program in Cancer Molecular Genetics at the University of Cincinnati, USA, under the supervision of Prof James A. Fagin. She is currently an Associated Professor of Medicine at the State University of Campinas- UNICAMP, in Campinas, São Paulo and the Chief of the Laboratory of Cancer Molecular Genetics in this University. Prof Ward published 109 articles in peer reviewed international medical journals, 91 included in the ISI database where they are quoted more than 800 times. She already was the editor of one book on thyroid diseases and helped editing three other books, wrote 40 books chapters and has participated with more than 200 presentations in both Brazilian and international congresses. In addition, teaching and supervising medical and research students represents an important aspect of her academic activities having supervised the accomplishment of 10 PhD`s and 21 Masters from UNICAMP. In the year 2011, Prof Ward was awarded the Latin American Thyroid Association prize.

Contents

Preface

Thyroid and parathyroid diseases are among the most frequent conditions we have to deal with in a clinical setting. Both nodular and autoimmune diseases affecting these glands have increased remarkably over the past decades. The widespread use of cross-sectional imaging and the introduction of neck ultrasonography have led to a thyroid nodule epidemics and the diagnostic of neck lesions in half of the population. Consequently, many patients with microscopic papillary thyroid cancers of uncertain clinical significance are submitted to surgeries that may, perhaps, be unnecessary. Differentiated thyroid cancer is the fastest-growing cancer in women; it increased 2.4% per year during 1980 to 1997 and 6.5% per year during 1997 to 2006 in the USA according to the National Cancer Institute's Surveillance Epidemiology and End Results (SEER). On the other hand, the refinement of new approaches for surveillance of patients with an established diagnosis of thyroid cancer is leading to the observation that many patients, previously thought to be cured, have evidence of minimal residual disease, a condition with which we still do not know how to manage properly.

Evaluating the Thyroid Gland and its Diseases section includes useful information into the anatomy and functions of the thyroid gland; the thyroid neoplasm and its most challenging type, the papillary thyroid microcarcinoma; the use and technical peculiarities of thyroglobulin dosages and fine aspiration citology. In addition, important articles approach basic aspects of thyroid carcinogenesis, namely growth factors, angiogenesis, and the importance of estrogen signaling on thyrocyte proliferation.

The increase in autoimmune thyroid diseases has been no less remarkable than that of thyroid nodules, but it is more difficult to document. However, there are evidences indicating that around 5-10% of the population suffers from a thyroid dysfunction, mostly autoimmune hypothyroidism. A beautiful article from Dr Cury explains to the reader how our immune system copes with the modifications associated to autoimmune thyroid diseases.

Thyroid disease can affect your mood, causing either anxiety or depression, and a second section of the book, **Psychiatric disturbances associated to thyroid diseases,** groups three very interesting articles approaching the psychiatric disturbances and the psychosocial aspects associated to thyroid diseases.

Finally, the third section, **Treatment of Thyroid and Parathyroid Diseases,** is designed mostly to the young practitioner. In fact, the field of thyroid and parathyroid surgery as well as thyroid diseases treatment modalities have undergone rapid change in the past few years with the advent of new techniques and the appearing of new basic and clinical evidences. Also, we need to understand how hormone analogs may affect our glands and a hole chapter is devoted to this subject.

The burden of thyroid and parathyroid diseases continue to increase and a better knowledge of these pathologies molecular, epidemiological and clinical behavior is essential in order to better manage our patients.

Thyroid and Parathyroid diseases aims to provide meaningful information to the practitioner through the eyes of though leaders in the discipline who have contributed their time and expertise to this effort. It is not a comprehensive textbook but rater a carefully chosen collection of very important topics written and illustrated in a form that hopefully will please all, the clinicians, the surgeons, the pathologists, the radiologists and all the fans of the head and neck diseases.

Hope you enjoy it!

Laura Sterian Ward
Associate Professor of Medicine at the Faculty of Medical Sciences,
State University of Campinas,
Brazil

Part 1

Evaluating the Thyroid Gland and Its Diseases

1

Introduction to Thyroid: Anatomy and Functions

Evren Bursuk
University of İstanbul
Turkey

1. Introduction

As it is known the endocrine system together with the nervous system enables other systems in the body to work in coordination with each other and protect homeostasis using hormones. Hormones secreted by the endocrine system are carried to target organs and cause affect through receptors.

2. Anatomy

The thyroid gland is among the most significant organs of the endocrine system and has a weight of 15-20g. It is soft and its colour is red. This organ is located between the C_5-T_1 vertebrae of columna vertebralis, in front of the trachea and below the larynx. It is comprised of two lobes (lobus dexter and lobus sinister) and the isthmus that binds them together (Figure 1a). Capsule glandular which is internal and external folium of thyroid

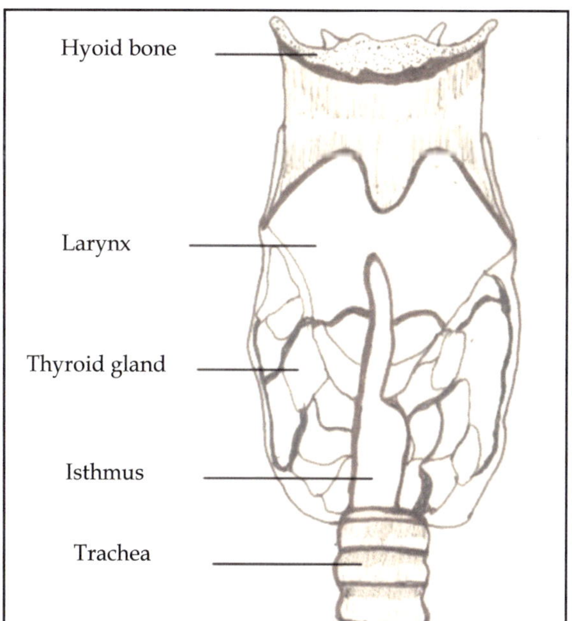

Fig. 1a. The thyroid gland anatomy

gland is wrapped up by a fibrosis capsule named thyroid. The thyroid gland is nourished by a thyroidea superior that is the branch of a. carotis external and a. thyroid inferior that is the branch of a. subclavia (Figure 1b) (Di Lauro & De Felice, 2001; Dillmann, 2004; Ganong, 1997; Guyton & Hall, 1997; Jameson & Weetman, 2010; Larsen et al., 2003; Lo Presti & Singer, 1997; Mc Gregor, 1996; Snell, 1995; Utiger, 1997).

In addition, there are 4 parathyroid glands in total, two of which are on the right and the other two are on the left in between capsule foliums and behind the thyroid gland lobes (Figure 1b) (Di Lauro & De Felice, 2001; Dillmann, 2004; Ganong, 1997; Guyton & Hall, 1997; Jameson & Weetman, 2010; Larsen et al., 2003; Lo Presti & Singer, 1997; Mc Gregor, 1996; Snell, 1995; Utiger, 1997).

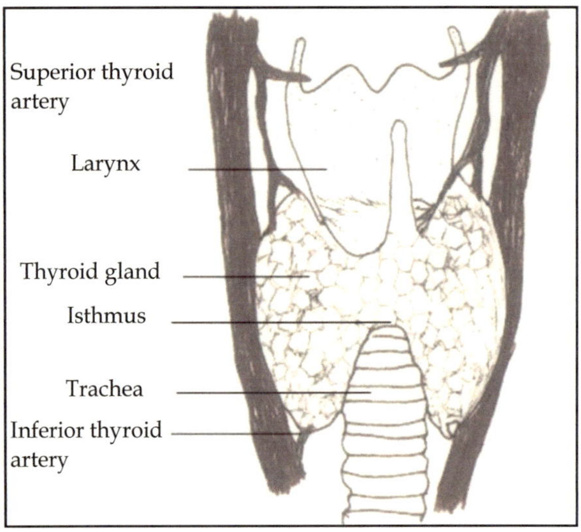

Fig. 1b. The thyroid gland anatomy with vessels

3. Embryology and histology

The thyroid gland develops from the endoderm by a merging of the 4th pouch parts of the primitive pharynx and tongue base median line in the 3rd gestational week. By fetus organifying iodine in the 10th gestational week and commencing the thyroid hormone synthesis, T_4 (L-thyroxin) and TSH (thyroid stimulating hormone) can be measured in fetal blood. Due to the fact that hormone and thyroglobulin syntheses in fetal thyroid increase in the 2nd trimester, an increase is also observed in T_4 and TSH amounts. In addition, the development of fetal hypothalamus contributes to the synthesizing of TRH (thyroid releasing hormone) and thus TSH increase. While TRH can be passed from mother to fetus through the placenta, TSH cannot. T_3 (3,5,3′-triiodo-L-thyronine) begins increasing at the end of the 2nd trimester and is detected in fetal blood in small amounts. Its synthesis increases after birth.

The development of the thyroid gland is controlled by thyroid transcription factor 1 (TTF-1 or its other name NKX2A), thyroid transcription factor 2 (TTF-2 or FKHL15) and paired homeobox-8 (PAX-8). (Di Lauro & De Felice, 2001; Dillmann, 2004; Ganong, 1997; Guyton & Hall, 1997; Jameson & Weetman, 2010; Larsen et al., 2003; Lo Presti & Singer, 1997; Mc Gregor, 1996; Scanlon, 2001; Snell, 1995; Utiger, 1997).

With these transcription factors working together, follicular cell growth and the development of such thyroid-specific proteins as TSH receptor and thyroglobulin is commenced. If any mutation occurs in these transcription factors, babies are born with hypothyroidism due to thyroid agenesis or insufficient secretion of thyroid hormones. (Di Lauro & De Felice, 2001; Dillmann, 2004; Ganong, 1997; Guyton & Hall, 1997; Jameson & Weetman, 2010; Larsen et al., 2003; Lo Presti & Singer, 1997; Mc Gregor, 1996; Scanlon, 2001; Snell, 1995; Utiger, 1997).

The fundamental functional unit of the thyroid gland is the follicle cells and their diameter is in the range of 100-300 μm. Follicle cells in the thyroid gland create a lumen, and there exists a protein named thyroglobulin that they synthesize in the colloid in this lumen (Figure 2a-b). The apical part of these follicle cells make contact with colloidal lumen and its basal part with blood circulation through rich capillaries. Thus, thyroid hormones easily pass into circulation and can reach target tissues. Parafollicular-c cells secreting a hormone called calcitonin that affects the calcium metabolism also exist in this gland (Di Lauro & De

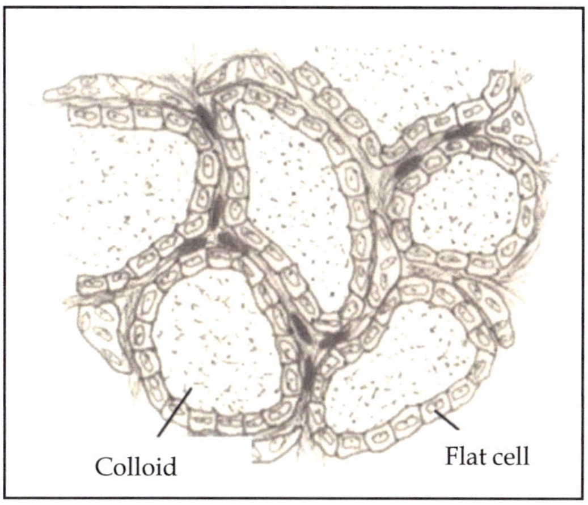

Fig. 2a. Thyroid follicule cell in the inactive state

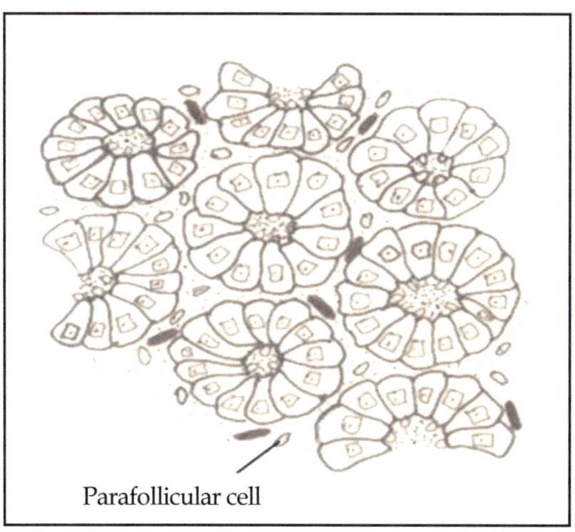

Fig. 2b. Thyroid follicule cell in the active state

Felice, 2001; Dillmann, 2004; Ganong, 1997; Guyton & Hall, 1997; Jameson & Weetman, 2010; Larsen et al., 2003; Lo Presti & Singer, 1997; Mc Gregor, 1996; Scanlon, 2001; Snell, 1995; Utiger, 1997).

4. Physiology

The thyroid gland synthesizes and secretes T_3 and T_4 hormones and these hormones play an important role in the functioning of the body.

4.1 Iodine metabolism

Chemicals in the organism are divided into two as organic and inorganic according to their carbon contents. Organic compounds always contain carbon and have covalent bonds. Carbohydrates, fats, proteins, nucleic acids, enzymes, and adenosine triphosphate (ATP) are the organic compounds. Inorganic compounds have simple structures and do not contain carbons except for carbon dioxide (CO_2) and bicarbonate ion (HCO_3^{-1}). They contain ionic and covalent bonds in their structures. Water, acid, base, salt, and minerals are the inorganic forms. Iodine that is a trace element important for life is among these minerals and is the fundamental substance for thyroid hormones (T_3 and T_4) synthesis. Iodine exists in 3 forms in the circulation. The first one is inorganic iodine (I^-) and is about 2-10 μg/L. Secondly, it exists sparingly in organic compounds before going into the thyroid hormone structure. And the third is the most important one and it is present as bound to protein in thyroid hormones (35-80 μg/L). About 59% and 65%, respectively, of the molecular weights of T_3 and T_4 hormones are comprised of iodine. This accounts for 30% of iodine in the body. The remaining iodine (approximately 70%) exists in a way disseminated to other tissues such as mammary glands, eyes, gastric mucosa, cervix, and salivary glands, and it bears great importance for the functioning of these tissues (Di Lauro & De Felice, 2001; Dillmann, 2004; Ganong, 1997; Guyton & Hall, 1997; Jameson & Weetman, 2010; Larsen et al., 2003; Lo Presti & Singer, 1997; Mc Gregor, 1996; Reed & Pangaro, 1995; Utiger, 1997).

The daily intake is recommended by the United States Institute of Medicine as in the range of 110-130 μg for babies up to 12 months, 150 μg for adults, 220 μg for pregnant women, and 290 μg for women in lactation (Di Lauro & De Felice, 2001; Dillmann, 2004; Ganong, 1997; Guyton & Hall, 1997; Jameson & Weetman, 2010; Larsen et al., 2003; Lo Presti & Singer, 1997; Mc Gregor, 1996; Reed & Pangaro, 1995; Utiger, 1997).

Iodine is taken into the body oral. Among the foods that contain iodine are seafood, iodine-rich vegetables grown in soil, and iodized salt. For this reason, iodine intake geographically differs in the world. Places that are seen predominantly to have iodine deficiency are icy mountainous areas and daily iodine intake in these places is less than 25 μg. Hence, diseases due to iodine deficiency are more common in these geographies. Cretinism in which mental retardation is significant was first identified in the Western Alps (Di Lauro & De Felice, 2001; Dillmann, 2004; Ganong, 1997; Guyton & Hall, 1997; Jameson & Weetman, 2010; Larsen et al., 2003; Lo Presti & Singer, 1997; Mc Gregor, 1996; Reed & Pangaro, 1995 Utiger, 1997).

4.2 Thyroid hormone synthesis

Iodine absorbed from the gastrointestinal system immediately diffuses in extracellular fluid. T_3 and T_4 hormones are fundamentally formed by the addition of iodine to tyrosine aminoacids. While the most synthesized hormone in thyroid gland is T_4, the most efficient hormone is T_3. (Dillmann, 2004; Dunn, 2001; Ganong, 1997; Guyton & Hall, 1997; Jameson & Weetman, 2010; Larsen et al., 2003; Lo Presti & Singer, 1997; Mc Gregor, 1996; Reed & Pangaro, 1995; Utiger, 1997). Basely, thyroid hormone synthesis occurs in 4 stages:

1st stage is the obtaining of iodine by active transport to thyroid follicle cells by utilizing Na^+/I^- symporter pump. Starting and acceleration of this transport is under the control of TSH. Organification increases as the iodine concentration of the cell rises, however, this pump slows down and stops after a point. For this reason, it is believed that a concentration-dependent autocontrol mechanism exists at this level. This stage of the synthesis that is the iodine transport can be inhibited by single-value anions such as perchlorate, pertechnetate, and thiocyanate. Pertechnetate (99mm) is also used in thyroid gland imaging due to its characteristic of being radioactive (Dillmann, 2004; Dunn, 2001; Ganong, 1997; Guyton & Hall, 1997; Jameson & Weetman, 2010; Larsen et al., 2003; Lo Presti & Singer, 1997; Mc Gregor, 1996; Reed & Pangaro, 1995; Utiger, 1997).

2nd stage is oxidation of iodine by NADPH dependent thyroperoxidase enzyme in the presence of H_2O_2 which, at this stage, occurs in follicular lumen. The drugs propylthiouracil and methimazole inhibit this step (Dillmann, 2004; Dunn, 2001; Ganong, 1997; Guyton & Hall, 1997; Jameson & Weetman, 2010; Larsen et al., 2003; Lo Presti & Singer, 1997; Mc Gregor, 1996; Reed & Pangaro, 1995; Utiger, 1997).

3rd stage is the binding of oxidized iodine with thyroglobulin tyrosine residues. This is called iodization of tyrosine or organification. Thus, monoiodotyrosine (MIT) or diiodotyrosine (DIT) is synthesized. These are the inactive thyroid hormone forms (Figure 3) (Dillmann, 2004; Dunn, 2001; Ganong, 1997; Guyton & Hall, 1997; Jameson & Weetman, 2010; Larsen et al., 2003; Lo Presti & Singer, 1997; Mc Gregor, 1996; Reed & Pangaro, 1995; Utiger, 1997).

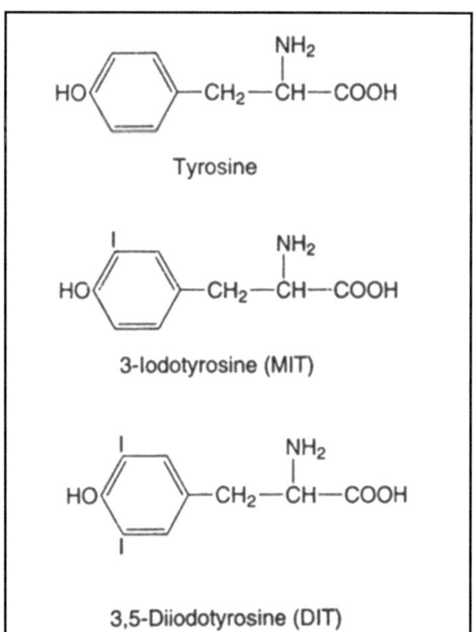

Fig. 3. Chemical structures of tyrosine, monoiodothyronine, and diiodothyronine

4th *stage* is the coupling and T_3 and T_4 are synthesized from MIT and DIT (Figure 4).

$$\text{MIT+DIT} \rightarrow \text{T}_3 \tag{1}$$

$$\text{DIT+DIT} \rightarrow \text{T}_4 \tag{2}$$

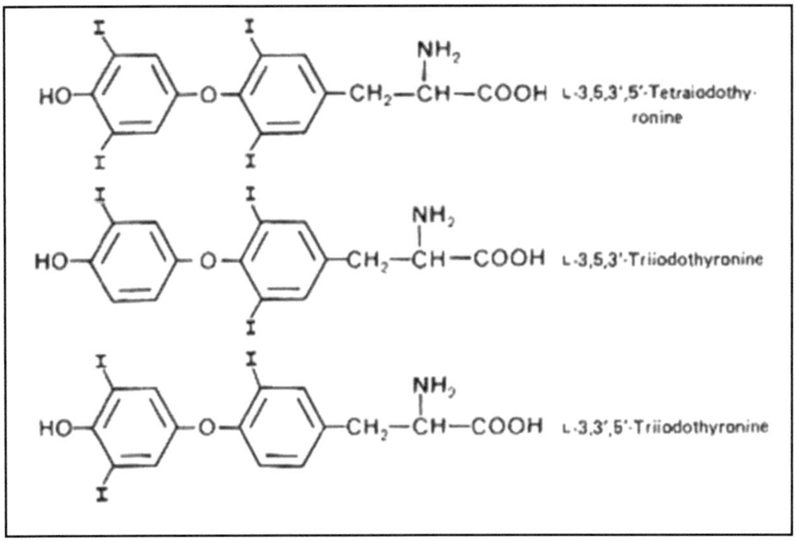

Fig. 4. Chemical structures of triiodothyronine, thyroxin, and revers T_3

In addition to synthesizing this way, the T_3 hormone is also created by the metabolization of T_4.

Almost the entire colloid found in each thyroid follicle lumen is thyroglobulin. Thyroglobulin that contains 70% of thyroid protein content is a glycoprotein with a molecular weight of 660 kDa. Each thryoglobulin molecule has 70 tyrosine aminoacids and contains 6 MIT, 4 DIT, 2 T_4, and 0.2 T_3 residues. Thyroglobulin synthesis is TSH-dependent and occurs in the granulose endoplasmic reticulum of the follicle cells of the thyroid gland. The synthesized thyroglobulin is transported to the apical section of the cell and passes to the follicular lumen through exocytose, and then joins thyroid hormone synthesis (Dillmann, 2004; Dunn, 2001; Ganong, 1997; Guyton & Hall, 1997; Jameson & Weetman, 2010; Larsen et al., 2003; Lo Presti & Singer, 1997; Mc Gregor, 1996; Reed & Pangaro, 1995; Utiger, 1997).

4.3 Thyroid hormone secretion

Thyroid hormones are stocked in the colloid of follicle cells lumen in a manner bound to thyroglobulin. With TSH secretion, apical microvillus count increases and colloid droplet is caught by microtubules and taken back to the apex of the follicular cell through pinocytosis. Lysosomes approach these colloidal pinocytic vesicles containing thyroglobulin and thyroid hormones. These vesicles bind with lysosomes and form fagolysosomes. Lysosomal proteases are activated while these fagolysosomes move towards the basal cell, and thus, thyroglobulin is hydrolyzed. Tyrosine formed as a result of this reaction is excreted by T_3

and T_4 facilitated diffusion (Dillmann, 2004; Dunn, 2001; Ganong, 1997; Guyton & Hall, 1997; Jameson & Weetman, 2010; Larsen et al., 2003; Lo Presti & Singer, 1997; Mc Gregor, 1996; Reed & Pangaro, 1995; Utiger, 1997).

Not all hormones separated from thyroglobulin can pass to the blood. Such iodotyronines as MIT and DIT cannot leave the cell and are reused as deiodonized. In addition, T_3 is formed from a certain amount of T_4 again by deiodonization. These reactions occur in the thyroid follicular cell and the enzyme catalyzing these reactions, in other words, deiodinizations is dehalogenase. Through this deiodinization, about 50% of iodine in the thyroglobulin structure is taken back and can be reused. Iodine deficiency in individuals lacking this enzyme, and correspondingly, hypothyroid goiter is observed. Such patients are given iodine replacement treatment (Dillmann, 2004; Dunn, 2001; Ganong, 1997; Guyton & Hall, 1997; Jameson & Weetman, 2010; Larsen et al., 2003; Lo Presti & Singer, 1997; Mc Gregor, 1996; Reed & Pangaro, 1995; Utiger, 1997).

4.4 Thyroid hormone transport

When thyroid hormones pass into circulation, all become inactive by reversibly binding to carrier proteins that are synthesized in the liver. While those being bound to proteins prevent a vast amount of hormones to be excreted in the urine, it also acts as a depository. Thus, free, in other words, active hormone exists in blood only as much as is needed. The main carrier proteins are thyroxin-binding globulin (TBG), thyroxin-binding prealbumin (transthyretin, TTR) and serum albumin (Table 1) (Benvenga, 2005; Dillmann, 2004; Dunn, 2001; Ganong, 1997; Guyton & Hall, 1997; Jameson & Weetman, 2010; Larsen et al., 2003; Lo Presti & Singer, 1997; Mc Gregor, 1996; Reed & Pangaro, 1995; Utiger, 1997).

TBG is the most bound protein by thyroid hormones. Its molecular weight is 54 kDa and is has the least concentration among others in circulations. The hormone that binds to this protein the most is T_4 and is about 75% of T_4 hormone. This is responsible for the diffusion of T_4 hormone in extracellular fluid in large amounts. However, T_3 is bound in fewer amounts. While TBG rise increases total T_3 and total T_4, it does not affect free T_3 and T_4 (Benvenga, 2005; Dillmann, 2004; Dunn, 2001; Ganong, 1997; Guyton & Hall, 1997; Jameson & Weetman, 2010; Larsen et al., 2003; Lo Presti & Singer, 1997; Mc Gregor, 1996; Reed & Pangaro, 1995; Utiger, 1997).

And TTR has a weight of 55kDa and has a lower rate of binding although its plasma concentration is less than TBG, and this value is more or less around 1/100 (Benvenga, 2005; Dillmann, 2004; Dunn, 2001; Ganong, 1997; Guyton & Hall, 1997; Jameson & Weetman, 2010; Larsen et al., 2003; Lo Presti & Singer, 1997; Mc Gregor, 1996; Reed & Pangaro, 1995; Utiger, 1997).

Serum albumin is a protein with a molecule weight of 65kDa and has a lower rate of binding even though its plasma concentration is the highest (Benvenga, 2005; Dillmann, 2004; Dunn, 2001; Ganong, 1997; Guyton & Hall, 1997; Jameson & Weetman, 2010; Larsen et al., 2003; Lo Presti & Singer, 1997; Mc Gregor, 1996; Reed & Pangaro, 1995; Utiger, 1997).

Due to the fact that T_3 binds to fewer proteins, it is more active in intracellular region. While they become free when needed because of the fact that the affinity of carrier proteins is more to T_4, the half-life of T_4 is about six days, whereas the half-life of T_3 is less than one day. T_3 is more active since T_4 binds to cytoplasmic proteins when they enter the cell are going to affect (Benvenga, 2005; Dillmann, 2004; Dunn, 2001; Ganong, 1997; Guyton & Hall, 1997; Jameson & Weetman, 2010; Larsen et al., 2003; Lo Presti & Singer, 1997; Mc Gregor, 1996; Reed & Pangaro, 1995; Utiger, 1997).

Proteins	Molecular weight (kDa)	Plasma concentration	Levels of binding
thyroxin-binding (TBG)	54	Lowest	Highest
thyroxin-binding prealbumin (TTR)	55	Higher	Lower
Albumin	65	Highest	Lowest

Table 1. Comparison of the binding of thyroid hormones to carrier proteins

4.5 Thyroid hormone metabolism

A 100 µg thyroid hormone is secreted from the thyroid gland and most of these hormones are T_4. About 40% of T_4 turn into T_3 which is 3 times stronger in periphery, especially in the liver and kidney with deiodinase enzymes (Dillmann, 2004; Dunn, 2001; Ganong, 1997; Guyton & Hall, 1997; Jameson & Weetman, 2010; Larsen et al., 2003; Lo Presti & Singer, 1997; Mc Gregor, 1996; Reed & Pangaro, 1995; Utiger, 1997).

Metabolically, in order for active T_3 to form, deiodination needs to occur in region 5′ of tyrosine. Instead, if it occurs in the 5th atom of inner circle, metabolically inactive reverse triiodothyronine (rT_3) is formed. Three types of enzymes that are Selenoenzyme 5′-deiodinase type I (5′-DI), the type II5′ iodothyronine deiodinase (5′-DII) and the 5, or inner circle deiodinase type III (5-DIII) catalyze these deiodinations (Dillmann, 2004; Dunn, 2001; Ganong, 1997; Guyton & Hall, 1997; Jameson & Weetman, 2010; Larsen et al., 2003; Lo Presti & Singer, 1997; Mc Gregor, 1996; Reed & Pangaro, 1995; Utiger, 1997).

5′-DI enzyme is especially found in the liver, kidneys, and thyroid, and 5′-DII enzyme exists in the brain, hypophysis, placenta, and keratinocytes. 5′-DIII is found in the brain, placenta, and epidermis. Both 5′-DI and 5′DII enzymes allow T_4 to transform into active T_3; but with one difference, that is, while 5′- DI enzyme provides the formed T_3 to plasma, T_3 formed by 5′-DII enzyme stays in the tissue and regulates local concentration. This enzyme is regulated by increases and decreases in thyroid hormones. For instance, hyperthyroidism inhibits enzyme and blocks the transformation from T_4 to T_3 in such tissues as the brain and hypophsis. Transformation from T_4 to T_3 is affected by such changes in the organism as hunger, systemic disease, acute stress, iodine contrating agents, and drugs such as propiltiourasil, propranolol, amiodaron, and glicocortikoid, but is not affected by metrmazol. 5′-DIII enzyme transforms T_4 into metabolically inactive reverse T_3 (rT_3) (Figure 5) (Dillmann, 2004; Dunn, 2001; Ganong, 1997; Guyton & Hall, 1997; Jameson & Weetman, 2010; Larsen et al., 2003; Lo Presti & Singer, 1997; Mc Gregor, 1996; Reed & Pangaro, 1995; Utiger, 1997). As mentioned earlier, 40% of T_4 is used for the formation of T_3. This constitutes 90% of T_3. Only 10% of T_3 is formed directly. Also, 40% of T_4 is used for the formation of reverse T_3 (rT_3). The remaining 20% is excreted with urine or feces.

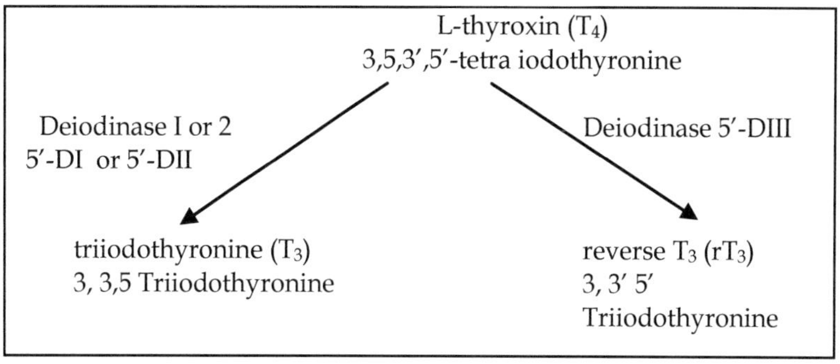

Fig. 5. Effects of deiodinase enzymes

4.6 Controlling the thyroid hormone synthesis and secretion

Synthesis and secretions need to be kept at a certain level in order for the liveliness of thyroid hormones to be maintained. In this respect, the most important mechanism in controlling the synthesis and secretion of thyroid hormones is the hypothalamus-hypophysis-thyroid axis. Another one is the autocontrol mechanism that is dependent on iodine concentration as noted earlier (Dillmann, 2004; Dunn, 2001; Ganong, 1997; Guyton & Hall, 1997; Jameson & Weetman, 2010; Larsen et al., 2003; Lo Presti & Singer, 1997; Mc Gregor, 1996; Reed & Pangaro, 1995; Santiseban, 2005; Utiger, 1997).

4.6.1 Hypothalamus-hypophysis-thyroid axe

Hormone synthesis and secretion of the thyroid gland is under the strict control of this axis. This event begins with TRH synthesis in the hypothalamus. TRH is carried from the hypothalamus to the hypophysis through portal circulation, and TSH hormone is secreted here following the interaction with TRH receptors in the hypophysis front lobe. TSH is then transferred by blood and stimulates the thyroid gland, and thus, thyroid hormone synthesis and secretion begins. However, if thyroid hormone and synthesis is too large an amount, the feedback system is activated and TSH and TRH are suppressed (Figure 6) (Dillmann, 2004, Dunn, 2001; Ganong, 1997; Guyton & Hall, 1997; Jameson & Weetman, 2010; Larsen et al., 2003; Lo Presti & Singer, 1997; Mc Gregor, 1996; Reed & Pangaro, 1995; Santiseban, 2005; Scanlon, 2001; Utiger, 1997).

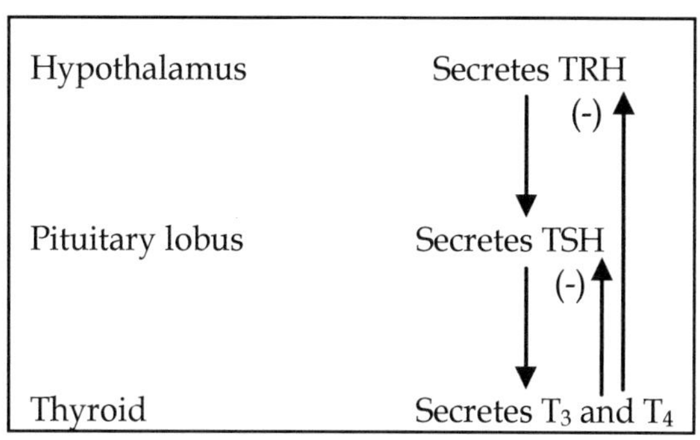

Fig. 6. Controlling of thyroid hormone secretion by the hypothalamus-hypothyroidism-thyroid axis

The thyrotrophin-releasing hormone (TRH) is a tripeptide synthesized in periventricular nucleus in the hypothalamus. The structure of TRH formed by the repetition of -Glu-H.5-Pro-Gly- series 6 times in the beginning turns into pyroglutamyl histidylprolinamide at the end of synthesis. As noted earlier, TRH is carried to the front hypophysis through hypophyseal portal system and provides the secretion of TSH from thyrotrope cells (Dillmann, 2004; Dunn, 2001; Ganong, 1997; Guyton & Hall, 1997; Jameson & Weetman, 2010; Larsen et al., 2003; Lo Presti & Singer, 1997; Mc Gregor, 1996; Reed & Pangaro, 1995; Santiseban, 2005; Scanlon, 2001; Utiger, 1997).

There are receptors specific to TRH on the surfaces of these cells. When TRH makes contact with these receptors, Gq protein is activated, and it then activates the phosphalipase C enzyme, fractionates membrane phospholipids and forms diacylglycerol (DAG) and inositole triphosphate (IP_3). These are secondary mesengers and cause the secretion of Ca^{+2} via IP_3 from endoplasmic reticulum, and DAG activates protein kinase C. The effect of TRH on TSH is provided through these secondary messengers (Dillmann, 2004; Dunn, 2001; Ganong, 1997; Guyton & Hall, 1997; Jameson & Weetman, 2010; Larsen et al., 2003; Lo Presti & Singer, 1997; Mc Gregor, 1996; Reed & Pangaro, 1995; Santiseban, 2005; Scanlon, 2001; Utiger, 1997).

TRH also increases the secretions of growth hormone (GH), follicle stimulating hormone (FSH), and prolactin (PRL). While the TRH secretion is increased by noradrenaline, somatostatin and serotonin inhibits it. (Dillmann, 2004; Dunn, 2001; Ganong, 1997; Guyton & Hall, 1997; Jameson & Weetman, 2010; Larsen et al., 2003; Lo Presti & Singer, 1997; Mc Gregor, 1996; Reed & Pangaro, 1995; Santiseban, 2005; Scanlon, 2001; Utiger, 1997).

The thyrotropin-stimulating hormone (TSH) is a hormone that has a glycoprotein structure comprised of α and β subunits and synthesized in 5% basophilic thyrotrope cells of frontal hypophysis. α subunit is almost the same as that found in such hormones as human chorionic gonadotropin (HCG), luteinizing hormone (LH), and follicle stimulating hormone (FSH). It is believed that the task of this subunit is the stimulation of adenilate cyclase that provides the formation of cAMP secondary precursor. β subunit is completely different to other hormones and is related with receptor specificity. Therefore, TSH is active when it possesses both subunits (Dillmann, 2004; Dunn, 2001; Ganong, 1997; Guyton & Hall, 1997; Jameson & Weetman, 2010; Larsen et al., 2003; Lo Presti & Singer, 1997; Mc Gregor, 1996; Reed & Pangaro, 1995; Santiseban, 2005; Scanlon, 2001; Utiger, 1997).

TSH activates Gs protein when it merges with the receptor in the membrane of thyroid gland follicle cell, and thus, the adenilat cyclase enzyme is activated as well. When this enzyme becomes activated, it increases the secondary messenger cAMP. Along with stimulating protein kinase A enzymes, it causes the development of thyroid follicular cell and the synthesis of thyroid hormone (Dillmann, 2004; Dunn, 2001; Ganong, 1997; Guyton & Hall, 1997; Jameson & Weetman, 2010; Larsen et al., 2003; Lo Presti & Singer, 1997; Mc Gregor, 1996; Reed & Pangaro, 1995; Santiseban, 2005; Scanlon, 2001; Utiger, 1997).

TSH is metabolized in kidneys and liver. It is released as pulsatile and demonstrates circadian rhythm, which means that the secretion begins at night, reaches a maximum at midnight, and decreases all day long (Dillmann, 2004; Dunn, 2001; Ganong, 1997; Guyton & Hall, 1997; Jameson & Weetman, 2010; Larsen et al., 2003; Lo Presti & Singer, 1997; Mc Gregor, 1996; Reed & Pangaro, 1995; Santiseban, 2005; Scanlon, 2001; Utiger, 1997).

The effects of TSH may be divided into three.

a. **Effects occurring within minutes**;
- Binding of iodine,
- T_3 and T_4 hormone synthesis
- Secretion of thyroglobulin into colloid
- Taking colloid back into the cell with endocytos,

b. **Effects occurring within hours**;
- Trapping iodine into the cell by active transport
- Increase in blood flow

c. **Chronic effects**,
- Hypertrophy and hyperplasia occurring in cells
- Gland weight increases.

Despite these effects, TSH does not affect the transformation from T_4 to T_3 in the periphery.

Although TSH secretion is stimulated by TRH and estradiol, it is inhibited by somatostatine, dopamine, T_3, T_4, and glucocorticoids. While α 1 adrenergics demonstrates inhibiting effects, α_2 adrenergics are stimulators (Dillmann, 2004; Dunn, 2001; Ganong, 1997; Guyton & Hall, 1997; Jameson & Weetman, 2010; Larsen et al., 2003; Lo Presti & Singer, 1997; Mc Gregor, 1996; Reed & Pangaro, 1995; Santiseban, 2005; Scanlon, 2001; Utiger, 1997).

4.6.2 Autoregulation of the thyroid

Changes in iodine concentrations in follicular cells of thyroid gland affect the iodine transport and form an autoregulation (Dillmann, 2004; Dunn, 2001; Ganong, 1997; Guyton & Hall, 1997; Jameson & Weetman, 2010; Larsen et al., 2003; Lo Presti & Singer, 1997; Mc Gregor, 1996; Reed & Pangaro, 1995; Santiseban, 2005; Scanlon, 2001; Utiger, 1997). Thyroid hormone synthesis is inhibited as the iodine amount increases in follicles, however, synthesis increases as the amount decreases. Wolf Chaikoff effect in which excessive iodine stops the thyroid hormone synthesis may also be mentioned. This effect is especially observed when individuals with hyperthyroidism take antithyroid along with iodine and become euthyroid (Dillmann, 2004; Dunn, 2001; Ganong, 1997; Guyton & Hall, 1997; Jameson & Weetman, 2010; Larsen et al., 2003; Lo Presti & Singer, 1997; Mc Gregor, 1996; Reed & Pangaro, 1995; Santiseban, 2005; Scanlon, 2001; Utiger, 1997).

In addition, the sensitivity of the thyroid gland also increases through a development of a response to TSH, although TSH does not have a stimulating effect in iodine deficiency. Along with the increase in sensitivity, follicular cells in the gland reach hypertrophy and hyperplasia, and increase the weight of the gland and create goiter. The effects of TSH decrease as the response to TSH decreases with the rise in iodine (Dillmann, 2004; Dunn, 2001; Ganong, 1997; Guyton & Hall, 1997; Jameson & Weetman, 2010; Larsen et al., 2003; Lo Presti & Singer, 1997; Mc Gregor, 1996; Reed & Pangaro, 1995; Santiseban, 2005; Scanlon, 2001; Utiger, 1997). In this case, all of the effects, such as binding of iodine, thyroid hormone synthesis, secretion of thyroglobulin into colloid, taking colloid back to cell by endocytosis, entrapment of iodine, and cell hypertrophy are decreased. However, blood flow to the thyroid glands is reduced. Iodine supplement before thyroid surgery is for the purpose of reducing the blood flow in the thyroid gland. (Dillmann, 2004; Dunn,

2001; Ganong, 1997; Guyton & Hall, 1997; Jameson & Weetman, 2010; Larsen et al., 2003; Lo Presti & Singer, 1997; Mc Gregor, 1996; Reed & Pangaro, 1995; Santiseban, 2005; Scanlon, 2001; Utiger, 1997).

4.7 Occurrence of the thyroid hormone effect

Thyroid hormone receptors exist within the cell. Most of these receptors are in the nucleus and show more affinity to T_3. Due to the fact that T_4 binds more to carrier proteins and exists more in extracellular region, it passes inside the cell, in other words, intracellular amount of T_4 is lesser. When they pass to the intracellular section, very few of them are free for receptors after they are bound to proteins. However, T_3 already exists more in intracellular section due to it binding to fewer amount of carrier proteins and receptors show more affinity to T_3 due to being free. As a result, T_3 is 3-8 times more potent compared to T_4. The reason for this difference in effect is that T_4 transforms into T_3 while T_4 exists in high amounts; the actual efficient one is T_3 (Dillmann, 2004; Dunn, 2001; Ganong, 1997; Guyton & Hall, 1997; Jameson & Weetman, 2010; Larsen et al., 2003; Lo Presti & Singer, 1997; Mc Gregor, 1996; Reed & Pangaro, 1995; Utiger, 1997; Usala, 1995).

Thyroid hormones easily pass through the cell membrane due to being lipid soluble and T_3 immediately binds to thyroid hormone receptor in nucleus. Thyroid hormone receptors are of two types as α (TR α) and β (TRβ). Although these receptors generally exist in all tissues, they differ in effects. While TR α is more efficient in the brain, kidneys, heart, muscles and gonads, TRβ is more efficient in liver and hypophysis. TR α and β are bind to a special DNA sequence that has thyroid response elements (TRE_s). Receptors bind and activate by retinoic acid X (RXR_s) receptors. They either stimulate transcription or inhibit it due to regulatory mechanisms in the target gene. When the transcription starts, various mRNAs are synthesized, and various proteins are synthesized by going through translation in ribosomes that are present in cell cytoplasm. Also, enzymes in the protein structure are synthesized and some of these play an active role in the formation of thyroid hormone effects (Dillmann, 2004; Dunn, 2001; Ganong, 1997; Guyton & Hall, 1997; Jameson & Weetman, 2010; Larsen et al., 2003; Lo Presti & Singer, 1997; Mc Gregor, 1996; Reed & Pangaro, 1995; Utiger, 1997; Usala, 1995).

4.8 Effects of thyroid hormones

The effects of thyroid hormones are varying. It can be divided into 4 as cellular level, and effects on growth, metabolism, and on systems.

4.8.1 Effects of thyroid hormones at the cellular level

The general cellular effect is the aforementioned T_3 synthesizing various proteins in which enzymes are also included by transcription and then translation in ribosomes in cytoplasm after interacting with receptor in nucleus. While, on one hand, protein synthesis increases, and on the other, a rise occurs in catabolism, and thus basal metabolism increases. Cell metabolism shows an increase of 60-100% when thyroid hormones are oversecreted (Dillmann, 2004; Dunn, 2001; Ganong, 1997; Guyton & Hall, 1997; Jameson & Weetman, 2010; Larsen et al., 2003; Lo Presti & Singer, 1997; Mc Gregor, 1996; Reed & Pangaro, 1995; Utiger, 1997; Usala, 1995).

Thyroid hormones accelerate mRNA synthesis in mitochondria by acting with intrinsic receptors in mitochondria inner and outer membranes and increases protein production. Due to these proteins produced here in mitochondria being respiratory chain proteins such as NADPH dehydrogenase, cytochrome-c-oxidase, and cytochrome reductase, the respiratory chain accelerates as the synthesis of these enzymes increases, and thus, ATP synthesis and oxygen consumption also increases. Therefore, it may be noted that ATP synthesis is dependent on thyroid hormone stimulation. In addition, the number of mitochondria increases due to the increase in mitochondria activity parallel to mitochondria protein synthesis (Dillmann, 2004; Dunn, 2001; Ganong, 1997; Guyton & Hall, 1997; Jameson & Weetman, 2010; Larsen et al., 2003; Lo Presti & Singer, 1997; Mc Gregor, 1996; Reed & Pangaro, 1995; Utiger, 1997; Usala, 1995).

Protein synthesis causes an increase in enzyme synthesis by increasing with the effect of thyroid hormones, and this affects the passage by increasing the production of transport enzymes in the cell membrane. Among these enzymes, the Na^+- K^+- ATPase pump provides Na^+ to exit and K^+ to enter by using ATP, thus, the rate of metabolism also increases (Dillmann, 2004; Dunn, 2001; Ganong, 1997; Guyton & Hall, 1997; Jameson & Weetman, 2010; Larsen et al., 2003; Lo Presti & Singer, 1997; Mc Gregor, 1996; Reed & Pangaro, 1995; Utiger, 1997; Usala, 1995).

Another membrane enzyme Ca^{+2}_ATPase acts more in the circulation system as intracellular Ca^{+2} decreases when this enzyme operates (Dillmann, 2004; Dunn, 2001; Ganong, 1997; Guyton & Hall, 1997; Jameson & Weetman, 2010; Larsen et al., 2003; Lo Presti & Singer, 1997; Mc Gregor, 1996; Reed & Pangaro, 1995; Utiger, 1997; Usala, 1995).

4.8.2 Effects on growth

Among the effects of thyroid is the effect it has on growth. This hormone has both specific and general effects on growth. Thyroid hormones are necessary for normal growth and muscle development. While children with hypothyroidism are shorter due to early epiphysis closure, children with hyperthyroidism are taller compared to their peers. Another important effect of the thyroid hormone is its contribution to the pre- and post-natal development of the brain. When in the mother's uterus, if the fetus cannot synthesize and secrete sufficient thyroid hormone and it is not replaced, growth and development retardation occurs in both pre- and post-natal periods (Dillmann, 2004; Dunn, 2001; Ganong, 1997; Guyton & Hall, 1997; Jameson & Weetman, 2010; Larsen et al., 2003; Lo Presti & Singer, 1997; Mc Gregor, 1996; Reed & Pangaro, 1995; Utiger, 1997; Usala, 1995). Normal serum levels are Total T_4 5-12µg/dl, Total T_3 80-200ng/dl, Free T_4 0,9-2ng/dl and free T_3 0,2-0,5ng/dl, respectively. If a thyroid hormone test is conducted on the baby after birth and hormone treatment is started immediately, a completely normal child is developed and a dramatic difference between early and late detection of the disease is clearly observed.

4.8.3 Metabolic effects

Thyroid hormones carry out their metabolic effects by carbohydrates, fat and protein metabolisms, vitamins, basal metabolic rate and its effect on body weight.

When the effects of thyroid hormones on carbohydrate metabolism are observed, it is established that it is both anabolic and catabolic. As a result of thyroid hormones increasing the enzyme synthesis due to protein synthesis in cells, enzymes in carbohydrate metabolism also increase their activities. Thus, thyroid hormones increase the entrance of glucose into the cell, absorption of glucose from the gastrointestinal system, both glycolysis and gluconeogenesis, and secondarily, insulin secretion (Dillmann, 2004; Dunn, 2001; Ganong, 1997; Guyton & Hall, 1997; Jameson & Weetman, 2010; Larsen et al., 2003; Lo Presti & Singer, 1997; Mc Gregor, 1996; Reed & Pangaro, 1995; Utiger, 1997; Usala, 1995).

The effect of thyroid hormone on fat metabolism are both anabolic and catabolic. Thyroid hormones have an especially lipolysis effect on adipose tissue ,and free fatty acid concentrations in plasma increase with the said effect, and in addition, fatty acid oxidation also increases (Dillmann, 2004; Dunn, 2001; Ganong, 1997; Guyton & Hall, 1997; Jameson & Weetman, 2010; Larsen et al., 2003; Lo Presti & Singer, 1997; Mc Gregor, 1996; Reed & Pangaro, 1995; Utiger, 1997; Usala, 1995). While, as a result of these effects, an increase is expected in the amounts of cholesterol and triglyceride, in contrast, their levels in blood are established to be low. This occurs due to two reasons. Firstly, thyroid hormones (especially T_3) cause an increase in receptor synthesis specific to LDL and cholesterol in liver, bind to lipoproteins, and decrease the triglyceride level in blood. Secondly, thyroid hormones accelerate the transformation of triglyceride to cholesterol with their effect. Cholesterol reaching the liver is used in the production of bile and the produced bile is excreted from the intestines with feces. Consequently, there occurs a decrease in adipose tissue, cholesterol and triglyceride in blood, and an increase in free fatty acids when thyroid hormone is oversecreted. The opposite occurs in individuals with hyperthyroidism. In a study by Bursuk et al., it was established by comparing the body composition in control, hypothyroidism, and hyperthyroidism groups with the bioelectrical impedance analysis method that body fat percentage and the amount decreased in cases with hyperthyroidism while they increased in cases with hypothyroidism (Bursuk et al., 2010; Dillmann, 2004; Dunn, 2001; Ganong, 1997; Guyton & Hall, 1997; Jameson & Weetman, 2010; Larsen et al., 2003; Lo Presti & Singer, 1997; Mc Gregor, 1996; Reed & Pangaro, 1995; Utiger, 1997; Usala, 1995).

As previously noted, thyroid hormones show an anabolic effect by increasing the protein syntheses and a catabolic effect by increasing the destruction when oversecreted. Thyroid hormones also regulate aminoacid transport due to the need for aminoacids in order to increase the protein synthesis. They also provide the synthesis for proteins specific to cell growth. Thyroid hormones provide a normal growth of the baby by increasing the syntheses of insulin-like factors in fetal period (Dillmann, 2004; Dunn, 2001; Ganong, 1997; Guyton & Hall, 1997; Jameson & Weetman, 2010; Larsen et al., 2003; Lo Presti & Singer, 1997; Mc Gregor, 1996; Reed & Pangaro, 1995; Utiger, 1997; Usala, 1995).

Hormones that provide growth and development are also under the control of thyroid hormones. As mentioned before, hypothyroidism causes growth-development retardation and can be reversed by hormone replacement treatment when diagnosed early. In hyperthyroidism in which thyroid hormones are oversecreted, muscle atrophies are observed as a result of an increase in protein catabolism (Dillmann, 2004; Dunn, 2001; Ganong, 1997; Guyton & Hall, 1997; Jameson & Weetman, 2010; Larsen et al., 2003; Lo Presti & Singer, 1997; Mc Gregor, 1996; Reed & Pangaro, 1995; Utiger, 1997; Usala, 1995).

Most of the enzymes need vitamins as co-factors in order to produce an effect. The need for the co-factor of thyroid hormones increases parallel to enzyme synthesis. Thiamine, riboflavin, B_{12}, folic acid and ascorbic acid (vitamin C) are predominantly used as co-factors. Therefore, deficiencies of these vitamins are common in cases with hyperthyroidism. In addition, vitamin D deficiency is also observed in these individuals due to an increase in excessive consumption and clearance. Also, thyroid hormones are necessary for carotene from food to be transformed into vitamin A. Vitamin A transformation does not occur in cases with hypothyroidism due to thyroid hormone deficiency and carotene is deposited under the skin giving it a yellow color. (Dillmann, 2004; Dunn, 2001; Ganong, 1997; Guyton & Hall, 1997; Jameson & Weetman, 2010; Larsen et al., 2003; Lo Presti & Singer, 1997; Mc Gregor, 1996; Reed & Pangaro, 1995; Utiger, 1997; Usala, 1995). Vitamin D deficiency is present in these cases due to a problem in A, E, and cholesterol metabolism. Thus, vitamin supplement is necessary in both hypothyroidism and hyperthyroidism cases.

Another effect of thyroid hormones is the acceleration of basal metabolism. As noted before, thyroid hormones increase the oxygen consumption and thus ATP synthesis by rising the count and activity of mitochondria. Thyroid hormones increase oxygen consumption except for the adult brain, testicles, uterus, lymph nodes, spleen, and front hypophysis. In addition, the increase of such enzymes as Na^{+}- K^{+}- ATPase, and Ca^{+}- ATPase contribute to it. Also, lipid catabolism lends to it. A high level of temperature is produced as a result (Dillmann, 2004; Dunn, 2001; Ganong, 1997; Guyton & Hall, 1997; Jameson & Weetman, 2010; Larsen et al., 2003; Lo Presti & Singer, 1997; Mc Gregor, 1996; Reed & Pangaro, 1995; Utiger, 1997; Usala, 1995).

A protein called thermogenin in brown adipose tissue is uncoupled, that is, ATP production and e^{-} - transport chain are separated from each other. An excessive temperature occurs as a result. All these effects provide acceleration of basal metabolism. The overworking thyroid gland increases the basal metabolism by 60-100% (Dillmann, 2004; Dunn, 2001; Ganong, 1997; Guyton & Hall, 1997; Jameson & Weetman, 2010; Larsen et al., 2003; Lo Presti & Singer, 1997; Mc Gregor, 1996; Reed & Pangaro, 1995; Utiger, 1997; Usala, 1995).

Due to the increase in basal metabolism, a decrease is observed in body weight. Thyroid hormones greatly reduce the fat deposit. Weight loss is observed in cases with hyperthyroidism although appetite increases in cases with hyperthyroidism. However, in cases with hypothyroidism, basal metabolism deceleration and weight gain occur in cases with hypothyroidism (Dillmann, 2004; Dunn, 2001; Ganong, 1997; Guyton & Hall, 1997; Jameson & Weetman, 2010; Larsen et al., 2003; Lo Presti & Singer, 1997; Mc Gregor, 1996; Reed & Pangaro, 1995; Utiger, 1997; Usala, 1995).

4.8.4 Effect of thyroid hormones on systems

The effect of thyroid hormones on circulation systems is predominantly through catecholamine. Thyroid hormones increase the β adrenergic receptor count without affecting catecholamine secretion. This causes an increase in heart rate, cardiac output, stroke volume, and peripheral vasodilation. Peripheral vasodilation causes the skin to be warm and humid. Warm and humid skin, sweating, and restlessness due to increased sympathetic activity are observed in cases with hyperthyroidism. However, the opposite is seen in hypothyroidism. The β adrenergic receptor count is decreased. In relation to this, heart rate, cardiac output, and stroke volume is also decreased and cold, dry skin is observed due to peripheral vasoconstriction. In a study by Bursuk et al., it was established by measuring and comparing the stroke volume, cardiac output, heart index, and blood flow in control, hypothyroidism, and hyperthyroidism groups with the bioelectrical impedance analysis method that these parameters significantly increased in cases with hyperthyroidism while they decreased in cases with hypothyroidism (Bursuk et al., 2010; Dillmann, 2004; Dunn, 2001; Ganong, 1997; Guyton & Hall, 1997; Jameson & Weetman, 2010; Larsen et al., 2003; Lo Presti & Singer, 1997; Mc Gregor, 1996; Reed & Pangaro, 1995; Utiger, 1997; Usala, 1995).

In addition, as metabolism products also increase due to an increase in oxygen consumption when thyroid hormones are oversecreted, vasodilation occurs in periphery. Thus, blood flow increases, and cardiac output can be observed to be 60% more than normal. The thyroid hormone also raises the heart rate due to its direct increasing effect on heart stimulation (Dillmann, 2004; Dunn, 2001; Ganong, 1997; Guyton & Hall, 1997; Jameson & Weetman, 2010; Larsen et al., 2003; Lo Presti & Singer, 1997; Mc Gregor, 1996; Reed & Pangaro, 1995; Utiger, 1997; Usala, 1995).

Thyroid hormones increase the contraction of heart muscles only when they raise it in small amounts. When thyroid hormones are oversecreted, a significant decrease occurs in muscle strength, and even myocardial infarction is observed in severely thyrotoxic patients (Dillmann, 2004; Dunn, 2001; Ganong, 1997; Guyton & Hall, 1997; Jameson & Weetman, 2010; Larsen et al., 2003; Lo Presti & Singer, 1997; Mc Gregor, 1996; Reed & Pangaro, 1995; Utiger, 1997; Usala, 1995).

Due to large amounts of oxygen thyroid hormones use during their increasing protein synthesis, hence the enzyme synthesis, and ATP synthesis as well, carbon dioxide amount is also increased. As a result of the carbon dioxide increase affecting the respiratory center of the brain, hyperventilation, that is, the rise in inhalation frequency and deepening of respiration is observed (Dillmann, 2004; Dunn, 2001; Ganong, 1997; Guyton & Hall, 1997; Jameson & Weetman, 2010; Larsen et al., 2003; Lo Presti & Singer, 1997; Mc Gregor, 1996; Reed & Pangaro, 1995; Utiger, 1997; Usala, 1995).

While appetite and food consumption increases, an increase has also been observed in digestive system fluids, secretions, and movements. Frequently, diarrhea occurs when the thyroid hormone is excessively secreted. In contrast, constipation is observed in the case of hypothyroidism (Dillmann, 2004; Dunn, 2001; Ganong, 1997; Guyton & Hall, 1997; Jameson & Weetman, 2010; Larsen et al., 2003; Lo Presti & Singer, 1997; Mc Gregor, 1996; Reed & Pangaro, 1995; Utiger, 1997; Usala, 1995).

When the effects of thyroid hormones on the skeletal system are checked, the first thing that needs to be examined is their effect on bones. The activities of osteoblast and osteoclast that are the main cells of bone structure increase parallel to thyroid hormones. In normal individuals, thyroid hormones possess direct proliferative effect on osteoblasts. In cases with hyperthyroidism, a decrease develops in the cortex of the bones due to increase in osteoclastic activities. Thus, the risk of post-menopausal osteoporosis development increases in these patients. While, in physiological cases, thyroid hormone creates an osteoblastic effect, it produces an osteoporotic effect in hyperthyroidism (Dillmann, 2004; Dunn, 2001; Ganong, 1997; Guyton & Hall, 1997; Jameson & Weetman, 2010; Larsen et al., 2003; Lo Presti & Singer, 1997; Mc Gregor, 1996; Reed & Pangaro, 1995; Utiger, 1997; Usala, 1995).

The thyroid also affects response to stimulants. When this hormone is excessively secreted, muscle fatigue occurs due to protein catabolism increase. The most typical symptom of hyperthyroidism is a faint muscle tremor. Such a tremor happening 10-15 times per second, occurs due to increase in activity of neuronal synapses in medulla spinalis regions that control muscle tone, and differs from tremors in Parkinson's disease. This tremor demonstrates the effects of thyroid hormones on central nervous system (Dillmann, 2004; Dunn, 2001; Ganong, 1997; Guyton & Hall, 1997; Jameson & Weetman, 2010; Larsen et al., 2003; Lo Presti & Singer, 1997; Mc Gregor, 1996; Reed & Pangaro, 1995; Utiger, 1997; Usala, 1995).

As mentioned above, muscle fatigue is observed in hyperthyroidism due to the accelerating effect of the thyroid hormone on protein catabolism. However, the excessive stimulant effect of this hormone on synapses leads to sleeplessness. In hypothyroidism, a sleepy state exists (Dillmann, 2004; Dunn, 2001; Ganong, 1997; Guyton & Hall, 1997; Jameson & Weetman, 2010; Larsen et al., 2003; Lo Presti & Singer, 1997; Mc Gregor, 1996; Reed & Pangaro, 1995; Utiger, 1997; Usala, 1995)..

Thyroid hormones play an important role in the development of the central nervous system. They are also responsible for the myelinization of the nerves. If there is thyroid hormone deficiency in fetus, it causes neuronal developmental disorders in the brain, myelinization retardation, decrease in vascularization, retardation in deep tendon reflexes, cerebral hypoxy due to decrease in cerebral blood flow, mental retardation, and lethargy. In cases with hyperthyroidism, the opposite occurs and hyperirritability, anxiety, and sleeplessness are observed in these children (Dillmann, 2004; Dunn, 2001; Ganong, 1997; Guyton & Hall, 1997; Jameson & Weetman, 2010; Larsen et al., 2003; Lo Presti & Singer, 1997; Mc Gregor, 1996; Reed & Pangaro, 1995; Utiger, 1997; Usala, 1995).

Thyroid hormones produce an effect by merging with their specific receptors in membrane and nuclei of hemopoietic stem cells. After T_3 and T_4 hormones bind with a receptor, erythroid stem cells go through mitosis and accelerate erythropoiesis. With the protein synthesis they caused to occur in these precursor cells, they provide the synthesis of enzymes at the beginning and at the end of hemoglobin synthesis (Dillmann, 2004; Dunn, 2001; Ganong, 1997; Guyton & Hall, 1997; Jameson & Weetman, 2010; Larsen et al., 2003; Lo Presti & Singer, 1997; Mc Gregor, 1996; Reed & Pangaro, 1995; Utiger, 1997; Usala, 1995).

In addition, when tissues are left without oxygen with the consumption of oxygen thanks to thyroid hormone effect, they stimulate the kidney and increase erythropoietin synthesis and secretion. Erythropoietin then stimulates the bone marrow and accelerates erythropoiesis. While polycythemia is not observed in patients with hyperthyroidism, anemia is quite prevalent among cases with hypothyroidism. Blood levels of cases with hyperthyroidism are generally within normal limits (Dillmann, 2004; Dunn, 2001; Ganong, 1997; Guyton & Hall, 1997; Jameson & Weetman, 2010; Larsen et al., 2003; Lo Presti & Singer, 1997; Mc Gregor, 1996; Reed & Pangaro, 1995; Utiger, 1997; Usala, 1995).

In a study by Bursuk et al., it has been established by measuring and comparing blood parameters and blood viscosity in control, hypothyroidism, and hyperthyroidism groups that blood viscosity was increased in cases with hypothyroidism due to blood count parameters being higher compared to cases with hyperthyroidism, blood lipids and fibrinogen were higher in cases with hypothyroidism, and in addition, blood viscosity was increased in cases with hypothyroidism due to high plasma viscosity (Bursuk et al., 2010; Dillmann, 2004; Dunn, 2001; Ganong, 1997; Guyton & Hall, 1997; Jameson & Weetman, 2010; Larsen et al., 2003; Lo Presti & Singer, 1997; Mc Gregor, 1996; Reed & Pangaro, 1995; Utiger, 1997; Usala, 1995).

Thyroid hormones regulate the actions of other endocrine hormones in order to accelerate basal metabolism. These hormones increase the absorption of glucose in gastrointestinal system, glucose reception into cells, and both glycolysis and gluconeogenesis by producing an effect on insulin and glucagon. Thyroid hormones enable the increase of insulin through secondary mechanism by occasionally rising blood sugar (Dillmann, 2004; Dunn, 2001; Ganong, 1997; Guyton & Hall, 1997; Jameson & Weetman, 2010; Larsen et al., 2003; Lo Presti & Singer, 1997; Mc Gregor, 1996; Reed & Pangaro, 1995; Utiger, 1997; Usala, 1995).

Due to the fact that both thyroid hormones and growth hormones are necessary for normal somatic growth, thyroid hormones increase the synthesis and secretion of growth hormone and growth factors (Dillmann, 2004; Dunn, 2001; Ganong, 1997; Guyton & Hall, 1997; Jameson & Weetman, 2010; Larsen et al., 2003; Lo Presti & Singer, 1997; Mc Gregor, 1996; Reed & Pangaro, 1995; Utiger, 1997; Usala, 1995).

Also, another effect is produced on prolactin. During hypothyroidism, TRH secretion stimulates prolactin secretion, and while galactorrhea and amenorrhea is observed in females, gynecomastia and impotence is found in males. The inhibiting effect of dopamine is of utmost importance in regulating the secretion of prolactin secretion (Dillmann, 2004; Dunn, 2001; Ganong, 1997; Guyton & Hall, 1997; Jameson & Weetman, 2010; Larsen et al., 2003; Lo Presti & Singer, 1997; Mc Gregor, 1996; Reed & Pangaro, 1995; Utiger, 1997; Usala, 1995).

Due to the fact that thyroid hormones regulate the secretion and use of all steroid hormones adrenal gland deficiency with such findings as lack of libido, impotence, amenorrhea, menorrhagia, and polymerrhea is observed in cases with hypothyroidism. Another cause for findings related to these sex steroids may be excessive prolactin (Dillmann, 2004; Dunn, 2001; Ganong, 1997; Guyton & Hall, 1997; Jameson & Weetman, 2010; Larsen et al., 2003; Lo Presti & Singer, 1997; Mc Gregor, 1996; Reed & Pangaro, 1995; Utiger, 1997; Usala, 1995).

Thyroid hormones affect bone metabolism in parallel with parathormone. Estrogen, vitamin D_3, TGF-β, PGE_2, parathormone (PTH), and all of the thyroid hormones are necessary for osteoblastic activity (Dillmann, 2004; Dunn, 2001; Ganong, 1997; Guyton & Hall, 1997; Jameson & Weetman, 2010; Larsen et al., 2003; Lo Presti & Singer, 1997; Mc Gregor, 1996; Reed & Pangaro, 1995; Utiger, 1997; Usala, 1995).

As noted earlier, thyroid hormones increase β adrenergic receptor count. Adrenaline and noradrenaline interact with these receptors and accelerates basal metabolism, stimulates the nervous system, and speeds up the circulation system just as in the effect of thyroid hormones (Dillmann, 2004; Dunn, 2001; Ganong, 1997; Guyton & Hall, 1997; Jameson & Weetman, 2010; Larsen et al., 2003; Lo Presti & Singer, 1997; Mc Gregor, 1996; Reed & Pangaro, 1995; Utiger, 1997; Usala, 1995).

For a normal sexual development and life, thyroid hormones are necessary. The reason for this is that thyroid hormones increase the use and secretion of sex steroids, and in addition, affect prolactin secretion. Lack of libido, impotence, gynecomastia, amenorrhea, menorrhagia, and polymenorrhea are observed due to sex steroid deficiency and excessive prolactin in cases with hypothyroidism (Dillmann, 2004; Dunn, 2001; Ganong, 1997; Guyton & Hall, 1997; Jameson & Weetman, 2010; Larsen et al., 2003; Lo Presti & Singer, 1997; Mc Gregor, 1996; Reed & Pangaro, 1995; Utiger, 1997; Usala, 1995).

5. Conclusion

Anatomy, histology and physiology of thyroid have been addressed in this chapter. In its physiology, its hormone synthesis, metabolism, effect generation mechanism and effects on the body has been explained. While mentioning these effects, the relationship between thyroid diseases and blood hemorheology has also been referred and relationship between disease groups (hyperthyroids and hypothyroids) has been analysed comparatively with these parameters.

6.References

Benvenga, S.(2005). Peripheral hormone metabolism thyroid hormone transport proteins and the physiology of hormone binding, In: *Werner&Ingbar's The Thyroid a Fundamental and clinical Text*, Braverman, LE.&Utiger, RD., pp. (97-105), Lippincott Williams&Wilkins Company, 0-7817-5047-4, Philadelphia.

Bursuk, E., Gulcur, H. & Ercan, M. (2010). The significance of body impedance and blood viscosity measurements in thyroid diseases, Proceedings of Biomedical Engineering Meeting (BIYOMUT), 15th National, 978-1-4244-6380-0, Antalya, April 2010 (http://ieeexplore.ieee.org/xpls/abs_all.jsp?arnumber=5479828&tag=1).

Di Lauro, R. & De Felice, M. (2001). Basic Physiology anatomy development, In: *Endocrinology*, DeGroot, LJ.&Jameson, JL., pp. (1268-1275), W.B. Saunders Company, 0-7216-7840-8, Philadelphia.

Dillmann, W.H. (2004). The thyroid, In: *Cecil Textbook of* Medicine, Goldman, L.&Ausrello, D., pp. (1391-1411), Saunders, Philadelphia.

Dunn, J.T. (2001). Biosynthesis and secretion of thyroid hormones, In: *Endocrinology*, DeGroort, LJ.,&Jameson, JL., pp. (1290-1298), W.B. Saunders Company, 0-7216-7840-8, Philadelphia.

Ganong, W.F. (1997). *Review of Medical Physiology* (eighteenth edition), Appleton&Lange, 0-8385-8443-8, Stamford.

Guyton, A.C. & Hall, JE. (2006). *Textbook of Medical Physiology* (eleventh edition), Elsevier Sanders, 0-7216-0240-1, Philadelphia.

Jameson, J.L. & Weetman, A.P. (2010). Disorders of the thyroid gland, In: *Harrison's Endocrinology*, Jameson, JL., pp. (62-69), The McGraw-Hill Companies, Inc., 978-0-07-174147-7, New York.

Larsen, P.R., Davies, T.F., Schlumberger, M.J. & Hay, I.D. (2003). Thyroid physiology and diagnostic evaluation of patients with thyroid disorders, In: *Williams Textbook of Endocrinology*, Larsen, PR., Kronenberg, HM., Melmed, S.&Polonsky, KS., pp. (331-353), Saunders, 0-7216-9184-6, Philadelphia.

Lo Presti, J.S. & Singer, P.A. (1997). Physiology of thyroid hormone synthesis, secretion, and transport, In: *Thyroid Disease Endocrinology, Surger, Nuclear Medicine and Radiotherapy.* Falk, SA, pp. (29-39), Lippincott-Raven Publishers, 0-397-51705-X, Philadelphia.

Mc Gregor, A.M. (1996). The thyroid gland and disorders of thyroid function, In: *Oxford Fextbook of Medicine,* Weatherall, DJ., Ledingham, JGG. & Warrell, DA, pp. (1603–1621), Oxford University Press, 0-19-262707-4, Oxford, Vol. 2.

Reed, L. & Pangaro, L.N. (1995). Physiology of the thyroid gland I: synthesis and release, iodine metabolism, and binding and transport, In: *Principles and Practice of Endocrinology and Metabolism,* Becher, KL., pp. (285-291), J.B. Lippincott Company, 0-397-51404-2, Philadelphia.

Santiseban, P. (2005). Development and anatomy of the hypothalamic – pituitary – thyroid axis, In: *Werner&Ingbar's The Thyroid a Fundamental and Clinical Text*, Braverman, LE.,&Utiger, RD., pp. (8-23), Lippincot Williams&Wilkins Company, 0-7817-5047-4, Philadelphia.

Scanlon, M.F. (2001). Thyrothropin releasing hormone and thyrothropin stimulating hormone, In: *Endocrinology,* DeGroot, LJ.&Jameson, JL., pp. (1279-1286), W.B. Saunders Company, 0-7216-7840-8, Philadelphia.

Snell, R.S. (1995). *Clinical Anatomy for my students* (fifth edition), Little, Brown and Company, 0-316-80135-6, Boston.

Usala, S.J. (1995). Physiology of the thyroid gland II: reseptors, postreceptor events, and hormone resistance syndromes, In: *Principle and Practice of Endocrinology and Metabolism,* Becker, KL., pp. (292-298), J.B. Lippincott Company, 0-397-51404-2, Philadelphia.

Utiger, R.D. (1997). Disorders of the thyroid gland, In: *Textbook of Intecnal Medrane,* Kelley, WN., pp. (2204–2219), Lippincott – Raven Publishers, 0-397-51540-5, Philadelphia.

2

The Thyroglobulin: A Technically Challenging Assay for a Marker of Choice During the Follow-Up of Differentiated Thyroid Cancer

Anne Charrié
Lyon University, INSERM U1060, CarMeN laboratory and CENS, Univ Lyon-1
Laboratory of Nuclear Technics and Biophysic, Hospices Civils de Lyon
France

1. Introduction

The thyroglobulin (Tg) is a normal secretory product of the thyroid gland. Tg is stored in the follicular light of the thyroid where it constitutes the majority of colloid proteins. It is the place of synthesis and storage of thyroid hormones.

This glycoprotein of high molecular weight (660 kDa) is constituted by two identical sub-units bound by disulphide-bridges. Each sub-unit contains 2 749 amino acids (Malthiery & Lissitzky, 1987 and Van de Graf et al., 1997). Its gene is situated on the chromosome 8 and different isoforms of Tg are secreted by alternative splicing. This molecule is heterogeneous by its degree of iodination (0.2 to 1.0%), of glycosylation, and by its contents in oses and in sialic acid (8 to 10%). The epitopic map of Tg revealed approximately about forty antigenic determinants, twelve epitopes grouped together in six domains (Piechaczyck et al., 1985). The central region of the Tg molecule is in majority immunoreactive (Henry et al, 1990).

Tg is not confined in the follicle, some molecules are co-secreted with thyroid hormones by a complex process which can modify it. Any conformational change entails a different antigenicity because some epitopes can be masked or on the contrary be exposed. Molecular forms of Tg found in the serum of patients with differentiated thyroid cancer correspond to dimeric Tg. It is little iodized and presents a change of the glycosylation (Sinadinovic et al., 1992 and Druetta et al., 1998). The heterogeneousness of Tg in the thyroid gland is increased in the cancer (Persani et al., 1998) and the changes of its conformation modifies its immunoreactivity (Kohno et al., 1985). All these structural characteristics are very important to know and can give some explanations about differences between Tg assays. It is not surprising to notice differences between Tg assays which use monoclonal antibodies by definition very specific. The follow-up of the differentiated thyroid cancers is the essential indication of the dosage of the serum Tg. Tg signs the presence of normal or pathological thyroid tissue. It is not possible to differentiate the normal tissue of the cancerous tissue thanks to serum Tg value. One reference point is mentioned in the laboratory medicine practice guidelines (Baloch et al., 2003): one gram of normal thyroid releases about 1µg/L Tg into the circulation when the serum thyroid stimulating hormone (TSH) is normal and 0.5 µg/L if the TSH value is suppressed below 0.1 mUI/L. Since its concentration is correlated with the size rather than with the nature of nodule of the thyroid gland, Tg is not used for the diagnosis of the thyroid cancer. Routine preoperative measurement of serum Tg for initial evaluation of thyroid nodules is not recommended (Cooper et al., 2006).

2. Thyroglobulin assay in serum

Serum Tg measurement is a technically challenging assay for a marker of choice during the follow-up of differentiated thyroid cancer. The use of the Tg assays requires a good knowledge of the technical difficulties. The quality of current Tg assay methods varies and influences the clinical utility of this test. All techniques are today immunometric assays with isotopic signal or not. Several methodological problems must be taken into account: standardization, functional sensitivity, precision, hook effects, interference by heterophile antibodies and interference by Tg antibodies (TgAb) (Spencer et al., 1996). Precision and hook effects are two parameters which are usual in biology when markers are used in the follow-up of cancer. Every laboratory scientist knows that it is sometimes better to measure stored serum samples from the patient in the same run as the current specimen to better appreciate the variability of the marker during the time. As regards the hook effect it is careful either to use a technique in 2 steps or to dilute systematically the serum suspected of very high values of Tg. Heterophile antibodies may cause falsely elevated serum Tg levels as in al immunometric assays. It is possible to reduce this interference by using heterophile blocking tubes when these antibodies are suspected (Preissner et al., 2003). Even if some solutions were studied for the other problems (standardisation, functional sensitivity and interference by TgAb) all persist always for more than fifteen years and guidelines have been published (Baloch et al., 2003; Pacini et al., 2006; Borson-Chazot et al., 2008).

2.1 Standardisation

Different guidelines and consensus (Baloch et al., 2003; Pacini et al., 2006; Borson-Chazot et al., 2008) recommended the use of the European human reference material CRM 457 (Feldt-Rasmussen U et al., 1996). Even if the use of this standard doesn't resolve all problems between different techniques it will be a minimal consensus that manufacturers would follow to get a homogenous basis of standardisation. The CRM 457 is produced from normal thyroid tissue. Now we know that tissular Tg is not strictly the one which circulates in the blood (Schulz et al., 1989). The ideal standard would be a preparation of thyroglobulin extracted from the blood. Because of a too small quantity of circulating Tg the manufacturing of such a reference was not possible. The actual recommendation is to use 1:1 CRM 457 standardisation. The configuration of the Tg molecule is not enough taken into account in the various Tg methods.

2.2 Functional sensitivity

Since Tg measurements have to detect very small amount of thyroid tissue, it is absolutely necessary to determine the sensitivity of the Tg assays. The definition of the functional sensitivity was established by Spencer for the TSH (Spencer et al., 1996 a). The same concept can be applied to Tg (Spencer et al, 1996 b): it is the Tg value that can be measured with 20% between-run coefficient of variation (CV), using a 1:1 CRM 457 standardisation. The proposed protocol is similar for Tg with the establishment of a profile of precision measuring human pool sera over 6 to 12 months (compatible deadline with the follow-up of the patients) with at least 2 batchs of reagents and 2 instrument calibrations (Baloch et al., 2003). The pools of serum used for this profile have to be TgAb negative. It must be repeated to the scientists how to verify the functional sensitivity of a Tg assay and not to take that given by the manufacturer. Analogous to TSH, Tg assay functional sensitivity permits a generational classification of Tg assays. Most current assays are actually first generation with a functional sensitivity about 0.5 to 1.0µg/L. The functional sensitivity is of a big importance to determine the «detectable Tg < institutional cut-off » mentioned in the European Consensus (Pacini et al., 2006) specially in the flow chart for the follow-up after initial treatment (6 to 12 months) and recombinant human thyrotropin (rhTSH). For example some authors (Kloos & Mazzaferri, 2005) considered a thyroglobulin cutoff level of 2.0µg/L highly sensitive for identifying persistent tumor after rhTSH stimulation in patients who had TSH-suppressed thyroglobulin undetectable with an assay functional sensitivity value of 1µg/L. This cut-off is also mentioned in the recommendations of the American Thyroid Association (Cooper et al., 2006).

In the European consensus, supersensitive Tg assays which have a higher sensitivity but at the expense of a much lower specificity are not currently recommended for routine use. Nevertheless some current assays are second generation with a ten-fold better functional sensitivity. An insufficient functional sensitivity is at the origin of most of false-negative results corresponding to an authentic recurrence of the disease with a value of Tg given undetectable. With a more sensitive second generation assay it would be possible to detect responses that will be undetectable with a first generation assay. At present this very low functional sensitivity for certain cases of dosages could allow to replace rhTSH stimulated Tg testing for the patients at low risk by a simple dosage of second generation Tg. Low risk patients are those with well-differentiated papillary or follicular thyroid cancer, patient age <45 years, thyroid tumor size ranging from 1 cm to <4 cm in diameter, no extension of the tumor beyond the thyroid capsule, no lymph-node involvement and no distant metastases (Schlumberger et al., 2007; Smallridge et al., 2007; Schlumberger et al., 2011).

2.3 Interference by TgAb

This type of analytical problem is completely characteristic of Tg assays and exists in no other immunoassay. It is connected to the fact that Tg is a major auto-antigen. All the actually methods are prone to interference by TgAb (Mariotti et al., 1995). The combined use of judiciously selected monoclonal antibodies directed against antigenic domains of Tg not recognized by most TgAb allowed to develop a Tg assay with minimal interference from TgAb (Marquet et al., 1996). In every case the presence of TgAb that mask certain epitopes can lead to underestimation of the Tg concentrations with the actuals immunometric methods.

We are however unable to evaluate the true interference of these TgAb: it is known that in some patients few Tgab can induce a major interference while in some others a lot of TgAb induce only a smooth interference. Everything depends on the affinity of these antibodies which we do not estimate. The various consensus recommend to measure antibodies by a enough sensitive method in a systematic way with any dosage of Tg. At first it had been suggested realizing a test of recovery to estimate the importance of the interference but this one was abandoned because of a bad standardization of the protocol

(Spencer et al, 1996c). When there is presence of TgAb and if Tg is found undetectable, its value is not interpretable. When the value of Tg is dosable with presence of antibodies, the returned value is then a "minimal" value knowing that she could be more raised in the absence of antibody. After thyroidectomy, TgAb will decrease and disappear in patients with remission but these antibodies may persist during 2-3 years after disappearance of Tg (Chiovato et al., 2003). During the follow-up of some patients persistence or reappearance of circulating TgAb may be regarded as an indicator of disease. More recently Spencer even concluded that TgAb trends can be used as a surrogate tumor marker in differentiated thyroid cancer in preference to Tg measurement, provided that the same method is used.

3. Thyroglobulin in fine needle aspiration biopsy

After surgery for differentiated thyroid cancer, cervical ultrasound is recommended to evaluate the thyroid bed and central and lateral cervical nodal compartments should be performed at 6 and 12 months and then annually for at least 3-5 years, depending on the patients' risk for recurrent disease and thyroglobulin status (Cooper et al., 2006). At present numerous studies describe the utility to look for thyroglobulin measurements in fine-needle aspiration biopsies (FNA-Tg) of lymph node (LN) during the follow-up of differentiated thyroid carcinoma. Although most patients have a long term survival rate, 5 to 20% of them will develop recurrence during follow-up, primarily in the cervical lymph nodes. An accurate distinction between metastatic and reactive benign lymph nodes (BLN) is essential in the management of thyroid cancer prior to surgery; it is necessary to specify the extent of surgery and identify early cervical relapse.

Cytological examination of fine-needle aspiration cytology (FNA-C) the reference method for the diagnosis of thyroid nodules has also been, until recently, the best method to diagnose a cervical LN in subjects with suspicion of thyroid cancer or patients followed for thyroid neoplasia. However, sensitivity of FNA-C is far from excellent, varying from 75 to 85% and altered by a high rate of non-diagnostic samples. Pacini was the first author who showed in 1992 high concentrations of thyroglobulin in metastatic LN of thyroid carcinoma. Although the performance of FNA-Tg is now well established, some methodological factors may influence the results and threshold value remains controversial. The first step is how to obtain the material from the fine needle aspiration. Ultrasound-guided fine-needle aspiration biopsy is carried out by a trained operator with a fine needle, preferably 25 to 27 gauges. After aspiration, the needle is rinsed.

3.1 The middle

The middle used to rinse the needle is variable according to the teams; it can be either physiological saline solution or a liquid supplied by the laboratory (assay buffer or Tg-free serum). Two studies show that some parasite effects are present in the dosage: some "noise" in the Tg assay was described by Baskin et al. (2004). Snozek et al. (2007) demonstrate with a recovery test (after an overload of exogenous Tg) that the values of Tg are 25% higher with the saline solution than with a serous matrix with his Tg assay. The nature of the buffer may have an influence on the conformation of proteins and affect antibody binding. The most important matrix effect is that due to the matrix used to prepare the calibration curve and the matrix to measure samples (Wild, 2005). We think that it is much better to use the Tg-free medium of the test kit to avoid bias in the determination of thyroglobulin in FNA wash samples (Bournaud et al., 2010). But for practical use the saline solution is often used and so it is recommended in the French good practice guide for cervical ultrasound scan and echo-guided techniques (Leenhardt et al., 2011) to check for the absence of matrix effect in the usual assay method. It is possible to validate the use of saline solution by comparing the results of Tg immunoreactivity obtained with Tg-free solution, saline solution and saline solution supplemented with serum albumin (Borel et al., 2008).

3.2 The volume

The quantity of the liquid used to rinse the needle varies between 0.5 to 1.0mL but is in general 1.0mL. All content of the needle is carefully removed by washing with from one to three pumping depending of the operator. Borel et al. (2008) shows that a triple pumping action of the 1 mL liquid through the needle was sufficient to wash out 97% of Tg out of the needle. If the needle has to be inserted several times into the same lymph node, the needle rinse can be poured into the same tube (Leenhardt et al., 2011).

3.3 The Tg method

The Tg method is the same used for the Tg serum assay. The problem of the interference by TgAb is however different. The presence of TgAb in fine needle aspiration biopsy washout can result of blood contamination when they are present or of active lymph node synthesis (Boi et al., 2006). But this interference seams to have small effect on the result of FNA-Tg. An explanation of this could be that the excessive high concentration of Tg is able to saturate TgAb binding sites. So it is not recommended to assay TgAb in the rinsing liquid (Leenhardt et al., 2011).

Another interference could be also evoked: the contamination with serum Tg. It seems that FNA-Tg is not affected by the circulating serum levels. In 2008 Borel et al calculate that the maximal contamination of FNA-Tg by serum Tg varied from 0.003 to 0.012% what is not significant. He measured also albumin in the LN washout to evaluate the contamination by plasma proteins. He concluded that serum Tg did not interfere in results of FNA-Tg and specially in negative controls (not thyroidectomized) who had undetectable FNA-Tg values.

3.4 The results and interpretation

The expression of the results varies according to studies. Some authors (Baskin, 2004; Boi et al, 2006; Kim et al, 2009) use the unit µg/L (or ng/ml), others (Pacini et al., 1992; Cignarelli et al., 2003; Borel et al., 2008; Bournaud et al., 2010) use µg/FNA. It is more suitable to use this type of result which reflects only the quantity of Tg present in the needle after rinsing and not a concentration of Tg in the LN.

We find here again the problem of functional sensitivity of the Tg method which directly affect the cut-off value. In the first study (Pacini et al., 1992), the cut-off value was 21.7µg/L but the functional sensitivity was only 3µg/L. This cut-off value was established as equal to the mean plus two standard deviations of the FNA-Tg values in patients with negative cytology. Other authors used the same type of cut-off (Cignarelli et al., 2003; Baskin, 2004;

Boi et al., 2006). In other studies of the literature threshold are sometimes the functional sensitivity (Cunha et al., 2007; Snozek et al., 2007) or study of sensitivity and specificity and choice of the better cut-off with a Receiver Operating Characteristic Curve (ROC) (Bournaud et al., 2010; Giovanella et al., 2011). For others again the FNA-Tg is compared with serum Tg: when the FNA-Tg value is greater than serum Tg value the LN is considered as metastasis (Uruno et al., 2005; Sigstad et al., 2007). However there is no correlation between serous Tg and FNA-Tg (Frasoldati et al., 1999). Kim et al. (2009) tested different threshold and propose a combination: the threshold values for FNA-Tg levels should be >10ng/ml if the serum Tg level or the mean plus two standard deviation in node-negative patients is not available for reference. Finally the French consensus (Leenhardt et al., 2011) recommends: Tg <1ng/FNA: normal result, Tg between 1 and 10 ng/FNA: to be compared with the results from cytology and Tg> 10 ng/FNA: suggest the presence of tumoral tissue.

FNA-Tg levels are significantly lower in subjects with metastatic poorly differentiated thyroid carcinoma than in subjects with differentiated thyroid cancer (Cignarelli et al., 2003) and may be nil (Boi et al., 2006), causing "false negatives" values.

Conversely FNA-Tg is particularly usefull for the diagnosis of LN metastasis when these LN have cystic changes (Cignarelli et al., 2003; Baloch et al., 2008). FNA-Tg is more sensitive for detecting metastasis when compared with FNA cytology (FNA-C) alone and allows the accurate diagnosis for samples with non conclusive cytology (Giovanella et al., 2011). For patients who received therapy with ^{131}I the delay between the treatment and FNA has to be enough long (more than 3 months) to allow definitive destruction of the metastatic LN because FNA-Tg value can be false-positive. Sensitivity of FNA-Tg in the different studies are comprise between 84% (Frasoldati et al., 1999) and 100% (Pacini et al., 1992; Snozek et al., 2007; Cunha et al., 2007; Sigstad et al., 2007). When FNA-Tg is combined with FNA-C 100% sensitivity and 100% specificity can be obtained (Bournaud et al., 2010; Giovanella et al., 2011). So FNA-C should remain combined with FNA-Tg (Leenhardt et al., 2011).

4. Conclusion

It seems that we can again progress in the evolution of the dosage of Tg in terms of quality. We underlined here the importance of analytical quality for a highly strategic parameter in the decision tree of the follow-up of differentiated thyroid cancer: the thyroglobulin. During these periods of great changes in laboratories with automation we have to remember ourselves another guideline: "choose a method Tg on the basis of its characteristics of performance not the costs". The biologist has to know all the difficulties of Tg assays to argue the choice of his method, to guarantee the quality of the dosage and to avoid serious medical errors especially in the follow-up of differentiated thyroid carcinoma. A good laboratory-physician dialogue is more than ever of great importance.

5. References

Baloch, Z.; Carayon, P.; Conte-Devolx, B.; Demers, L.M.; Feldt-Rasmussen, U.; Henry, J.F.; LiVosli, V.A.; Niccoli-Sire, P.; John, R.; Ruf, J.; Smyth, P.P.; Spencer, C.A.; Stockigt, J.R. & Guidelines Committee, National Academy of Clinical Biochemistry.(2003).

Laboratory medicine practice guidelines. Laboratory support for the diagnosis and monitoring of thyroid disease. *Thyroid,* Vol. 13, pp.3-126.

Baloch, ZW.; Barroeta, JE.; Walsh, J.; Gupta, PK.; Livolsi, VA.; Langer, JE & Mandel, SJ. (2008). Utility of thyroglobulin measurement in fine needle aspiration biopsy specimens of lymph nodes in the diagnosis of recurrent thyroid carcinoma. *Cytojournal* Vol.5, pp.1-5.

Baskin, HJ. (2004).Detection of recurrent papillary thyroid carcinoma by thyroglobulin assessment in the needle washout after fine-needle aspiration of suspicious lymph nodes. *Thyroid,* Vol. 14, pp.959-63.

Boi, F.; Baghino, G.; Atzeni, F.; Lai, ML.; Faa, G. & Mariotti, S. (2006). The diagnostic value for differentieted thyroid carcinoma metastases of thyroglobulin (Tg) measurement in washout fluid from fine-needle aspiration biopsy of neck lymph nodes is maintained in the presence of circulating anti-Tg antibodies. *J Clin Endocrinol Metab,* Vol.91, N0.4, pp.1364-9.

Borel, AL.; Boizel, R.; Faure, P.; Barbe, G.; Boutonnat, J.; Sturm, N.; Seigneurin, D.; Bricault, I.; Caravel, JP.; Chaffanjon, P. & Chabre, O. (2008). Significance of low levels of thyroglobulin in fine needle aspirates from cervocal lymph nodes of patients with a history of differentiated thyroid cancer. *Eur J Endocrinol,* Vol. 158, pp.691-8.

Borson-Chazot, F.; Bardet, S.; Bournaud, C.; Conte-Devolx, B.; Corone, C.; D'Herbomez, M.; Henry, JF.; Leenhardt, L.; Peix, JL.; Schlumberger, M.; Wemeau, JL.; Baudin, E.; Berger, N.; Bernard, MH.; Calzada-Nocaudie, M.; Caron, P.; Catargi, B.; Chabrier, G.; Charrié, A.; Franc, B.; Hartl, D.; Helal, B.; Kerlan, V.; Kraimps, JL.; Leboulleux, S.; Le Clech, G.; Menegaux, F.; Orgiazzi, J.; Perie, S.; Raingeard, I.; Rodien, P.; Rohmer, V.; Sadoul, JL.; Schwartz, C.; Tenenbaum, F.; Toubert, ME.; Tramalloni, J.; Travagli, JP. & Vaudrey, C. (2008). Guidelines for the management of differentiated thyroid carcinoma of vesicular origin. *Ann Endocrinol (Paris)* Vol. 69, pp.472-86.

Bournaud, C; Charrié, A.; Nozières, C.; Chikh, K.; Lapras, V.; Denier, ML.; Paulin, C.; Decaussin-Petrucci, M.; Peix, JL.; Lifante, JC.; Cornu, C.; Giraud, C.; Orgiazzi, J. & Borson-chazot, F. (2010). Thyroglobulin measurement in fine-needle aspirates of lymph nodes in patients with differentiated thyroid cancer: a simple definition of the threshold value, with emphasis on potential pitfalls of the method. *Clin Chem Lab Med,* Vol.48, N0.8, pp.1171-7.

Chiovato, I.; Iatrofa, F.; Braverman, LE. ; Pacini, F.; Capezzone, M.; Masserini, I.; Grasso, L. & Pinchera, A. (2003). A disappearance of humoral thyroid autoimmunity after complete removal of thyroid antigens. *Ann Intern Med* Vol.139, pp.346-51.

Cignarelli, M.; Ambrosi, A.; Marino, A.; Lamacchia, O.; Campo, M.; Picca, G. & Giorgino, F. (2003). Diagnostic utility of thyroglobulin detection in fine-needle aspiration of cervical cystic metastatic lymph nodes from papillary thyroid cancer with negative cytology. *Thyroid* Vol.13, N012, pp.1163-7.

Cooper,DS.; Doherty, GM.; Haugen, BR.; Kloos, RT.; Lee, SL.; Mandel, SJ.; Mazzaferri, EL.; McIver, B.; Sherman, SI. & Tuttle, RM. (2006). Management guidelines for patients with thyroid nodules and differentiated thyroid cancer. *Thyroid* Vol.16, No.2, pp.109-42

Cunha, N.; Rodrigues, F.; Curado, F.; Ilheu, O.; Cruz, C.; Naidenov, P.; Rascao, MJ.; Ganho, J.; Gomes, I.; Pereira, H. Real, O.; Figueiredo, P.; Campos, B. & Valido, F. (2007). Thyroglobulin detection in fine-needle aspirates of cervical lymph nodes: a technique for the diagnosis of metastatic differentiated thyroid cancer. *Eur J Endocrinol* Vol.157, pp.101-7.

Druetta, L.; Croizet, K.; Bornet, H. & Rousset, B. (1998). Analyses of the molecular forms of serum thyroglobulin from patients with Graves' disease, subacute thyroiditis or differentiated thyroid cancer by velocity sedimentation on sucrose gradient and Western blot. *Eur J Endocrinol.* Vol.139, pp.498-507.

Feldt-Rasmussen, U.; Profilis, C.; Colinet, E.; Black, E.; Bornet, H.; Bourdoux, P.; Carayon, P.; Ericsson, UB.; Koutras, DA.; Lamas de Leon, L.; DeNayer, P.; Pacini, F.; Palumbo, G.; Santos, A.; Schlumberger, M.; Seidel, C.; Van

Herle, AJ. & De Vijlder, JJ. (1996) (a). Human thyroglobulin reference material (CRM 457). 1st Part: Assessment of homogeneity, stability and immunoreactivity. *Ann Biol Clin (Paris)* Vol.54, pp.337-42. (b) a human thyroglobulin reference material (CRM 457). 2nd Part: Physicochemical characterization and certification. *Ann Biol Clin (Paris)* Vol.54, pp.343-8.

Frasoldati, A.; Toschi, E.; Zini, M.; Flora, M.; Caroggio, A.; Dotti, C. & Valcavi, R. (1999). Role of thyroglobulin measurement in fine-needle aspiartion biopsies of cervical lymph nodes in patients with differantiated thyroid cancer. *Thyroid.* Vol.9, pp.105-11.

Henry, M.; Malthiery, Y.; Zanelli, E. & Charvet, B. (1990). Epitope mapping of human thyroglobulin Heterogeneous Recognition by thyroid pathologic sera. *J Immunol* Vol.145, pp.3692-8.

Kim, MJ.; Kim, EK.; Kim, BM.; Kwak, JY.; Lee, EJ.; Park, CS.; Cheong, WY. & Nam, KH. (2009). Thyroglobulin measurement in fine-needle aspirate washouts: the criteria for node dissection for patients with thyroid cancer. *Clin Endocrinol* Vol.70, pp.145-51.

Kloos, RT. & Mazzaferri, EL. (2005). A single recombinant human thyrotropin-stimulated serum thyroglobulin measurement predicts differentiated thyroid carcinoma metastases three to five years later. *J Clin Endocrinol Metab.* Vol.90, pp.5047-57.

Kohno, Y.; Tarutani, O.; Sakata, S. & Nakajima, H. (1985).Monoclonal antibodies to thyroglobulin elucidate differences in protein structure of thyroglobulin in healthy individuals and those with papillary adenocarcinoma. *J Clin Endocrinol Metab* Vol.61, pp.343-50.

Leenhardt, L.; Borson-Chazot, F.; Calzada, M.; Carnaille, B.; Charrié, A.; Cochand-Priolet, B. ; Cao, CD.; Leboulleux, S.; Le CLech, G.; Mansour, G.; Menegaux, F.; Monpeyssen, H.; Orgiazzi, J.; Rouxel, A.; Sadoul, JL.; Schlumberger, M.; Tramalloni, J.; Tranquart, F.; Wemeau, JL.; (2011).Good practice guide for cervical ultrasound scan and echo-guided techniques in treating differentiated thyroid cancer of vesicular origin. *Ann Endocrinol* Vol. 72, pp.173-97.

Malthiery, Y. & Lissitzky, S. (1987). Primary structure of human thyroglobulin deduced from the sequence of its 8448-base complementary DNA *Eur J Biochem* Vol.165, pp.491-8.

Mariotti, S.; Barbesino, G.; Caturegli, P.; Marino, M.; Manetti, L.; Pacini, F.; Centoni, R. & Pinchera, A. (1995). Assay of thyroglobulin in serum with Tg antibodies: un obtainable goal? *J Clin Endocrinol Metab* Vol.90, pp.5566-75.

Pacini, F.; Fugazzola, I.; Lippi, F.; Ceccarelli, C.; Centoni, R. & Miccoli, P. (1992). Detection of thyroglobulin in fine needle aspirates of nonthyroidal neck masses: a clue to diagnosis of metastasis differentiated thyroid cancer. *J Clin Endocrinol Metab* Vol.74, pp.1401-4.

Pacini, F. Schlumberger, M.; Dralle, H.; Elisei, R.; Smit, JWA.; Wiersinga, W.& the European Thyroid Cancer Taskforce (2006). European consensus for the management of patients with differentiated thyroid carcinoma of the follicular epithelium. *Eur J Endocrinol* Vol.154, pp.787-803.

Persani, L.; Ferrari, M.; Borgato, S.; Bestagno, M.; Faglia, G. & Beck Peccoz, P. (1998). Concanavalin A affinity chromatography can distinguish serum thyroglobulin (Tg) from normal subjects or patients with differentiated thyroid cancer. *J Endocrinol Invest* Vol.21 No.Suppl 4, pp.4.

Piechaczyck, M.; Chardès, T.; Cot, C.; Pau, B. & Bastide, JM. (1985). Production and characterisation of monoclonal antibodies against human thyroglobulin *Hybridoma* Vol.4, pp.361-7.

Preissner, CM.; O'Kane, DJ.; Singh, RJ.; Morris, JC. & Grebe, SK. (2003). Phantoms in the assay tube: heterophile antibody interferences in serum thyroglobulin assays. *J Clin Endocrinol Metab* Vol.88, pp.3069-74.

Schlumberger, M.; Hitzel, A.; Toubert, ME.; Corone, C.; Troalen, F.; Schlageter, MH.; Claustrat, F.; Koscielny, S.; Taieb, D.; Toubeau, M.; Bonichon, F.; Borson-Chazot, F.; Leenhardt, L.; Schwartz, C.; Dejax, C.; Brenot-Rossi, I.; Torlontano, M.; Tenenbaum, F.; Bardet, S.; Bussière, F.; Girard, JJ.; Morel, O.; Schneegans, O.; Schlienger, JL.; Prost, A.; So, D.; Archambaud, F.; Ricard, M. & Benhamou, E. (2007). Comparison of seven serum thyroglobulin assays in the follow-up of papillary and follicular thyroid cancer. *J Clin Endocrinol Metab* Vol.92, pp.2487-95.

Schlumberger, M.; Borget, I.; Nascimento, C.; Brassard, M. & Leboulleux S (2001). Treatment and follow-up of low-risk patients with thyroid cancer. *Nat Rev Endocrinol* Vol7, pp.625-8.

Schultz, R.; Bethauser, H.; Stempka, L.; Heilig, B.; Moll, A. & Hufner, M. (1989). Evidence for immunological differences between circulating and tissue-derived thyroglobulin in men. *Eur J Clin Invest* Vol.19, pp.459-63.

Sigstad, E.; Heilo, A.; Paus, E.; Holgersen, K.; Groholt, KK.; Jorgensen, LH.; Bogsrud, TV.; Berner, A. & Bjoro, T. (2007). The usefulness of detecting thyroglobulin in fine-needle aspirates from patients with neck lesions using a sensitive thyroglobulin assay. *Diagn Cytopathol* Vol.35, pp.761-7.

Sinadinovic, J.; Cvejic, D.; Savin, S.; Jancic-Zuguricas, M. & Micic, JV. (1992). Altered terminal glycosylation of thyroglobulin in papillary thyroid carcinoma. *Exp Clin Endocrinol.* Vol.100, pp.124-8.

Smallridge, RC.; Meek, SE.; Morgan, MA.; Gates, GS.; Fox, TP.; Grebe, S. & Fatourechi, V. (2007). Monitoring thyrogloulin in a sensitive immunoassay has comparable sensitivity to recombinant human TSH stimulated thyroglobulin in follow-up of thyroid cancer patients. *J Clin Endocrinol Metab* Vol.92, pp.82-7.

Snozek, CL.; Chambers, EP.; Reading, CC. ; Sebo, TJ.; Sistrunk, JW. ; Singh, RJ. & Grebe, SK. (2007). Serum thyroglobulin, high resolution ultrasound and lymph node thyroglobulin in diagnosis of differentiated thyroide carcinoma nodal metastases. *J Clin Endocrinol Metab*, Vol. 92, pp. 4278-81.

Spencer, C.; Takeuchi, M. & Kazarosyan, M. (1996), (a) Current status and performance goals for serum thyrotropin (TSH) assays. *Clin Chem* Vol42, pp.140-45 (b) Current status and performance goals for serum thyroglobulin assays. *Clin Chem* Vol.42, pp.164-73 (c) Recoveries cannot be used to authenticate thyroglobulin (Tg) when sera contain Tg autoantibodies. *Clin Chem* Vol.42, pp.661-3.

Uruno, T.; Miyauchi, A.; Shimizu, K.; Tomoda, C.; Takamura, Y.; Ito, Y.; Miya, A.; Kobayashi, K.; Matsuzukz, F.; amino, N. & Kuma, K. (2005). Usefulness of thyroglobulin measurement in fine-needle aspiration biopsy specimens for diagnosing cervical lymph node metastasis in patients with papillary thyroid cancer. *World J Surg* Vol.29, pp.483-5.

Van de Graf, SA.; Pauws, E.; de Vijlder, JJ. & Ris-Stalpers, C. (1997). The revised 8307 base pair coding sequence of human thyroglobulin transiently expressed in eukaryotic cells. *Eur J Endocrinol* Vol.136, pp.508-15.

Wild, D. (Ed). (2005). *The immunoassay handbook*, Third edition, Elsevier Ltd Publisher, ISBN-10: 0080445268, London

3

Papillary Thyroid Microcarcinoma – Do Classical Staging Systems Need to Be Changed?

Carles Zafon
Dept. of Endocrinology, Vall d'Hebron University Hospital
Autonomous University of Barcelona, Barcelona
Spain

1. Introduction

It has been broadly demonstrated that there has been a dramatic, worldwide, increase in the incidence of papillary thyroid carcinoma (PTC). Leenhardt *et al.* [2004] showed that there was approximately a 10-fold increase in the ratio of thyroid cancer for the cohort born in 1978 compared to those born in 1928. Davies & Welch [2006] found that the incidence of thyroid cancer in the United States had more than doubled from 1973 to 2002 and that this augmentation was virtually entirely due to an increase in PTC. However, it is uncertain whether this increase is a real phenomenon, or whether it is simply due to an increased rate of detection. Practices for management of thyroid diseases were deeply modified over the past few decades. The wide availability of ultrasonography (US) and fine needle aspiration biopsy (FNAB), as well as the improved accuracy of histopathological examination of surgical samples (that is the thinness of the anatomical slice of the thyroid specimen) are indicated as causes of this so-called spreading of the epidemic [Grodski & Delbridge, 2008]. Furthermore, the characteristics of PTCs, especially its size at diagnosis, have changed over time.

According to the World Health Organization, papillary microcarcinoma (PTMC) of the thyroid is defined as a papillary carcinoma measuring 1 cm or less [Lloyd et al., 2004]. PTMC is not recognized as a specific entity in the Tumor, Node and Metastasis (TNM) classification, and it is included in the T1 category, which has tumors as large as 2 cm.

The aim of the present article is to highlight how PTMC is changing the classical point of view of PTC and how, in the next few years, we must be able to incorporate the new phenotypic characteristics of PTC in the staging systems.

2. PTMC has changed the classical features of PTC

Several authors described a temporal trend toward decreasing tumor size in PTC. Chow *et al.* [2003] found that the percentage of PTMC has increased from 11.9% of all PTCs before the year 1980 to 25.5% in the decade 1990-1999. In an epidemiologic study carried out in a Brazilian region, Cordioli *et al.* [2009] reported that the average size of thyroid tumors decreased from 1.51 cm in the year 2000 to 1.02 cm in the year 2005. Moreover, in 2000 36.9% of cancers were smaller than 1 cm, whereas in 2005 PTMC accounted for 61.48% of all thyroid carcinomas. In the USA there was a 49% increase in the incidence of PTC, consisting of cancers measuring 1 cm or smaller [Davies & Welch, 2006]. In a large study Hay *et al.* [2008] found that PTMC represented 31% of the total patients with PTC. Additionally, during the decade 1945-1954 PTMC accounted for only 19% of the total patients with PTC, whereas in the decade 1995-2004 the percentage rose to 35%. Leenhardt *et al.* [2004] showed that the proportion of PTMC among cancers, which were operated on, increased form 18.4% in the period 1883 to 1987 to 43.1% in the period 1998 to 2001. Furthermore, in the most recent literature, especially those that analyzed cases from the last decade, PTMC comprises almost half of all papillary cases [D. Lim et al., 2007; Pakdaman et al., 2008].

3. Staging systems

There exist different scoring systems currently used to stratify patients with differentiated thyroid carcinoma (DTC). With the identification of certain clinicopathological parameters, associated with indolent or aggressive tumor behavior, patients may be separated in to risk groups based on these parameters, such as age, gender, size of tumor, and cancer extension. Consequently, treatment and follow-up decisions should be based on the analysis of these risk groups. Although they are broadly accepted, prognostic significance of the scoring systems is limited for several reasons [Sherman, 1999]. For example, all the systems are based on retrospective studies and the vast majority of them were published more than 20 years ago using historical cases. Thus, the age, grade, extent, size (AGES) scoring system was verified in a cohort of subjects with papillary thyroid carcinoma treated in the Mayo Clinic from 1946 through 1970 [Hay et al., 1987]. The age, distant metastases, extent, and size (AMES) staging proposal was developed in a controlled study of 821 patients with differentiated thyroid carcinoma (including both PTC and follicular thyroid carcinoma, FTC) between 1941 and 1980 [Cady et al., 1988]. The Clinical Class staging system, proposed by deGroot, was based on 269 patients with PTC treated during the interval of 1968-1980 [DeGroot et al., 1990]. The Ohio State University (OSU) study first enrolled 1355 patients (including PTC and FTC), treated between 1950 and 1993 [Mazzaferri & Jhiang, 1994].

It is interesting to note that treatment of PTC has significantly changed from those early years. Radioiodine ablation was introduced some years later. In the aforementioned cohort study of the Mayo Clinic only 3% of patients underwent postoperative ablation [Hay et al, 1987]. Moreover, the utilization of thyroglobulin levels as a tumor marker was introduced in 1975 [Van Herle & Uller, 1975]. Tubiana et al.[1985] showed that patients treated after 1960 had a better outcome than patients treated earlier, though they did not differ in age, histological characteristics, sex ratio or incidence of palpable lymph nodes. In addition, it has been said that most of the scoring systems do not take in to consideration the clinical status of the patient or the treatment procedure [Duntas & Grab-Duntas, 2006]. Moreover, it was proposed that different staging systems should be evaluated and validated independently for PTC and FTC [Lang et al., 2007a]. Finally, PTMCs are excluded from some studies [Schindler et al., 1991].

Some authors compared the utility of several staging systems in their series of patients, with the aim to find out the one that is the most predictive [Kingma et al., 1991; Lang et al., 2007b; Passler et al., 2003; Voutilainen et al, 2003]. Results do not confirm that any of them are better than the other. However, the TNM staging system, employed by the American Joint Committee on Cancer (AJCC) and the International Union Against Cancer (UICC) is currently the most widely used.

3.1 PTMC in the staging systems

PTMCs are considered a subset of PTCs that behave more benign. They follow an indolent course and carry an excellent prognosis. Distant metastases and mortality rates were reported to be less than 0.5% [Hay et al., 2008; Roti et al., 2008]. However, some authors suggest that there exists a subgroup of PTMCs that can be aggressive, requiring therapeutic management similar to larger tumors [Page et al., 2009]. Unfortunately, within this set of patients, prognostic factors have not been well defined. However, in recent years some specific markers for aggressiveness were identified, including sizes larger than 5 mm, multifocality, capsular invasion, tumor extension beyond the parenchyma, lymph node involvement, tumor non-incidentally discovered, and the extent of primary surgery [Küçük et al., 2007; S. Le et al., 2008; Mercante et al., 2009; Paget et al., 2009; Pelizzo et al., 2006; Roti et al, 2006]. Probably, three of the most accepted factors are multifocality, lymph node metastasis, and the mode of diagnosis.

Multiple foci were reported in approximately 7-56% of PTMCs [Dietlein et al., 2005; Hay et al., 2008; J. Lee et al., 2006; Roti et al., 2008]. A number of clinical studies showed that patients with ≥ two foci had a higher recurrence rate and cancer mortality than those with unifocal PTMCs [Baudin et al., 1998; Hay et al., 2008; J. Lin et al., 2009]. Moreover, multifocality is an independent risk factor for metastases [Gülben et al., 2008]. Hence, multifocal PTMCs have been considered to have a poor prognosis.

PTMCs also showed a high incidence of regional lymph node metastasis, occurring in 12--64% of patients [Besic et al., 2008; Choi et al, 2008; Chung et al., 2009; J. Lee et al., 2006; S. Lee et al., 2008; Y. Lim et al., 2009; Roh et al., 2008]. It was demonstrated that cases with positive lymph nodes had a higher risk of recurrence [Chow et al., 2003]. Kim et al. [2008] found that lateral cervical node metastasis was the most powerful independent predictor of clinical recurrence.

More than 70% of PTMCs are diagnosed incidentally (in specimens of the thyroid removed for benign thyroid disease) [Chow et al., 2003; Roti et al., 2008]. It has been suggested that clinical and biological behaviors may differ between incidental and non-incidental PTMCs [Barbaro et al., 2005; Chow et al., 2003; J. Lin et al., 2008]. Overt tumors are associated with a higher incidence of multicentricity, extrathyroidal involvement, lymphovascular invasion, higher stage, risk of relapse, and death [Besic et al., 2009; Chow et al., 2003; J. Lin et al., 2008; Lo et al., 2006; Noguchi et al., 2008; Pisanu et al., 2009].

4. Immunohistological markers

The knowledge of the molecular basis of cancer has changed dramatically, and what is more important, the accuracy of the diagnosis has changed as well [Chan, 2000]. The diagnosis of cancer in pathology is mainly based on the morphology of tissues and cells. Immunohistochemistry allows us to detect molecules in these tissues, including cell components, cell products, tumor markers or molecules, which help to predict the tumor behavior. The immunological reaction that takes place with this technique has remarkable sensitivity and specificity and it is applicable to routinely processed tissues, including fixed tissues. A great advantage of immunohistochemistry is the fact that we can simultaneously visualize the morphology of the cells and the immunostaining, so that we can locate the antigen we are detecting, in a particular subcellular localization or in a specific subtype of cells. Another advantage of the technique is that it is applicable to several types of material including tissue sections and cytological specimens [Chess & Hajdu, 1986].

In PTC, immunohistochemistry could be a useful tool to help not only in identifying the subset of patients at high risk, but also in those cases with no clear histological diagnosis [Rezk & Khan, 2005]. Several novel markers were tested, but, unfortunately, none of them were proved to be useful enough in clinical diagnosis [Asa, 2005]. At present, it is thought that their utility depends on the use of a panel of markers that include various combinations of them [Zafon et al., 2010]. For example, simultaneous immunohistochemical expression of HBME-1 and galectin-3 differentiates papillary carcinomas from hyperfunctioning lesions of the thyroid [Rossi et al, 2006].

Also in PTMC several possible immunohistological markers were proposed to assess the biological aggressiveness of the cancer [Boucek et al., 2009; Cvejic et al., 2008; Khoo et al., 2002; D. Lim et al., 2007] (table). Some authors compared molecular expression in PTMCs and PTCs of larger size. For example, Cvejic et al [2009] reported differences in the expression of the apoptotic molecule Bax and in the ratio Bcl-2/Bax between PTMC and larger tumors. Batistatou ***et al*** [2008] found a negative correlation between E-cadherin and dysadherin expression and the tumor size. Other authors attempted to define molecular characteristics of aggressiveness. For instance, D. Lim et al. [2007] showed that the absence of EGFR expression was correlated with extrathyroid extension and lymph node metastases. Lantsov et al. [2005] found a significant association between Cyclin D1 expression and both tumor size and lymph node metastases. Khoo et al. [2002] obtained similar results. Finally, Ito et al. [2005] reported that expression of proliferating markers such as Ki-67, Cyclin D1 and the retinoblastoma gene product (pRb) increased in PTMCs with clinically apparent metastases.

Molecule	Size	Aggressiveness	Reference
E-Cadherin	--		Batistatou *et al* [2008]
Dysadherin	--		Batistatou *et al* [2008]
Bcl-2/Bax ratio	+		Cvejic *et al* [2009]
MUC4	+		Nam *et al.* [2011]
Cyclin- D1	+	+	Lantsov *et al.* [2005]
		+	Khoo *et al.* [2002]
		+	Ito *et al.* [2005]
Ki-67		+	Ito *et al.* [2005]
pRb		+	Ito *et al.* [2005]
S100A4		+	Min *et al.* [2008]
EGFR		--	D. Lim *et al.* [2007]
Galectin-3		0	Cvejic *et al* [2005]

Table 1. Correlation (+ positive, - negative, 0 no correlation) between molecular markers and papillary thyroid microcarcinoma features.

5. The age factor

Some studies failed to identify independent prognostic factors, arguing that to distinguish PTC on the basis of size alone may be clinically irrelevant [Arora et al., 2009; Sugino et al., 1998]. Moreover classical scoring systems seem to be less accurate when the PTC is of a smaller size. Additionally, the role of age, as the paradigm of prognostic factors, remains to be established.

Most reports in the literature show that older patients with PTC have a worse prognosis. In DTC age is the most important factor and this parameter is included in the TNM staging system as well as in the vast majority of the other scores. Older age is especially significant in patients with advanced tumors [Pelizzo et al., 2005]. However, once again, though articles recognize the age factor, most of them are retrospective studies that include cases without current standardized therapeutic protocols. Moreover, few reports specifically analyze the behavior of thyroid cancer in the elderly. Vini et al. [2003] studied the biological behavior in 111 patients with DTC, who were older than 70. The authors found that older age was an important risk factor for overall survival. It is noteworthy that only 52% of patients had PTC, total thyroidectomy was performed in only 41% of cases and postoperative radioiodine was administered in the 72%. Furthermore, investigators showed that the probability of survival changed significantly according to the decade in which the patient was treated. Thus, median survival improved from 4.7 years before 1970, to more than 10 years after 1990 [Vini et al., 2003]. J. Lin et al. [2000] analyzed thyroid cancer in patients age 60 or older. Less than half of all the cases were papillary. They concluded that one important difference with respect to younger subjects was the delay in the diagnosis.

The increased aggressiveness of PTC in elderly patients may be attributed to a variety of factors. It is assumed that older subjects have tumors with a higher percentage of histological types with less favorable prognosis [Hundahl et al., 1998]. Also, effectiveness of radioiodine therapy decreases in the elderly. Schlumberger et al. [1996] found that metastases of DTC uptake iodine in 90% of patients less than 40 years of age and in 56% of patients over 40. Mihailovic et al. [2009] found that age is related with the radiodione avidity of distant metastases. Moreover, aged patients show a higher rate of large tumors. Biliotti et al. [2006] found that in subjects, who were older than 70, with thyroid tumors > 2 cm in diameter, the survival rates were markedly lower than rates among patients with a tumor diameter of < 2 cm. Other factors have been proposed such as the sexual hormone status and the impaired immune response, which accompanies older individuals [Haymart, 2009a]. Accordingly, it appears that thyroid cancer in the elderly and in younger patients could have a different behavior [Biliotti et al, 2006].

5.1 Age in PTMC

Some reports also demonstrate the importance of age in PTMCs [J. Lin et al, 2005]. H. Lin & Bhattacharyya [2009] examined the Surveillance, Epidemiology and End Results (SEER) registry, a database from the National Cancer Institute of the USA. The authors analyzed 7,818 cases of PTMC, which presented without local or distant metastasis. They found that only an increased age at diagnosis predicted decreased disease-specific survival. In a recent report, Elisei et al. [2010] showed that though patients diagnosed during the last two decades have smaller tumors, older age still represents the most important prognostic factor for survival.

However, despite the fact that older age is a universally identified poor prognostic factor in PTC, other investigators failed to find that age affects the outcome of patients with PTMC. In the aforementioned report of Chow et al. [2003], the authors found that, in PTMC, age was not a significant factor in predicting disease recurrence or survival. Gülben et al. [2008] found that mean age was higher in patients with lymph node metastases but the difference was not significant. In the large study reported by Pakdaman et al. [2008] investigators showed that the prevalence of PTMC was higher in patients 45 years and older, than in patients under 45. However, age was not related with multifocality, bilaterality and extrathyroid extension, risk factors shown to increase recurrences. Of particular interest is the recent article of Besic et al. [2009], which reported that in PTMC, lymph node metastases were more common in patients over 45 years of age. The same authors also showed that there was no correlation between the duration of the disease-free interval and the age of patients [2008]. Moreover, in an adjusted model, Noguchi et al. [2008] found that age was not a risk factor for recurrence in PTMC. Mercante et al. [2009], in their large study of 445 cases demonstrated that age was not a significant risk factor for neck recurrence or distant metastasis. Another study reported that patients with lymph node metastasis were younger than those without lymph node metastases [Chung et al., 2009]. Y. Lim et al. [2009] also found that in patients under 45 there was a higher incidence of ipsilateral central lymph node metastases. Previously, Baudin et al. [1998] described that patients with non-incidental PTMC were significantly younger. Non-incidental diagnosis was proposed as a criterion for a poor outcome. Another study reported that patients with PTMC were significantly older that patients with larger tumors. Moreover, in the PTMC group lymph node metastasis at diagnosis was correlated with a younger age [Tzvetov et al., 2009]. Jacquot-Laperrière et al. [2007] found that age did not become a prognostic factor for the risk of metastatic spread.

In the meta-analysis carried out by Roti et al. [2008] a younger age (< 45 years) was significantly associated with cancer recurrence. Haymart et al. [2009b] found that patients who received radioiodine ablation were younger that those not receiving this treatment. Recently, we reported that PTMCs in older patients were associated with less multifocality, bilaterality, fewer lymphadenectomies and a decreased rate of non-incidental tumors than in younger patients [Zafon et al, 2011].

In summary, several data suggest that age is not a significant factor in predicting disease recurrence or survival for PTMC. On the contrary, some reports suggest that younger age could be a worse prognostic factor. It is conceivable that in older patients there exist two different forms of PTMC. One form is the "clinical PTMC" which behaves as PTC. The second form is a "silent PTMC," a tumor incidentally discovered that will never be apparent and that may be in concordance with the occult carcinoma detected in thyroid glands from autopsies. In this regard, it is interesting to note that gender distribution of PTMC found in autopsies shows differences as compared to clinical papillary tumors [Kovács et al, 2005]. It is well established that the incidence of PTC in women is significantly higher than that in men (with a female to male ratio greater than 2 to 1) [Yao et al, 2011]. However, several authors have not found any significant gender-related differences in PTMC found at autopsies [Lang et al, 1988; Neuhold et al, 2001; Kovács et al, 2005].

6. Conclusions

The rising incidence of PTMC demands the identification of specific prognostic factors for cancers measuring 1.0 cm or less, to differentiate those truly aggressive neoplasms from the clinically insignificant tumors. For that, it is mandatory to reevaluate the classic prognostic scores with the aim to define their usefulness in the management of PTMC. To date, the clinical significance of many of these variables is yet to be established. As a consequence, there is no agreement about the optimal treatment of smaller tumors [Küçük et al, 2007]. Whereas some authors argue for an aggressive approach, others suggest that no further treatment is needed after lobectomy or thyroidectomy. Moreover, some even propose observation, without surgical treatment [Ito et al, 2003]. In the next few years, we will need to improve the role of the staging systems in accordance with the new phenotypic characteristics of PTC. Finally, age, as a prognostic factor, must be cautiously interpreted in PTCs less than 1 cm.

7. References

Arora, N.; Turbendian, H.; Kato, M.; Moo, T.; Zarnegar, R. & Fahey III, T. (2009). Papillary thyroid carcinoma and microcarcinoma: is there a need to distinguish the two? *Thyroid*, Vol. 19, No. 5, pp. 473-477.

Asa, S. (2005). The role of immunohistochemical markers in the diagnosis of follicular-patterned lesions of the thyroid. *Endocrine Pathology*, Vol. 16, No. 4, pp. 295-309.

Barbaro, D.; Simi, U.; Meucci, G.; Orsini, P. & Pasquini, C. (2005). Thyroid papillary cancers: microcarcinoma and carcinoma, incidental cancers and non-incidental cancers - are they different diseases? *Clinical Endocrinology*, Vol. 63, pp. 577-581.

Batistatou, A.; Charalabopoulos, K.; Nakanishi, Y.; Vagianos, C.; Hirohashi, S.; Agnantis, N. & Scopa, C. (2008). Differential expression of dysadherin in papillary thyroid carcinoma and microcarcinoma: correlation with E-cadherin. *Endocrine Pathology*, Vol. 19, No. 3, pp. 197-202.

Baudin, E.; Travagli, J.; Ropers, J.; Mancusi, F.; Bruno-Bossio, G.; Caillou, B.; Cailleaux, A.; Lumbroso, J.; Parmentier, C. & Schlumberger, M. (1998). Microcarcinoma of the thyroid gland. The Gustave-Roussy institute experience. *Cancer*, Vol. 83, No. 3, pp. 553-559.

Besic, N.; Pilko, G.; Petric, R.; Hocevar, M. & Zgajnar, J. (2008). Papillary thyroid microcarcinoma: prognostic factors and treatment. *Journal of Surgical Oncology*, Vol. 97, pp. 221-225.

Besic, N.; Zgajnar, J.; Hocevar, M. & Petric, R. (2009). Extent of thyroidectomy and lymphadenectomy in 254 patients with papillary thyroid microcarcinoma: A single-institution experience. *Annals of Surgical Oncology*, Vol. 16, pp. 920-928.

Biliotti, G.; Martini, F.; Vezzosi, V.; Seghi, P.; Tozzi, F.; Castagnoli, A.; Basili, G. & Peri, A. (2006). Specific features of differentiated thyroid carcinoma in patients over 70 years of age. *Journal of Surgical Oncology*, Vol. 93, pp. 194-198.

Boucek, J.; Kastner, J.; Skrivan, J.; Grosso, E.; Gibelli, B.; Giugliano, G. & Betka, J. (2009). Occult thyroid carcinoma. *Acta Otorhinolaryngologica Italica*, Vol. 29, No. 6, pp. 296-304.

Cady, B. & Rossi, R. (1988). An expanded view of risk-group definition in differentiated thyroid carcinoma. *Surgery*, Vol. 104, No. 6, pp. 947-953.

Chan, J. (2000). Advances in immunohistochemistry: impact on surgical pathology practice. *Seminars in Diagnostic Pathology*, Vol. 17, No. 3, pp. 170-177.

Chess, Q. & Hajdu, S. (1986). The role of immunoperoxidase staining in diagnostic cytology. *Acta Cytologica*, Vol. 30, No. 1, pp. 1-7.

Choi, S.; Kim, T.; Lee, J.; Shong, Y.; Cho, K.; Ryu, J.; Lee, J.; Roh, J & Kim, S. (2008). Is routine central neck dissection necessary for the treatment of papillary thyroid microcarcinoma? *Clinical and Experimental Otorhinolaryngology*, Vol. 1, No. 1, pp. 41-45.

Chow, S.; Law, S.; Chan, J.; Au, S.; Yau, S. & Lau, W. (2003). Papillary microcarcinoma of the thyroid - prognostic significance of lymph node metastasis and multifocality. *Cancer*, Vol. 98, No. 1, pp. 31-40.

Chung, Y.; Kim, J.; Bae, J.; Song, B.; Kim, J.; Jeon, H.; Jeong, S.; Kim, E. & Park, W. (2009). Lateral lymph node metastasis in papillary thyroid carcinoma: results of the therapeutic lymph node dissection. *Thyroid*, Vol. 19, No. 3, pp. 241-246.

Cordioli, M.; Canalli, M. & Coral, M. (2009). Increase incidence of thyroid cancer in Florianopolis, Brazil: comparative study of diagnosed cases in 2000 and 2005. *Arquivos Brasileiros de Endocrinologia e Metabologia*, Vol. 53, No. 4, pp. 453-460.

Cvejic, D.; Savin, S.; Petrovic, I.; Paunovic, I.; Tatic, S.; Krgovic, K. & Havelka, M. (2005). Galectin-3 expression in papillary microcarcinoma of the thyroid. *Histopathology*, Vol. 47, No. 2, pp. 209-214.

Cvejic, D.; Selemetjev, S.; Savin, S.; Paunovic, I.; Petrovic, I. & Tatic, S. (2008). Apoptosis and proliferation related molecules (Bcl-2, Bax, p53, PCNA) in papillary microcarcinoma versus papillary carcinoma of the thyroid. *Pathology*, Vol. 40, No. 5, pp. 475-480.

Cvejic, D.; Selemetjev, S.; Savin, S.; Paunovic, I. & Tatic, S. (2009). Changes in the balance between proliferation and apoptosis during the progression of malignancy in thyroid tumours. *European Journal of Histochemistry*, Vol. 53, No. 2, pp. 65-71.

Davies, L. & Welch, H. (2006). Increasing incidence of thyroid cancer in the United States, 1973-2002. *Journal of the American Medical Association*, Vol. 295, No. 18, pp. 2164-2167.

DeGroot, L.; Kaplan, E.; McCormick, M. & Straus, F. (1990). Natural history, treatment, and course of papillary thyroid carcinoma. *Journal of Clinical Endocrinology and Metabolism*, Vol. 71, No. 2, pp. 414-424.

Dietlein, M.; Luyken, W.; Schicha, H. & Larena-Avellaneda, A. (2005). Incidental multifocal papillary microcarcinomas of the thyroid: is subtotal thyroidectomy combined with radioiodine ablation enough? *Nuclear Medicine Communications*, Vol. 26, No. 1, pp 3-8.

Duntas, L. & Grab-Duntas, B. (2006). Risk and prognostic factors for differentiated thyroid cancer. *Hellenic Journal of Nuclear Medicine*, Vol. 9, No. 3, pp. 156-162.

Elisei, R.; Molinaro, E.; Agate, L.; Bottici, V.; Masserini, L.; Ceccarelli, C.; Lippi, F.; Grasso, L.; Basolo, F.; Bevilacqua, G.; Miccoli, P.; Di Coscio, G.; Vitti, P.; Pacini, F. & Pinchera, A. (2010). Are the clinical and pathological features of differentiated thyroid carcinoma really changed over the last 35 years? Study on 4187 patients from a single Italian institution to answer this question. *Journal of Clinical Endocrinology and Metabolism*, Vol 95, No. 4, pp. 1516-1527.

Grodski, S. & Delbridge, L. (2008). An update on papillary microcarcinoma. *Current Opinion in Oncology*, Vol. 21, pp. 1-4.

Gülben, K.; Berberoglu, U.; Çelen, O. & Mersin, H. (2008). Incidental papillary microcarcinoma of the thyroid - factors affecting lymph node metastasis. *Langenbeck's Archives of Surgery*, Vol. 393, pp. 25-29.

Hay, I.; Grant, C.; Taylor, W. & McConahey, W. (1987). Ipsilateral lobectomy versus bilateral lobar resection in papillary thyroid carcinoma: A retrospective analysis of surgical outcome using a novel prognostic scoring system. *Surgery*, Vol. 102, No. 6, pp. 1088-1095.

Hay, I.; Hutchinson, M.; Gonzalez-Losada, T.; McIver, B.; Reinalda, M.; Grant, C.; Thompson, G.; Sebo, T. & Goellner, J. (2008). Papillary thyroid microcarcinoma: A study of 900 cases observed in a 60-year period. *Surgery*, Vol. 144, No. 6; pp. 980-988.

Haymart, M. (2009a). Understanding the relationship between age and thyroid cancer. *Oncologist*, Vol. 14, pp. 216-221.

Haymart, M.; Cayo, M. & Chen, H. (2009b). Papillary thyroid microcarcinoma: big decisions for a small tumor. *Annals of Surgical Oncology*, Vol. 16, No. 11, pp. 3132-3139.

Hundahl, S.; Fleming, I.; Fremgen, A. & Menck, H. (1998). A National Center Data Base report on 53,856 cases of thyroid carcinoma treated in the U.S., 1985-1995. *Cancer*, Vol. 83, No. 12, pp. 2638-2648.

Ito, Y.; Uruno, T.; Nakano, K.; Takamura, Y.; Miya, A.; Kobayashi, K.; Yokozawa, T.; Matsuzuka, F.; Kuma, S.; Kuma, K. & Miyauchi, A. (2003). An observation trial without surgical treatment in patients with papillary microcarcinoma of the thyroid. *Thyroid*, Vol. 13, No. 4, pp. 381-387.

Ito, Y.; Uruno, T.; Takamura, Y.; Miya, A.; Kobayashi, K.; Matsuzuka, F.; Kuma, K. & Miyauchi, A. (2005). Papillary microcarcinomas of the thyroid with preoperatively detectable lymph node metastasis show significantly higher aggressive characteristics on immunohistochemical examination. *Oncology*, Vol. 68, No. 2-3, pp. 87-96.

Jacquot-Laperrière, S.; Timoshenko, A.; Dumollard, J.; Peoc'h, M.; Estour, B.; Martin, C. & Prades, J. (2007). Papillary thyroid microcarcinoma: incidence and prognostic factors. *European Archives of Otorhinolaryngology*, Vol. 264, No. 8, pp. 935-939.

Khoo, M.; Ezzat, S.; Freeman, J. & Asa, S. (2002). Cyclin D1 protein expression predicts metastatic behavior in thyroid papillary microcarcinomas but is not associated with gene amplification. *Journal of Clinical Endocrinology and Metabolism*, Vol. 87, No. 4, pp. 1810-1813.

Kim, T. Hong, S.; Kim, J.; Kim, W.; Gong, G.; Ryu, J.; Kim, W.; Yun, S. & Shong, Y. (2008). Prognostic parameters for recurrence of papillary thyroid microcarcinoma. *BMC Cancer*, Vol. 8, No. 296.

Kingma, G.; van der Bergen, H. & de Vries, J. (1991). Prognostic scoring systems in differentiated thyroid carcinoma: which is the best? *Netherlands Journal of Surgery*, Vol. 43, No. 3, pp. 63-66.

Kovács, G.; Gonda, G.; Vadász, G.; Ludmány, E.; Uhrin, K.; Görömbey, Z.; Kovács, L.; Hubina, E.; Bodó, M.; Góth, M. & Szabolcs, I. (2005). Epidemiology of thyroid microcarcinoma found in autopsy series conducted in areas of different iodine intake. *Thyroid*, Vol. 15, No. 2, pp. 152-157.

Küçük, N.; Tari, P.; Tokmak, E. & Aras, G. (2007). Treatment for microcarcinoma of the thyroid - clinical experience. *Clinical Nuclear Medicine*, Vol. 32, No. 4, pp. 279-281.

Lang, B.; Lo, C.; Chan, W.; Lam, K. & Wan, K. (2007a). Prognostic factors in papillary and follicular thyroid carcinoma: their implications for cancer staging. *Annals of Surgical Oncology*, Vol. 14, No. 2, pp. 730-738.

Lang, B.; Lo, C.; Chan, W & Lam, K. (2007b). Staging systems for papillary thyroid carcinoma. A review and comparison. *Annals of Surgery*, Vol. 245, No. 3, pp. 366-378.

Lang, W.; Borrusch, H. & Bauer, L. (1988). Evaluation of 1020 sequential autopsies. *American Journal of Clinical Pathology*, Vol. 90, pp. 72 - 76.

Lantsov, D.; Meirmanov, S.; Nakashima, M.; Kondo, H.; Saenko, V.; Naruke, Y.; Namba, H.; Ito, M.; Abrosimov, A.; Lushnikov, E.; Sekine, I. & Yamashita, S. (2005). Cyclin D1 overexpression in thyroid papillary microcarcinoma: its association with tumor size and aberrant beta-catenin expression. *Histopathology*, Vol. 47, No. 3, pp. 248-256.

Lee, J.; Rhee, Y.; Ahn, C.; Cha, B.; Kim, K.; Lee, H.; Kim, S.; Park, C. & Lim, S. (2006). Frequent, Aggressive behaviors of thyroid microcarcinoma in korean patients. *Endocrine Journal*, Vol. 53, No. 5. pp. 627-632.

Lee, S.; Le, S.; Jin, S.; Kim, J. & Rho, Y. (2008). Predictive factors for central compartment lymph node metastasis in thyroid papillary microcarcinoma. *Laryngoscope*, Vol. 118, No. 4, pp. 659-662.

Leenhardt, L.; Grosclaude, P. & Chérié-Challine, L. (2004). Increased incidence of thyroid carcinoma in France: a true epidemic or thyroid nodule management effects? Report from the French thyroid cancer committee. *Thyroid*, Vol. 14, No. 12, pp. 1056-1060.

Lim, D.; Baek, K.; Lee, Y.; Park, W.; Kim, M.; Kang, M.; Jeon, H.; Lee, J.; Yun-Cha, B.; Lee, K.; Son, H. & Kang, S. (2007). Clinical, Histopathological, and molecular characteristics of papillary thyroid microcarcinoma. *Thyroid*, Vol. 17, No. 9, pp. 883-888.

Lim, Y.; Choi, E.; Yoon, Y.; Kim, E. & Koo, B. (2009). Central lymph node metastases in unilateral papillary thyroid microcarcinoma. *British Journal of Surgery*, Vol. 96, pp. 253-257.

Lin, H & Bhattacharyya, N. (2009). Survival impact of treatment options for papillary microcarcinoma of the thyroid. *Laryngoscope*, Vol. 119, No. 10, pp. 1983-1987.

Lin, J.; Chao, T.; Chen, S.; Weng, H & Lin, K. (2000). Characteristics of thyroid carcinomas in aging patients. *European Journal of Clinical Investigation*, Vol. 30, No. 2, pp. 147-153.

Lin, J.; Chen, S.; Chao, T.; Hsueh, C. & Weng, H. (2005). Diagnosis and therapeutic strategy for papillary thyroid microcarcinoma. *Archives of Surgery*, Vol. 140, pp. 940-945.

Lin, J.; Kuo, S.; Chao, T. & Hssue, C. (2008). Incidental and nonincidental papillary thyroid microcarcinoma. *Annals of Surgical Oncology*, Vol. 15, No. 8, pp. 2287-2292.

Lin, J.; Chao, T.; Hsueh, C. & Kuo, S. (2009). High recurrent rate of multicentric papillary thyroid carcinoma. *Annals of Surgical Oncology*, Vol. 16, No.9, 2609-2616.

Lloyd, R.; De Lellis, R.; Heitz, P. & Eng, C. (2004). World Health Organization classification of tumors: Pathology and genetics of tumors of the endocrine organs. Lyon, France: IARC Press.

Lo, C.; Chan, W.; Lang, B.; Lam, K. & Wan, K. (2006). Papillary microcarcinoma: is there any difference between clinically overt and occult tumors? *World Journal of Surgery*, Vol. 30, pp. 759-766.

Mazzaferri, E. & Jhiang, S. (1994). Long-term impact of initial surgical and medical therapy on papillary and follicular thyroid cancer. *American Journal of Medicine*, Vol. 97, No. 5, pp. 418-428.

Mercante, G.; Frasoldati, A.; Pedroni, C.; Formisano, D.; Renna, L.; Piana, S.; Gardini, G.; Valcavi, R. & Barbieri, V. (2009). Prognostic factors affecting neck lymph node recurrence and distant metastasis in papillary microcarcinoma of the thyroid: results of a study in 445 patients. *Thyroid*, Vol. 19, No. 7, pp. 707-716.

Mihailovic, J.; Stefanovic, L.; Malesevic, M. & Markoski, B. (2009). The importance of age over radioiodine avidity as a prognostic factor in differentiated thyroid carcinoma with distant metastases. *Thyroid*, Vol. 19, No. 3, pp. 227-232.

Min, H.; Choer, G.; Kim, S.; Park, Y.; Park do, J.; Youn, Y.; Park, S.; Cho, B. & Park, S. (2008). S100A4 expression is associated with lymph node metastasis in papillary microcarcinoma of the thyroid. *Modern Pathology*, Vol. 21, No. 6, pp. 748-755.

Nam, K.; Noh, T.; Chung, S.; Lee, S.; Lee, M.; Hong, S.; Chung, W.; Lee, E. & Park, C. (2011). Expression of the membrane mucins MUC4 and MUC15, potential markers of malignancy and prognosis, in papillary thyroid carcinoma. *Thyroid*, Vol. 21, No. 7, pp. 745-750.

Neuhold, N.; Kaiser, H. & Kaserer, K. (2001). Latent carcinoma of the thyroid in Austria: a systematic autopsy study. *Endocrine Pathology*, vol. 12, pp. 23 - 31.

Noguchi, S.; Yamashita, H.; Uchino, S. & Watanabe, S. (2008). Papillary microcarcinoma. *World Journal of Surgery*, Vol. 32, pp. 747-753.

Page, C.; Biet, A.; Boute, P.; Cuvelier, P. & Strunski, V. (2009). "Aggressive papillary" thyroid microcarcinoma. *European Archives of Otorhinolaryngology*, Vol. 266, No. 12, pp. 1959-1963.

Pakdaman, M.; Rochon, L.; Gologan, O.; Tamilia, M.; Garfield, N.; Hier, M.; Black, M. & Payne, R. (2008). Incidence and histopathological behavior of papillary microcarcinomas: Study of 429 cases. *Otolaryngology Head and Neck Surgery*, Vol. 139, No. 5, pp 718-722.

Passler, C.; Prager, G.; Scheuba, C.; Kaserer, K.; Zettinig, G. & Niederle, B. (2003). Application of staging systems for differentiated thyroid carcinoma in an endemic goiter region with iodine substitution. *Annals of Surgery*, Vol. 237, No. 2, pp. 227-234.

Pelizzo, M.; Toniato, A.; Boschin, I.; Piotto, A.; Bernante, P.; Pagetta, C.; Palazzi, M.; Maria Guolo, A.; Preo, P.; Nibale, O. & Rubello, D. (2005). Locally advanced differentiated thyroid carcinoma: a 35-year mono-institutional expericence in 280 patients. *Nuclear Medicine Communications*, Vol. 26, No. 11, pp. 965-968.

Pelizzo, M.; Boschin, I.; Toniato, A.; Piotto, A.; Bernante, P.; Pagetta, C.; Rampin, L. & Rubello, D. (2006). Papillary thyroid microcarcinoma (PTMC): prognostic factors, management and outcome in 403 patients. *European Journal of Surgical Oncology*; Vol. 32, No. 10, pp. 1144-1148.

Pisanu, A.; Reccia, I.; Nardello, O. & Uccheddu, A. (2009). Risk factors for nodal metastasis and recurrence among patients with papillary thyroid microcarcinoma: differences in clinical relevance between nonincidental and incidental tumors. *World Journal of Surgery*, Vol. 33, No. 3, pp. 460-468.

Rezk, S. & Khan, A. (2005). Role of immunohistochemistry in the diagnosis and progression of follicular epithelium-derived thyroid carcinoma. *Applied Immunohistochemistry and Molecular Morphology*, Vol. 13, No. 3, pp. 256-264.

Roh, J.; Kim, J. & Park, C. (2008). Central cervical nodal metastasis from papillary thyroid microcarcinoma: pattern and factors predictive of nodal metastasis. *Annals of Surgical Oncology*, Vol. 15, No. 9, pp. 2482-2486.

Rossi, E.; Raffaelli, M.; Miraglia, A.; Lombardi, C.; Vecchio, F. & Fadda, G. (2006). Simultaneous immunohistochemical expression of HBME-1 and galectin-3 differentiates papillary carcinomas from hyperfunctioning lesions of the thyroid. *Histopathology*, Vol. 48, No. 7, pp. 795-800.

Roti, E.; Rossi, R.; Trasforini, G.; Bertelli, F.; Ambrosio, M.; Busutti, L.; Pearce, E.; Braverman, L. & Uberti, E. (2006). Clinical and histological characteristics of papillary thyroid microcarcinoma: results of a retrospective study in 243 patients. *Journal of Clinical Endocrinology and Metabolism*, Vol. 91, No. 6, pp. 2171-2178.

Roti, E.; Uberti, E.; Bondanelli, M. & Braverman, L. (2008). Thyroid papillary microcarcinoma: a descriptive and meta-analysis study. *European Journal of Endocrinology*, Vol. 159, pp. 659-673.

Schindler, A.; van Melle, G.; Evequoz, B. &, Scazziga, B. (1991). Prognostic factors in papillary carcinoma of the thyroid. *Cancer*, Vol. 68, No. 2, pp. 324-330.

Schlumberger, M.; Challeton, C.; De Vathaire, F.; Travagli, J. ; Gardet, P. ; Lumbroso, J.; Francese, C.; Fontaine, F.; Ricard, M. & Parmentier, C. (1996). Radioactive iodine treatment and external radiotherapy for lung and bone metastases from thyroid carcinoma. *Journal of Nuclear Medicine*, Vol. 37, No. 4, pp. 598-605.

Sherman, S. (1999). Toward a standard clinicopathologic staging approach for differentiated thyroid carcinoma. *Semininars in Surgical Oncology*, Vol. 16, No. 1, pp. 12-15.

Sugino, K.; Ito, K.J.; Ozaki, O.; Mimura, T.; Iwasaki, H. & Ito, K. (1998). Papillary microcarcinoma of the thyroid. *Journal of Endocrinological Investigation*, Vol. 21, No. 7, pp. 445-448.

Tubiana, M.; Schlumberger, M.; Rougier, P.; Laplanche, A.; Benhamou, E.; Gardet, P.; Caillou, B.; Travagli, J. & Parmentier, C. (1985). Long-term results and prognostic factors in patients with differentiated thyroid carcinoma. *Cancer*, Vol. 55, No. 4, pp. 794-804.

Tzvetov, G.; Hirsch, D.; Shraga-Slutzky, I.; Weinstein, R.; Manistersky, Y.; Kalmanovich, R.; Lapidot, M.; Grozinsky-Glasberg, S.; Singer, J.; Sulkes, J.; Shimon, I. & Benbassat, C. (2009). Well-differentiated thyroid carcinoma: comparison of microscopic and macroscopic disease. *Thyroid*, Vol. 19, No. 5, pp. 487-494.

Van Herle, A. & Uller, R. (1975). Elevated serum thyroglobulin. A marker of metastases in differentiated thyroid carcinomas. *Journal of Clinical Investigation*, Vol. 56, pp. 272-277.

Vini, L.; Hyer, S.; Marshall, J.; A´Hern, R. & Harmer, C. (2003). Long-term results in elderly patients with differentiated thyroid carcinoma. *Cancer*, Vol. 97, No.11, pp. 2736-2742.

Voutilainen, P.; Siironen, P.; Franssila, K.; Sivula, A.; Haapiainen, R. & Haglund, C. (2003). AMES, MACIS and TNM prognostic classifications in papillary thyroid carcinoma. *Anticancer Research*, Vol. 23, No. 5b, pp. 4283-4288.

Yao, R.; Chiu, C.; Strugnell, S.; Gill, S. & Wiseman, S. (2011). Gender differences in thyroid cancer. *Expert Review of Endocrinology and Metabolism*, Vol. 6, No. 2, pp. 215 - 243.

Zafon, C.; Castellvi, J. & Obiols, G. (2010). Usefulness of the immunohistochemical analysis of several molecular markers in the characterization of papillary thyroid carcinoma with initial lymph node mestastasis. *Endocrinologia y Nutricion*, Vol. 57, No. 4, pp. 165-169.

Zafon, C.; Baena, J.; Castellvi, J.; Obiols, G.; Monroy, G. & Mesa, J. (2011). Differences in the form of presentation between papillary microcarcinomas and papillary carcinomas of larger size. *Journal of Thyroid Research*, ID 639156.

4

Thyroid Neoplasm

Augusto Taccaliti, Gioia Palmonella,
Francesca Silvetti and Marco Boscaro
Politecnic University of Marche, Ancona
Italy

1. Introduction

Thyroid gland comprises 2 types of cells: Follicular cells (or thyrocytes) which produce and secrete thyreoglobulin and thyroid hormones, thyroxine (T_4) and triiodothyronine (T_3) and Parafollicular cells (or C cells), secrete calcitonin. Papillary Thyroid Carcinoma (PTC) and Follicular Thyroid Carcinoma (FTC) are tumors originating by thyrocytes and are referred as Differentiated Thyroid Carcinomas (DTCs). Anaplastic Thyroid Carcinoma (ATC) is the undifferentiate tumor which may arises from DTCs or may be undifferentiated to origin. Medullary Thyroid Carcinoma (MTC), is the tumor arising to C cell. Rare tumors of non-epithelial thyroid origin are lymphoma, fibrosarcoma, squamous cell carcinoma, malignant teratoma and metastasis of other tumors.

2. Differentiated thyroid carcinomas (DTCs)

2.1 Epidemiology

Thyroid tumor represent about 1% of all human malignancy and about 90% of all endocrine tumor. PTC represents about 90% and FTC the 10% of DTCs. The annual incidence of thyroid cancer has been reported to range between 1.2 and 2.6 cases per 100.000 in men and 2.0-3.8 cases per 100.000 in women. Recently epidemiological studies have shown an increased incidence of DTCs in worldwide (Kosary, 2007; Kilfoy et al., 2009). PTC and microPTC (size < 1cm) represents the cancer prevalently increased. Reasons of increased incidence are not completely understood and controversies exist whether this increase is real or only apparent due to an increase in diagnostic activity. Probably the increased incidence may reflect the increased detection of small tumors through the use of imaging, particularly ultrasonografy (US), and increased use of fine needle aspiration citology (FNAC). Mortality records in the SEER database from 1997-2006 show relatively stable or slightly improved mortality rates for thyroid cancer (Edwards et al, 2010). However, over the same period, SEER mortality rates measured in terms of relative survival show reduced mortality rates in women respect to in men (Kosary, 2007).

2.2 Risk factors

2.2.1 Ionizing radiation

Ionizing radiations interacting with DNA produce mutations. thyroid was a tissue sensitive to ionizing radiation as demonstrate by the increased incidence in thyroid cancer after

Chernobyl accident. Children and young people were affected by DTCs and PTC was the histotype prevalently. Moreover, WHO has reported that newborn and children below 5 years old have high risk to develop thyroid cancer respect to adolescent and adults (Papadopoulou et al., 2009; Williams, 2008).

2.2.2 Iodine intake

Iodine is essential for T_4 and T_3 production. iodine deficient or inadequate intake induces low t4 levels and TSh increase and chronic tsh stimuli promotes growth goiter and nodules. thyroid nodules represent a clinical condition to develop thyroid cancer and especially FTC histotype. Studies have show a reduction of PTC/FTC ratio in iodine deficient area (Farahati et al., 2004; Lind et al., 1998).

2.3 Familial thyroid cancer syndromes

Non Medullary Familial Thyroid Cancer represents a rare disease where thyroid cancer is the only manifestation or thyroid cancer may represent a component of a complex syndrome.

Familial thyroid cancer PTC may have familial factors in 3.2 and 6.2%of cases. in fact, has been reported an increased incidence in relatives of patients with PTC of 4-10 fold (Pal et all, 2001). Some studies have found an association between altered telomere length (TL) and cancer phenotype (Capezzone et al, 2011). In these cases, the tumors are PTC with onset at an earlier age, with reversed gender distribution and with a more aggressive phenotype (Hemminki et al., 2005) with anticipation of neoplasia.

2.4 Familial tumour syndromes with thyroid cancer

1. Polyposis coli and Gardner's syndrome: Familial Adenomatous Polyposis (FAP) and Gardner's syndrome are inherited diseases characterized by colonic polyposis the former, and osteomas, lipomas and fibromas plus colonic polyposis the latter. Both syndromes show 5–10-fold increase in the incidence of PTC and tumor is multicentric. Germline mutations of tumor suppressor gene APC (Adenomatosis Polyposis Coli) are described in both syndromes. PTC in familial polyposis syndromes often harbours RET/PTC rearrangements (see below) in addition to the APC deletion (Cetta et al., 1998).
2. Cowden's disease: Patients with Cowden's disease have breast carcinoma and hamartomas. Cowden's disease is caused by germ-line mutations in the phosphatase and tensin homologue (PTEN) tumour suppressor gene inheritance in autosomal dominant pattern. Cowden's disease increases the incidence of follicular tumours of the thyroid, but the incidence is hard to estimate (Hemmings, 2003). Papillary cancer is also found with increased frequency.
3. Carney complex: The Carney complex consists of spotty skin pigmentation, myxomas, schwannomas, pigmented nodular adrenal hyperplasia, pituitary and testicular tumors and an increased incidence of follicular adenoma and FC. It is due to a mutation in the type 1 alpha regulatory subunit of the protein kinase A (PRKAR1A) which leads to constitutively activated protein kinase A (PKA) (Boikos & Stratakis, 2006) PRKAR1A mutations have been found in sporadic thyroid tumors and are more common in FC than follicular adenoma.

2.5 Somatic genetic alterations

DTCs frequently have somatic mutations that constitutively activated the mitogen-activated protein kinase (MAPK) pathway and PI3K-AKT pathway. These pathways include cell surface receptors such as RET and NTK, and intracellular signal transduceds , RAS gene and kinases RAF. Ultimately, this leads to increased nuclear translocation of phosphorylated MAPK and altered transcriptional regulation of target genes. Although the characteristic genetic alterations in PTC are all capable of activating the MAPK pathway, the histological phenotype and the expression profile are not identical between the different genetic alterations suggesting that other pathways such as the phosphoinositide-3-kinase (PI3K), protein kinase C and Wnt signalling pathways may be variously involved (figure 1).

2.5.1 Thyrosine kinase receptors

Tyrosine kinase receptors function as receptors for many growth factors and carry growth signals into the cell through tyrosine autophosphorylation and the initiation of kinase cascades. Tyrosine kinase receptors implicated on thyroid oncogenesis include RET and TRK:

1. RET: RET proto-oncogene is a 21-exons gene located on the proximal long arm of chromosome 10 that encodes a tyrosine kinase receptor. It is involved in the regulation of growth, survival, differentiation, and migration of cells of neural crest origin. It is not normally expressed in the follicular cell. The interaction extracellular ligand-binding domain and RET receptor leads the activation of a serine/threonine kinase pathway including RAS, BRAF and MAPK. This ultimately leads to a proliferative signal as well as inhibiting apoptosis and increasing genetic instability.

RET/PTC rearrangement: Rearrangements of RET gene in papillary thyroid carcinoma (PTC) are known as RET/PTC. Low-level expression may be seen in non-malignant follicular cells especially in Hashimoto's thyroiditis (Nikiforov, 2006). Although more than 10 rearrangements have been described, RET/PTC1 (60-70%), RET/PTC2 (20-30%), and RET/PTC3 (10%) account for most of the rearrangements found in PTC. Other RET/PTC rearrangements are rare (Santoro et al., 2006). In each of these rearrangements, the upstream (5′) component of a "housekeeping" (or ubiquitously expressed) gene drives the expression of the tyrosine kinase domain of RET. Two of the most common rearrangement types are RET/PTC1 and RET/PTC3. Both type of rearrangement paracentric intrachromosomal inversions, as all fusion partners reside on the long arm of chromosome 10. By contrast, RET/PTC2 and nine more RET/PTC rearrangements are all intrachromosomal rearrangements formed by RET fusion to genes located on different chromosomes. In the adult population, the RET rearrangements have been found in 2.6% to 34% of PTC. This variation is due to true differences in the prevalence of this alteration in PTC in specific age group in individuals exposed to ionizing radiation. Other causes might be represented by heterogeneous distribution of this rearrangements within the cancer and the various sensibilities of the detention methods used. In the pediatric population RET/PTC1 and RET/PTC3 have been found in up to 80% of the cases. These mutations are found in children exposed to radiation after the Chernobyl nuclear accident or to external irradiation for treatment of benign diseases of the head and neck. There are evidences that RET/PTC rearrangements represent an early genetic changes leading to the development of PTC (Nikiforov, 2002; Xing, 2005).

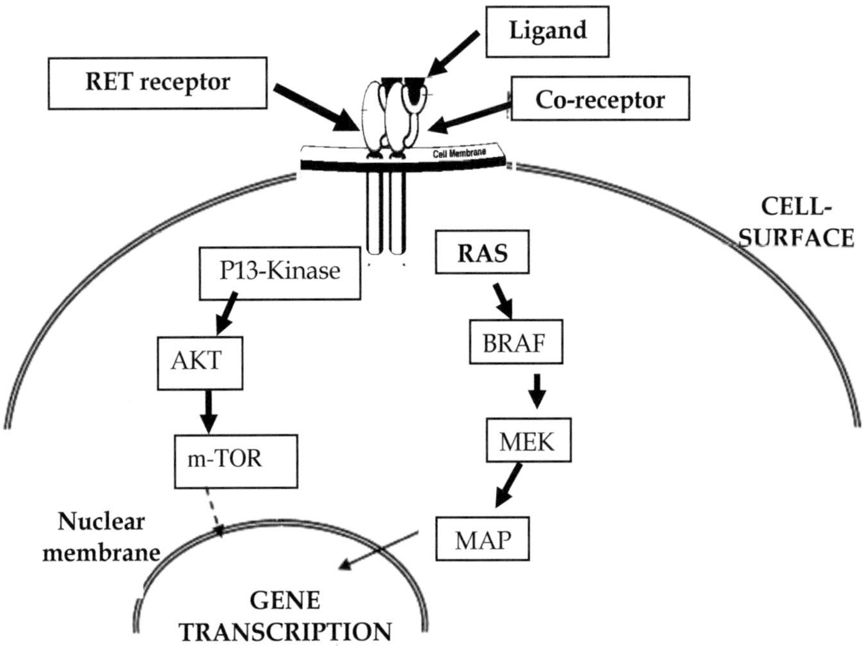

Fig. 1. RET receptor with MAP-Kinase and PI3-Kinase-AKT pathways in thyroid cell.

2. Trk: Trk proto-oncogene is located on chromosome 1q22 and encodes a tyrosine kinase receptor for nerve growth factor (27). It is expressed in the neurons in both peripheral and central nervous system, and is involved in the regulation of growth, differentiation and survival of these cells.

Trk rearrangements: occur in DTCs with lower prevalence than RET/PTC rearrangements. In thyroid follicular cells, the gene is activated through chromosomal rearrangement, with juxtaposes the intracellular thyrosine kinase domain of NTRK1 to the 5′ terminal sequence of different genes. Various genes combine with TRK gene forming chimeric genes. The main ones are tropomyosin gene (TPM3) gene and the translocated gene promoter (TPR). Trk rearrangements have been identified in 2-5% of PTC. (Musholt et al., 2000).

2.5.2 BRAF mutations

The RAF proteins are serine/threonine kinases involved in intracellular signalling via the MAPK pathway (Davies et al., 2002). Point mutations in BRAF leading to mutant proteins that mimic the conformation of the phosphorylated form and are therefore constitutively activated are involved in several of human malignancies including melanoma, ovarian and colorectal cancers. Mutations in the BRAF gene are the most common genetic alteration seen in PTC. BRAF mutations occur in 30–60% of PTC and are 100% specific. BRAF point mutations are rarely associated with radiation-induced PTC. A paracentric inversion involving BRAF (AKAP9-BRAF) was found in 11% of post Chernobyl tumors BRAF and RET/PTC are mutually exclusive, not occurring in the same tumor. The presence of BRAF mutations appears to be associated with poor prognosis, reduced iodine uptake and failure of radioiodine ablation. Poorly differentiated and ATC harbour BRAF mutations, but not RET/PTC rearrangements, suggesting that BRAF mutations may predispose PTC to de-differentiation (Xing et al., 2005a; Nikiforova et al., 2003).

2.5.3 RAS mutations

Three RAS genes, H-RAS, K-RAS, and N-RAS, synthesize a family of 21-kDa proteins that play an important role in tumorigenesis. Their function is to convey signals originating from tyrosine kinase membrane receptors to a cascade of mitogen-activated protein kinases (MAPK). This activates the transcription of target genes involved in cell proliferation, survival, and apoptosis. The RAS proteins exist in two different forms: an inactive form that is bound to guanosine diphosphate (GDP) and an active form that exhibits guanosine triphosphatase (GTPase) activity. Oncogenic RAS activation results from point mutations, affecting the GTP-binding domain (codons 12 or 13) in exon 1 or the GTPase domain (codon 61) in exon 2, which fix the protein in the activated state and thus resulting in chronic stimulation of downstream targets, genomic instability, additional mutations, and malignant transformation. Mutations in all three cellular RAS genes have been identified in benign and malignant thyroid tumors. They seem to be common in follicular carcinoma (50%) (Di Cristofaro et al., 2006), PDTC, and ATC and occur less frequently in PTC (<10%) (Meinkoth, 2004). Some studies have shown a similar prevalence of RAS mutations in benign and malignant thyroid neoplasms, suggesting that RAS activation may represent an early event. Other studies have shown that RAS mutations, specifically mutations at codon 61 of N-RAS, are involved with tumor progression and aggressive clinical behavior. The presence of RAS mutations predicted a poor outcome for WDTC independent of tumor stage. Furthermore, they found that PDTC and ATC often harbor multiple RAS mutations. These mutations probably represent an intermediate event in the progression of thyroid carcinoma.

2.5.4 PAX8-PPARγ

The PAX8 gene encodes a transcription factor essential for the genesis of thyroid follicular cell lineages and regulation of thyroid specific gene expression. The Peroxisome Proliferator-Activated Receptor γ (PPARγ) is a member of the nuclear hormone receptor superfamily that includes thyroid hormone, retinoic acid, and androgen and estrogen receptors. The PAX8-PPARγ rearrangement leads to in-frame fusion of exon 7, 8, or 9 of PAX8 on 2q13 with exon 1 of PPARγ on 3p25. It appears as though the PAX8-PPARγ chimeric protein inactivates the wild-type PPARγ, which is a putative tumor suppressor (Ying et al., 2003) As with RAS mutations, PAX8-PPARγ rearrangement has also been shown to be involved in the development of FTC. The PAX8-PPARγ rearrangement is found in FTC (26–63%) and in the follicular variant of PTC, where it occurs in approximately 33% of all tumors (Castro et al., 2006) The role of this rearrangement in the progression and dedifferentiation of follicular thyroid cancer to PDTC and ATC has not been well defined.

2.5.5 PI3K/AKT mutations

The PI3K/Akt pathway is a key regulator of cell proliferation and inhibitor of apoptosis. This pathway can be activated by the upstream stimulatory molecules (i.e. RAS), through the loss of function of PTEN protein that normally inhibits PI3K signaling, or as a results of activating mutations or amplification of gene coding for the effectors of this pathway. Inactivating mutations in PTEN are seen in Cowden's disease, a familial tumour syndrome associated with FC. In sporadic FC, the incidence of PTEN mutations is low (7%). Activating mutations of the catalytic subunit of PI3K have been found in small numbers of FC and FA (Wang et al., 2007; Hou et al., 2007).

2.6 Clinical features

The thyroid carcinoma manifesting as thyroid nodule. Palpable thyroid nodules are present in approximately 4-7% while high-resolution ultrasonography thyroid nodules are described in 19-67% of the general population. Most thyroid nodules are benign and only 5-10% are malignant. Thyroid nodule of large or small size have the same risk of malignancy. Solitary nodules in patients older more than 60 years and in young patients of less 30 years old are more frequently malignant. Male subjects have more risk of thyroid cancer than women. Rapid growth of a nodule may suggest malignancy.

2.6.1 Papillary carcinoma

Women develop PTC 3 times more frequently than men do, and the mean age at presentation is 34-40 years.

1. *Pathology:* Macroscopically the PTC are whitish nodules, without capsule and with ill-defined margins compared to the surrounding thyroid tissue. Microscopically the tumor cells of PTC typically grow with papillae and are characterized by ground-glass nuclei with pseudoinclusios, rare mitosis, and psammoma bodies (in 50% of papillary carcinomas). Beyond this classic PTC other variants of PTC may be present as Oxyphilic, Tall Cell, Columnar cell invade the thyroid capsule and surrounding extrathyroidal structures such as trachea, laryngeal, Follicular variant and diffuse sclerosing
2. *Local invasion* → Cancer can nerves, and airways. In these cases the patient may present with hemoptysis, hoarse voice and dysphagia.
3. *Regional and metastatic disease* → PTC spreads to the cervical lymph nodes. Clinically evident lymph node metastases are present in approximately one third of patients at presentation. Microscopic metastases are present in one half. The most common site of lymph node involvement is central compartment (level 6). The jugular lymph node chains (levels 2-4) are the next most common sites of cervical node involvement. Lymph nodes in the posterior triangle of the neck (level 5) may also develop metastases. This finding has important implications on the treatment algorithm for patients in this situation (Figure 2). Approximately 5-10% of patients develop distant metastases. Distant spread of PTC typically affects the lungs and bone

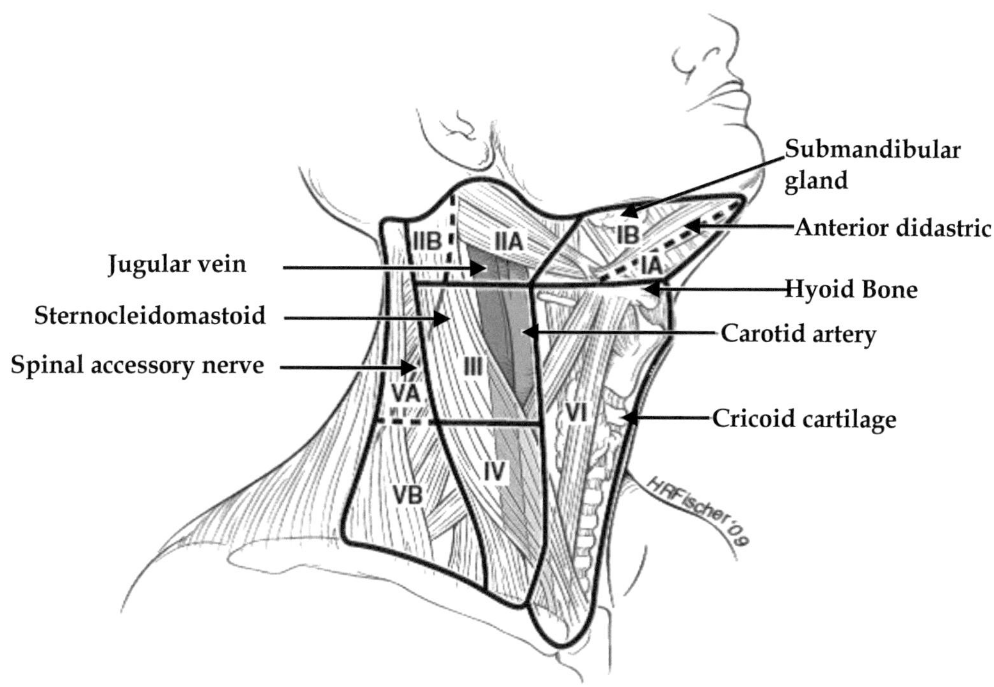

Fig. 2. Shows the lymph nodes in 6 neck clustered in compartments.

2.6.2 Follicular carcinoma

FTC represents thyroid cancers in area with insufficient iodine intake. As PTC, FTC occurs 3 times more frequently in women than in men. The mean age range at diagnosis is late in the fifth to sixth decades.

1. *Pathology.* Macroscopically, FTC appears as encapsulated nodule. Microscopically, tumor cells may show an increase solid, trabecular or follicular, which may invade the tumor capsule or the surrounding vascular structures. The tumors are divided into minimally invasive and widely invasive lesions depending on the histologic evidence of capsule and vascular invasion.
2. *Local invasion.* Local invasion can occur as PTC (see Local invasion for Papillary Carcinoma, above).
3. *Cervical and distant metastases.* Cervical metastases might be present at diagnosis. However, the rate of distant metastasis is significantly increased (approximately 20%) respect to PTC. Lung and bone are the most common sites.

2.7 Diagnosis

Clinical presentation of thyroid cancer is a thyroid nodule. Suspicious criteria of malignancy are: 1) Age: <20 or> 60 years 2) Sex: male> female; 3) Irradiation of head and/or neck; 4) Family history of papillary carcinoma 5) Rapid growth of the nodule 6) Growth during suppressive therapy with LT4 (L-thyroxine); 7)Fixed, hard consistency 8) Lymphadenopathy

2.7.1 Laboratory and thyroid scintigraphy

TSh evaluation allows to identify hyperfunction nodule. The TSH determination should be performed in nodule with large size > 2.5-3 cm. Tc^{99} thyroid scintiscan allows to confirm the uptake of large nodule. Hyperfunctioning nodules rarely are malignant, therefore no other diagnostic procedure should be performed.

2.7.2 Thyroid ultrasound (US)

US is a widespread technique that is used as a first-line diagnostic procedure for detecting and characterizing nodular thyroid disease. US permit to distinguish solid, cystic or mixed nodule, to evaluate ultrasound characteristic as hyperechogenicity , hypoechogenicity or isoechogenicity. the presence of some US aspects in the same thyroid nodule might have a higher likelihood of malignancy. These include: hypoechogenicity, irregular margins, microcalcifications, an absent halo, increased intranodular vascularity (Moon et al., 2008).

Elastography is an emerging and promising sonographic technique that requires additional validation with prospective studies (Machens et al., 2005; Rago et al., 2007).

2.7.3 Fine-needle aspiration cytology (FNAC)

Fine-needle aspiration cytology (FNAC) is the most accurate and cost-effective method for evaluating thyroid nodules. FNAC is not recommended in all nodules. The presence in the same nodule of 2 or more US characteristics above reported, recommended FNAC.

Cytology results should be included in the following diagnostic categories (Fadda et al., 2010**)**: THYR 1: non diagnostic; THYR 2: negative for malignant cells; THYR 3: inconclusive /indeterminate (follicular proliferation); THYR 4: suspicion of malignancy; THYR 5: positive for malignant cells

THYR 1:.The "non diagnostic" can be classified as inadequate and/or non representative, depending on technical factor. *Operative suggestion.* FNAC repetition after at least one month from the previous one, according to the clinician's opinion.

THYR 2.This category accounts for 60-75% of all cytologic samples. Operative suggestion. FNAC repetition to reduce the false negative results, .if nodule growing during L-T4 treatment or modified US aspects

THYR 3.This category encompasses all follicular-patterned lesions: About 80% of the TIR 3 diagnoses are benign lesions whereas only 20% of them result as malignant tumors after surgery and histologic examination. Some immunohistochemical markers such as Galectin-3, HBME-1, Cytokeratin 19 may improve the accuracy of the cytologic diagnosis. Operative suggestion. Surgical excision of the lesion and histological examination. The surgical option should be evaluated in the clinical and imaging setting.

THYR 4.It represents an heterogeneous group of lesions. Are included in this category samples without a sufficient amount of malignant cells or without cytological atypias sufficient for a diagnosis of cancer. Operative suggestion. Surgery

THYR 5.All cases with a diagnosis of malignant neoplasm (papillary, medullary and anaplastic carcinomas, lymphomas and metastasis) are included in this category Operative suggestion. Surgery for differentiated carcinomas. The results of FNAC are very sensitive for the differential diagnosis of benign and malignant nodules although there are limitations: inadequate samples and follicular neoplasia. In these cases the definitive diagnosis can be made only by histological examination

2.8 Treatment

2.8.1 Neartotal or total thyroidectomy

Near-total or total thyroidectomy is recommended if the primary thyroid carcinoma is >1 cm, multinodular goiter, regional or distant metastases at diagnosis, patient with personal history of radiation therapy to the head and neck, or patient with family history of DTCs. Older age (>45 years) may also be a criterion for recommending near-total or total thyroidectomy even with tumors <1-1.5 cm, because of higher recurrence rates in this age group. Increased extent of primary surgery may improve survival for high-risk patients and low-risk patients (Bilimoria et al., 2007)

2.8.2 Lymph node dissection

Regional lymph node metastases are frequently at diagnosis ranging from 20 to 90%. Although lymph node metastases in PTC patients are reported no clinically relevance on outcome in low risk patients, recently SEER registry study concluded that cervical lymph node metastases are a poor prognostic factor on survival in patients with FTC and in patients with PTC over 45 years (Zaydfudim et al., 2008). In experienced hands, therapeutic or prophylactic central compartment dissection can be achieved with low morbidity. In addition, selective unilateral paratracheal central compartment node dissection increases the proportion of patients who appear disease free.

2.8.3 Risk staging

Postoperative staging for thyroid cancer is used: 1) to permit prognostication for an individual patient with DTC; 2) to tailor decisions regarding postoperative adjunctive therapy, including RAI therapy and TSH suppression, to assess the patient's risk for disease recurrence and mortality; 3) to make decisions regarding the frequency and intensity of follow-up, directing more intensive follow-up towards patients at highest risk; and 4) to enable accurate communication regarding a patient among health care professionals. Varius risk definition for thyroid carcinoma have been evaluated. The American Joint Committee on Cancer (AJCC)/International Union Against Cancer (UICC) tumor-node-metastasis (TNM) classification has been used in clinical practice for DTC. This classification has also been evaluated to determine its utility in discriminating patients who have distinct outcomes. The fifth edition AJCC/UICC TNM classification (1997) was revised as the sixth edition in 2002 (Table 1).

In 2009, ATA has developed classes of risk in DTCs patients, to predict risk for recurrence, not death (ATA Surgery Working Group, 2009):

1. Low-risk patients have the following characteristics: 1) no local or distant metastases; 2) all macroscopic tumor has been resected; 3) there is no tumor invasion of locoregional tissues or structures; 4) the tumor does not have aggressive histology (e.g., tall cell, insular, columnar cell carcinoma) or vascular invasion; 5) and, if 131I is given, there is no 131I uptake outside the thyroid bed on the first post-treatment whole-body RAI scan (RxWBS)
2. Intermediate-risk patients have any of the following:1) microscopic invasion of tumor into the perithyroidal soft tissues at initial surgery; 2) cervical lymph node metastases or 131I uptake outside the thyroid bed on the RxWBS done after thyroid remnant ablation or 3) tumor with aggressive histology or vascular invasion
3. High-risk patients have:1) macroscopic tumor invasion, 2) incomplete tumor resection, 3) distant metastases, and possibly 4) thyroglobulin out of proportion to what is seen on the post-treatment scan

T0	Failure to evidence of primary tumor
T1	Tumor diameter ≤ 2 cm, limited to the thyroid
T2	Tumor diameter > 2 cm but < 4 cm, limited to the thyroid
T3	Tumor diameter > 4 cm, limited to the thyroid
	Any tumor size with minimal extrathyroidal extention (soft perithyroid tissue or sternocleidomastoid muscle)
T4a	Any tumor size with extension beyond the thyroid capsule to invade subcutaneous soft tissues, larynx, trachea, esophagus or recurrent laryngeal nerve
T4b	Tumor invades prevertebral fascia or encases carotid artery or mediastinal vessels
Nx	Regional lymph nodes can not be assessed
N0	Absence of lymph nodes metastases
N1	Metastasis to regional lymph nodes
N1a	Metastasis to level IV (pretracheal, paratracheal and prelaryngeal lymph nodes)
N1b	Ipsilateral, controlateral or bilateral cervical lymph nodes metastases or superior mediastinal lymph nodes metastases
Mx	Distant metastasis can not be assessed
M0	No distant metastasis
M1	Presence of distant metastasis

Table 1. TMN 6th edition (IUCC 2002)

The TNM classification allows to stratify patients into four classes according to risk of death at 10 years (Table 2).

	Age < 45 years			Age ≥ 45 years		
Stage	**T**	**N**	**M**	**T**	**N**	**M**
I	Any T	Any N	M0	T1	N0	M0
II	Anny T	Any N	M1	T2	N0	M0
III				T3	N0	M0
				T1 - T3	N1a	M0
IVA				T4a	N0	M0
				T4a	N1a	M0
				T1 - T4a	N1b	M0
IVB				T4b	Any N	M0
IVC				Any T	Any N	M1

Table 2. TMN classification

Tuttle (Tuttle et al., 2008a) stratified risk of death into four categories: very low risk, low risk, intermediate risk and high risk (table 3).

	Very low	**Low**	**Intermediate**	**High**
Age at diagnosis	< 45 years	< 45 years	< 45 years Classic PTC > 4 cm or vascular invasion, or extrathyroidal extention, or worrisome histology of any size	> 45 years
Primary tomor size	<1 cm	1-4 cm	>45 years Classic PTC > 4cm or extrathyroidal extention, or worrisome histology < 1-2 cm confined to the thyroid	> 4 cm classic PTC
Histology	Classic PTC, confined to the thyroid gland	Classic PTC, confined to the thyroid gland	Histology in conjunction with age as above	Worrisome histology > 1-2 cm
Completennes of resection	Complete resection	Complete resection	Complete resection	Incomplete tumor resection
Lymph node involvement	None apparent	Present or absent	Present or absent	Present or absent
Distant metastasis	None apparent	None apparent	None apparent	Present

Table 3. Risk of death.

In accordance with this system, a European Consensus Report (ETA) defined three categories of risk to establish the indication for radioiodine ablation therapy (Pacini et al., 2006):

1. very low-risk: unifocal T1 (<1 cm) N0 M0, no extension beyond the thyroid capsule, favourable histology], no indication for radioiodine ablation,
2. low-risk : T1 (>1 cm) or T2 N0 M0 or multifocal T1 N0 M0, or unfavourable histology, probable indication
3. high-risk: any T3 and T4 or any T, N1, or any M1, definite indication

Recently, has been proposed an 'ongoing risk stratification' which takes into account the response to therapy (Tuttle et al., 2008). Patients can be classified as having an excellent, acceptable or incomplete response to therapy:

1. Excellent response (undetectable basal and stimulated Tg, negative AbTg and negative neck US) patients should have a very low risk of recurrence and their long-term follow-up will be based on yearly physical examination and suppressed Tg value.
2. Acceptable response (undetectable basal Tg, stimulated Tg <10 ng/ml, trend of Tg in decline, AbTg absent or declining, substantially negative neck US) patients require a closer follow-up reserving additional treatment in the case of evidence of disease progression.
3. Incomplete response (detectable basal and stimulated Tg, trend of Tg stable or rising, structural disease present, persistent or recurrent RAI-avid disease present) patients require continued intensive follow-up with neck ultrasound, cross-sectional imaging, RAI imaging and FDG-PET imaging. The majority of these patients will require additional therapy such as surgical resection, RAI therapy, external beam irradiation and systemic therapies.

2.8.4 Radioiodine ablation

Surgery is usually followed by the administration of ^{131}I activities aimed at ablating any remnant thyroid tissue and potential microscopic residual tumour. This procedure decreases the risk of locoregional recurrence and facilitates long-term surveillance based on serum Tg measurement and diagnostic radioiodine whole body scan (WBS). In addition the high activity of ^{131}I allows obtaining a highly sensitive post-therapeutic WBS. Radioiodine ablation is recommended for all patients except those at very low risk. FTC and Hurthle cell cancer are generally regarded as higher risk tumors. On the contrary, "minimally invasive FTC", characterized only by capsular invasion, has an excellent prognosis with surgery alone and RAI ablation may not be required. Effective thyroid ablation requires adequate stimulation by TSH. The method of choice for preparation to perform radioiodine ablation is based on:

1. Endogenous TSH elevation: can be achieved by thyroid hormone withdrawal, increasing serum TSH levels >30mU=L in more than 90% of patients. Patients affected by chronic kidney failure, heart failure, panhypopituitarism, ecc...might worse their clinical status with thyroid hormone withdrawal
2. Administration of recombinant human TSH (rhTSH) rhTSH is helpful in patients with chronic diseases, able to increase tSH levels after L-T4 withdrawal, or intollerant hypothyroidism (Tuttle et al., 2008b).

Recent studies demonstrated ablation with lower doses than 100 mCi of I131. In fact the same ablation rate might be performed with 50 (Chianelli et al., 2009) and 30 mCi (Maenpaa et al., 2008) with rhTSh stimuli. These low doses reduce the radiation exposure to the whole body. Body weight or surface area should be evaluated for ablation in pediatric patients (Franzius et al., 2007).

2.8.5 Levo-thyroxine (L-T4) therapy

Thyroid hormone suppression therapy has an important role during follow-up blocking the recurrence and metastasis progression. Several reports have shown that L-T4 suppressive treatment has usefull in patients with high-risk decreasing progression, recurrence rates, and cancer-related mortality (Mc Griff et al., 2002; Hovens et al., 2007). On the other hand, in patients with low-risk no significant improvement has been obtained by L-T4 suppressive therapy. The duration of suppression therapy is currently being debated. According to the current guidelines, low-risk patients free at the first follow-up might have replacement L-T4 therapy, with the goal of maintaining serum TSH level within the normal range. On the contrary, high risk patients even free at the follow-up should continue with suppressive L-T4 doses for the high risk of relapse (Jonklaas et al., 2006; Cooper et al., 2009)

2.9 Prognosis

2.9.1 Tumour factors

1. Histology Histological characteristics have critical role of patient outcomes. The variants of PTC include the following:
    - Encapsulated tumor: About 10% of PTC are completely surrounded by a dense fibrous capsule. The prognosis for this subtype is better than unencapsulated PTC.
    - Diffuse sclerosing variant: Occurs in PTC of younger age, the diffuse sclerosing variant constitutes 2% of PTC. Prognosis for this subtype is less favorable than typical PTC.
    - Oxyphilic (Hürthle) cell type: The oxyphilic (Hürthle) cell type may be more aggressive than usual PTC.
    - Follicular variant: The follicular variant is less favorable than typical PTC.
    - Tall-cell carcinoma: Tall-cell carcinoma is a more aggressive form of thyroid carcinoma that differs from the usual form by showing tall columnar cells.
    - Columnar cell carcinoma: Columnar cell carcinoma is a distinctly more aggressive form of PTC that occurs more often in older men and is associated with a poor prognosis.

FTC is encapsulated, and invasion of the capsule and vessels is the key feature distinguishing follicular carcinomas from follicular adenomas. The subtypes are: 1) minimally invasive: good prognosis is a cancer with very low aggressiveness; widely invasive: cancer with poor prognosis for quick spreading of metastasis; 3) Hurthle-cell (oxyphilic follicular or oncocytic) carcinoma is a cytological variant of FTC with poor outcome

2. Tumour size: Tumor size correlates with outcome in patients with PTC; larger tumours are more likely to present with locoregional and/or distant metastases. However, the risk of recurrent disease and cancer-specific mortality increases linearly with tumour size.
3. Lymph node metastases: Cervical lymph nodes are involved in 20–50% of DTC, particularly PTC, and may be the first presentation. The frequency of micrometastases may approach 90%. Preoperative US identifies suspicious cervical adenopathy in 20–31% of cases, (Stulak et al., 2006). Confirmation of malignancy in lymph nodes with a suspicious sonographic appearance is achieved by US-guided FNA aspiration for cytology. Malignant lymph nodes are much more likely to occur in levels III, IV, and VI than in level II (Figure 2). Controversy exists over the clinical importance of lymph node metastases. Several studies have found no difference in survival between patients with and without lymph node metastases. Other studies have found that their presence leads to an increased risk of recurrence and reduced survival (Lee et al., 2009). The presence of lymph node metastases in patients <45 years has no effect on survival. On the contrary lymph nodes metastasis in patient ≥45 years are associated an increased risk of death.
4. Extrathyroidal extension: The extension of cancer outside the thyroid into the surrounding tissues may be found in about 30% of patients with PTC (Mazzaferri, 2007). The massive extension out thyroid into the surrounding musculature, oesophagus or trachea is associated with a high-risk of locoregional disease recurrence. It requires massive surgical debulking and may benefit from external beam radiotherapy. Microscopic extension beyond the thyroid capsule is associated with a higher risk of recurrent disease, greater likelihood of lymph node metastases and a higher mortality rate than in patients without such extracapsular spread (Lee et al., 2009).
5. Distant metastases The main cause of death from DTC is distant metastases; fortunately, only 5–10% of patients have distant metastases at initial presentation. Over 50% have lung involvement alone, 25% have bone involvement alone, 20% have both lung and bone involvement, and about 5% develop distant metastases in other sites (Lee & Soh, 2010). Mortality is high with distant disease, with 50% survival at 3.5 years. Less frequently are liver metastasis.
6. Oncogenes The study of oncogenes and their ability to predict the clinical behaviour of thyroid cancers has been an exciting and intensely investigated field. Moreover, these researches have resulted in the creation of several new therapeutic agents to target these genetic aberrations.
   - BRAF: The presence of a *BRAF* mutation is associated with extrathyroidal invasion, multicentricity, presence of nodal metastases, higher-stage disease, older age at initial presentation, and higher likelihood of recurrent or persistent disease. (Elisei et al., 2008). Further study is needed to clarify this complex issue.
   - RAS: Numerous studies have show that ras mutations define a subset of thyroid carcinoma characterized by aggressive behavior. This is indicated by the close relationship between oncogenic ras and the loss of those histologic features that characterize well-differentiated thyroid tumor phenotypes. Remarkably, oncogenic K-ras correlates with the loss of tumor differentiation, presence of distant

metastases, and is associated with poor prognosis among DTC independently tumor stage (Garcia-Rostan et al., 2003).

- RET/PTC: Ret/PTC1 is the most frequent (60–70%), while ret/PTC3 (20-30%) and ret/PTC2 are the least common (10%). RET/PTC rearrangements are associated with PTC that lacks evidence of progression to PDTC or ATC demonstrating a low potential for de-differentiation.

2.9.2 Patient variables

1. Age: Age at diagnosis and therapy is a critical predictor of patient outcome; patients aged >45 years have increased recurrence rates and reduced mortality. Children and adolescents (age <20 years) tend to present with higher-stage disease and greater likelihood of locoregional and distant metastases. Despite late-stage presentation of tumors, children generally have excellent survival rates. The exception to this rule is when the disease presents in children aged ≤10 years; in this age group, the disease is notably more aggressive. Mortality is high in this group (Fugazzola et al., 2004).
2. Gender: As discussed above, mortality rates are higher among men than women even DTCs are more frequent in woman. Recurrence rates are also higher in men.

2.10 Follow-up

The aim of the follow-up is the early discovery of persistent disease. Local recurrences develop in the first 5 years mainly, and only in a minority of cases local or distant recurrences develop 20 years after the initial treatment. Thyroid hormone FT3, FT4, TSH, should be evaluated 2-3 months after initial treatment to check the adequacy of LT4 suppressive therapy. At 6–12 months the first follow-up is aimed to ascertain whether the patient is free of disease.

Disease-free status comprises all of the following:

1. no clinical evidence of tumor,
2. no imaging evidence of tumor (no uptake outside the thyroid bed on the initial posttreatment WBS, or, if uptake outside the thyroid bed had been present, no imaging evidence of tumor on a recent diagnostic scan and neck US), and
3. undetectable serum Tg levels during TSH suppression and stimulation in the absence of interfering antibodies.

In the absence of Tg antibody the measurement of serum Tg levels is an important modality to monitor patients for residual or recurrent disease. Serum Tg has a high degree of sensitivity and specificity to detect thyroid cancer recurrences during thyroid hormone withdrawal or stimulation using rhTSH. Serum Tg measurements obtained during L-T4suppression therapy may fail to identify patients with relatively small amounts of residual tumor (Hovens et al., 2007). Nevertheless, a single rhTSH-stimulated serumTg<0.5 ng/mL in the absence of anti-Tg antibody has an approximately 98–99.5% likelihood of identifying patients completely free of tumor on follow-up (67). On the contrary, diagnostic-therapeutic procedures should be performed in patients with basal or after rhTSH stimuli Tg detectable values (value>2ng/ml). Diagnostic procedures comprise neck US, diagnostic I131 Whole Body Scan, Computer Tomography. Negative radiological imagines require a therapeutic dose of I131 to identified recurrences and the subsequent follow-up will be evaluated on post dose scintiscan. PET- TC 18 FDG sholud be performed in all patients with detectable Tg values and negative post therapeutic I 131 dose scintiscan. The identification of PET-TC positive lesions implies the de-differentation of metastasis.

The long-term follow-up differs on class of risk of recurrence. Very low-risk patients should be followed through physical examination, basal serum Tg measurement on substitutive LT4 therapy and neck US yearly if Tg values was undetectable at first follow-up. Low risk, Intermediate Risk and High-risk require Tg evaluation after rhTSH stimuli, neck US. Radiological techniques imagines if Tg increased up the cut-off, as above described. However, the recent introduction of an ultrasensitive Tg assay might reduce the need to perform Tg measurements after rhTSH-stimuli (Robert et al., 2007). About 25% of DTCs shows anti-Tg antibodies that could falsely lower serum Tg in immunometric assays (Cooper et al., 2009). Serial serum anti-Tg antibody quantification using the same methodology may serve as an imprecise surrogate marker of residual normal thyroid tissue or tumor. Patients with anti Tg antibodies should perform follow-up with I 131 Whole Body Scan. Suppressive doses of L-T4 with TSH levels under 0.1 mU/l reduce recurrence or progression of disease only in patients with high risk. Therefore, TSH levels <0.1 mU/l should be maintained until first follow-up and in high risk patients. Patients disease free and very low risk should take replacement doses.

3. Poor differentiate thyroid carcinoma (PDTC)

PDTC includes tumors of follicular origin that retain sufficient differentiation to produce Tg, histologically show scattered small follicular structures, but generally lack the usual morphologic characteristic of PTC or FTC. PDTC could be considered as an intermediate form of thyroid cancer with a prognosis that falls between DTCs and ATC (Sobrinho-Simoes et al., 2002). It is noteworthy that in the north half of Italy about 15% of thyroid cancer are PDTC whereas in North America the PDTC comprise only 2-3% of thyroid malignancy. These observations demonstrate that environmental factors may play a significant role in the genesis of these lesions, including iodine deficiency. PDTC may occur in a recurrence of a previously treated DTCs or at the time of diagnosis PDTC parts of tumor may show characteristics histological characteristics of PTC more rarely FTC. Clinically PDTC can produce Tg but do not respond to radioactive iodine. Therefore, therapy of PDTC can be inefficient by radioiodine. PDTC with extracapsular extension, massive lymph nodes involvement and no radioiodine up-take benefits of external radiotherapy (RT) after surgery, but no advantage to adjuvant RT to the neck in PDTC with diffuse metastasis. PDTC has poor sensitive to chemotherapy using different drugs as methotrexate, adriamycin, bleomycin and vinblastin. Response ranging from 55 to 70% when chemotherapy is associated to RT.

4. Anaplastic thyroid carcinoma (ATC)

Anaplastic thyroid carcinoma (ATC) is the most aggressive and lethal form of thyroid cancer with a median survival of 4 to 12 months from the time of diagnosis.

4.1 Epidemiology

ATC accounts for less than 2% of all thyroid malignancies, it is responsible for 14%-39% of deaths related to malignant thyroid tumors. The female/male ratio is 5 to 1 and the peak of incidence is in the sixth and seventh decades of life. The age at diagnosis of ATC is over 70 years. The incidence of ATC is estimated at 1 to 2 cases per million population per year, and the trend has been decreasing even though the incidence of well-differentiated subtypes (e.g., papillary and follicular) of thyroid cancer has been increasing.

4.2 Risk factors

Patients with ATC show goiter in 25% of cases, in 10% a family history of goiter. Therefore, ATC is more common in places with endemic goiter and iodine supplementation has decrease the incidence of ATC in these countries (Besic N, 2010).

4.3 Genetic alteration

ATC may derive from DTCs, including PTC, FTC or Hurthle cell or may be "de novo". Several mutations are identified in ATC, some occurring in PTC and FTC (e.g., RAS and BRAF). Late mutations include p53, catenin (cadherin-associated protein), beta 1, and PIK3CA, suggesting that one or more of these mutations contribute to the extremely aggressive behavior of ATC. By contrast, the RET/PTC rearrangements found in childhood and radiation-induced PTCs, and the PAX8/PPARG fusion protein detected in follicular carcinoma, are not observed in poorly differentiated and ATCs. RAS and BRAF are the same described in DTCs. p53 is a tumor suppressor gene located in chromosome 17p that increases the cyclin kinase inhibitor, p21, promoting cell cycle arrest at G1/S. Mutations impair p53 transcriptional activity, and occur in 55% of ATC. Polymorphism in codon 72, identify only in ATC, but in no benign nodules or differentiated thyroid cancers, could be considered as a risk factor (Boltze C, 2002). Other gene as Wnt, a catenin beta 1 gene is involved in signaling and cell-cell adhesion, was detected in ATC and PDTC but not in PTC and FTC.

4.4 Clinical presentation

Clinical manifestation of ATC is a nodule with a rapidly growth, enlarging anterior neck mass, accompanying dysphagia (40%), voice change or hoarseness (40%), and stridor (24%). Regional symptoms included a noticeable lymph node mass (54%) and neck pain (26%). Systemic symptoms include anorexia, weight loss, and shortness of breath with pulmonary metastases. ATC is usually advanced at diagnosis and frequently surgically unresectable. Around 20%-50% of patients present with distant metastases, most often pulmonary, and another 25% develop new metastasis during the rapid course of the disease, lungs (80%), bone (6–16%), and brain (5–13%) were the most common sites of metastasis.

4.5 Prognosis

The median survival rate from 4 to 12 months. On multivariate analysis, distant or metastatic disease, tumor size greater than 7 centimeters, and treatment with surgery with or without radiotherapy were statistically significant prognostic markers(Chen et al.,

2008). Age, sex, size of the tumor, resectability, and the extent of disease has been shown to affect the course of the disease. Age less than 60 years, female sex, tumor size less than 7 centimeters, were the most favourable prognostic markers (Kim et al., 2007). A recent study from France based on 26 patients with ATC, univariate analysis showed that age above 75, capsular invasion, lymph nodes metastasis, tumor residue after surgery, and lack of multimodal treatment (particularly radiotherapy in patients without tumor residue) are poor prognosistic factors. Multivariate analysis in the same cohort showed age above 75, followed by node invasion, capsular invasion, and female sex to be poor prognosticators (Roche B, 2010).

4.6 Therapeutic approach

Patients with ATC even in the absence of metastatic disease are considered to have systemic disease at the time of diagnosis. ATC is considered stage IV by the International Union Against Cancer (UICC)—TNM staging and American Joint Commission on Cancer (AJCC) system. Multimodality treatment consisting of surgery when feasible combined with radiation and chemotherapy is generally recommended.

4.6.1 Surgery

The aim of surgery in ATC, whether it is removal of all gross disease or palliation, remains controversial. Complete resection has been identified as a prognostic factor in several clinical trials. When feasible, surgery must aim at a radical intent. The categories of patients that may be most suitable for this approach are young patients (< 65 years old) with small lesions (< 6 cm) and no distant metastasis. However, surgery also plays an important role for palliation. Partial resection of the tumor followed by radiotherapy and chemotherapy may delay or avoid airway obstruction, although it can improve survival only by a few months (Miccoli et al., 2007). It is theoretically possible that, in selected patients, even in the setting of metastatic disease, surgery may result in an improved quality of life and prevent death from suffocation (Yau et al., 2008). Since surgery alone is not able to control the disease even in patients with small intra-thyroidal masses, adjuvant therapy is always required, and can be administered either with radiotherapy (RT) or chemoradiotherapy.

4.6.2 Systemic treatment

Chemotherapy: ATC cannot be regarded as a very chemo-sensitive tumor. Doxorubicin is not able to achieve more than a 20% response rate. A study (Shimaoka et al., 1985) has observed that combination chemotherapy based on doxorubicin (60 mg/m2) and cisplatin (40 mg/m2) was more effective than doxorubicin alone and provided a higher complete response rate. More recently, single drug docetaxel was tested as first-line chemotherapy in patients with advanced ATC. In a prospective phase II clinical trial of paclitaxel, showed a remarkable response rate of 53% (Schoenberger et al., 2004). In a preclinical experiment only paclitaxel, gemcitabine and vinorelbine appeared to be active in ATC (Bauer et al., 2003) and the combinations of vinorelbine/gemcitabine and paclitaxel/gemcitabine seemed to act synergistically. These results should receive confirmation in clinical trials.

4.6.3 Radiation

Achieving local control is important since death from ATC is usually a consequence of uncontrolled local disease. The indication for RadioTherapy (RT) range from providing palliation to improving survival. RT is used alone or in combined with surgery and chemotherapy. Intensity-modulated radiation therapy (IMRT) based on computerized treatment planning and delivery is able to generate a dose distribution that delivers radiation accurately with sparing of the surrounding normal tissue (Lee et al., 2007). Higher doses of radiation can be given over a shorter time with less toxicity by employing hyperfractionation techniques. Toxicity can be a limiting factor with radiation. Kim and Leeper reported complications particularly, pharyngoesophagitis and tracheitis in their series. Wong also noted skin changes, esophageal toxicity, and radiation myelopathy (Wong et al., 2001). Daily doses of greater than 3 Gy should be cautiously used as it can increase the incidence of myelopathy.

5. New treatments

PDTC and ATC are poor sensitive to radioiodione, chemotherapy and RT alone or associate. The knowledges on genetic transformation and the intracellular pathway involved in thyroid cancer transformation has permitted to develop target drugs. Therefore, interest arose in the therapeutic potential of target-specific kinase inhibitors for these diseases. Angiogenesis plays a critical role to support tumor cell growth and metastasis, supplying nutrients and oxygen, removing waste products, and facilitating distant metastasis.

5.1 Targeting signaling kinases

RET and VEGFR kinases have considerable similarity structural and multitargeted kinase inhibitors are capable of affecting both kinases. A wide variety of kinase inhibitors have entered clinical trials for patients with advanced thyroid cancers, PDTC or ATC. Because of the targeting similarities of many of these agents, common toxicities exist among these agents, including hypertension, diarrhea, skin rashes, and fatigue.

1. Motesanib (AMG706): is an oral, tyrosine kinase inhibitor targeting the VEGF receptors 1, 2, and 3.
2. Sorafenib (BAY 43-9006): is an oral, small molecule tyrosin-kinase inhibitor (TKI) and targeting VEGF receptors 2 and 3, RET and BRAF. Like other agents that inhibit BRAF, sorafenib also has been associated with development of cutaneous squamous cell carcinomas in up to 5% of treated patients, and a similar frequency of keratoacanthomas and other premalignant actinic lesions (Dubauskas et al., 2009). In a recent retrospective series, sorafenib therapy was associated with prolongation of median progression-free survival by at least 1 year, compared with patients' rate of disease progression prior to initiation of therapy (Cabanillas et al., 2010). A randomized, placebo-controlled phase III study of sorafenib as first-line therapy for progressive metastatic DTC has been initiated. Although not specifically approved for thyroid carcinomas, sorafenib is being used in selected patients with PDTC and medullary thyroid carcinoma for whom clinical trials are not appropriate

(Waguespack et al., 2009). Compared with patients' rate of disease progression prior to initiation of therapy, sorafenib may prolong progression-free survival in DTC by at least 1 year (Cabanillas et al., 2010). The drug may also be appropriate in selected pediatric cases; in 1 report, treatment with sorafenib yielded a marked response in a child whose lung metastases from PTC were progressing despite radioiodine therapy (Waguespack et al., 2009).

3. Sunitinib (SU11248): is an oral, small molecule TKI of all 3 VEGF receptors, RET, and RET/PTC subtypes 1 and 3 (Pasqualetti et al., 2011)
4. Axitinib (AG-013736): is an oral inhibitor that effectively blocks VEGF-1, -2 and -3. Partial response was seen in patients refractory radioiodine. Currently ongoing is a multicenter, open-label phase II study to determine the efficacy of axitinib in patients with metastatic DTC refractory to doxorubicin, or for whom doxorubicin therapy is contraindicated.
5. Pazopanib: is a potent small molecule inhibitor of all VEGFR subtypes as well as PDGFR. Like axitinib, it has insignificant inhibitory activity against the oncogenic kinases RET, RET/PTC, or BRAF, and therefore its actions are expected to be primarily anti-angiogenic in thyroid carcinoma.
6. Gefitinib (ZD1839): is an oral, small molecule inhibitor of the EGF receptor, was initially introduced for treatment of non-small cell lung carcinoma. Because many PDTC and ATC display activated EGFR signaling, and inhibitors have had demonstrated efficacy in preclinical models, an open-label phase II study was initiated, examining the effectiveness of gefitinib in a mixed cohort of thyroid cancer patients (Mrozek et al., 2006).

5.2 Other drugs

Beyond direct inhibitors of angiogenic kinases such as VEGFR, other drugs are capable of either inhibiting angiogenesis or disrupt existing tumor vasculature. Two of these agents, thalidomide and fosbretabulin (combretastatin A4 phosphate), have been of particular interest following reported responses in individual patients with ATC .

1. **Thalidomide and lenalidomide** Thalidomide was found to be an angiogenesis inhibitor decades after it achieved notoriety as a teratogenic cause of neonatal dysmelia. Eligibility was limited to PDTC patients whose measured tumor volumes had increased by at least 30% in the past year.
2. **Combretastatin** A4 phosphate (CA4P): is a tubulin-binding vascular disrupting agent that inhibits tumor blood flow. In a phase I trial, one patient with ATC showed a progression-free survival of 30 mo, however, the drug was found to be associated with significant cardiovascular side effects at the escalating doses employed.
3. **Romidepsin** The cyclic peptide romidepsin (previously known as depsipeptide) selectively inhibits four isotypes of histone deacetylases. Toxicities were primarily hematologic, nausea, and vomiting. A phase II trial was initiated in patients with radioiodine-unresponsive, PDTC. Romidepsin induces stable disease and in few subjects exhibited restoration of uptake permitting therapeutic radioiodine administration.
4. **Vorinostat and valproic acid (VPA)** The orally available histone deacetylase (HDAC) inhibitor vorinostat, derived from hydroxamic acid, inhibits all known classes of HDAC

enzymes. An ongoing phase II trial is evaluating the effect of monotherapy with VPA on tumor size and radioiodine uptake in patients with radioiodine-refractory PDTC. One PTC patient had prolonged stable disease beyond 1 year, but no objective responses were identified in any tumor type.

5. **Azacytidine and decitabine →** A broad array of tumor suppressor genes is hypermethylated in PTC and FTC leading to their decreased expression, including *PTEN*, tissue inhibitor of metalloproteinase-3, and death-associated protein kinase . A phase II trial of 5-azacytidine monotherapy to restore radioiodine uptake was initiated, but results were never reported. Given the greater potency and tolerance of the azacytidine derivative decitabine, a phase II trial of this latter agent has been underway, evaluating the ability to restore radioiodine uptake in radioiodine-non-avid metastases; results of this multicenter trial are expected shortly.

6. Medullary thyroid carcinoma (MTC)

6.1 Epidemiology

MTC arises from C cells o parafollicular cells which produce and secrete Calcitonin (Ct) . MTC represents about 5-10% of all thyroid cancers and 13.4% of all thyroid-related deaths. Survival rates for MTC are impacted by age of diagnosis and stage of disease

6.2 Secretory products

Several biochemical features typical of normal C cells (production of Ct) are retained by neoplastic C cells and represent specific and sensitive diagnostic markers. Ct is a small peptide (32 amino acids) coded by a gene located on the short arm of chromosome 11, the gene codes a second peptide called CT-gene-related peptide (CGRP). Carcinoembryonic antigen (CEA) is produced by neoplastic C cells. There is no close relationship between serum concentrations of CEA and CT. Serum CEA concentration is normal in patients with preclinical MTC and does not increase after pentagastrin stimulation. Measurement of serum CEA concentration is useful during follow-up because high concentrations or rapidly increasing concentrations indicate disease progression.

6.3 Clinical presentation

MTC is mainly in sporadic form, but an hereditary pattern is present in 20–30% of cases, transmitted as an autosomal-dominant trait (Schlumberger & Pacini, 2006).The hereditary form is also referred to as 'multiple endocrine neoplasia type 2' (MEN 2), characterized by MTC in combination with pheochromocytoma and hyperparathyroidism (MEN 2A), or MTC in combination with pheochromocytoma, multiple mucosal neuromas and marfanoid habitus (MEN 2B). The occurrence of familial MTC (FMTC) in the absence of other neoplasias is also possible.

6.3.1 Sporadic MTC

Patients with sporadic MTC usually present with a palpable thyroid nodule indistinguishable from any other thyroid nodule. Clinical neck lymph node metastases are detected in at least 50% of patients and may reveal the disease. Metastases outside the neck, in liver, lungs or bones, are initially present in 10–20% of cases. Flushing and diarrhea might occur in the presence of liver metastasis. FNAC has made it possible to diagnose MTC prior to surgery. However, cytology may be misleading and, in case of doubt, positive immunocytochemical staining for Ct, Ct measurement in the washout fluid of FNAC or both (Kudo et al., 2007) will confirm the diagnosis. Patients with clinical MTC have elevated basal circulating Ct concentrations. Whenever MTC is suspected, staging and careful clinical screening for pheochromocytoma and hyperparathyroidism should be carried out before surgery.

6.3.2 Hereditary MTC

1. **Multiple Endocrine Neoplasia Type 2A (MEN2A):** MEN 2A is a syndrome characterized by MTC, pheochromocytoma and hyperparathyroidism. Clinically MTC develops in about 100% of patients affected by this syndrome. Pheochromocytoma occurs in about 50% of *MEN 2A* patients depending on the type of gene mutation. Hyperparathyroidism occurs in 10–25% of known *MEN 2A* gene carriers with a mutation in codon 634, usually after the third decade of life (Leboulleux et al., 2002). Clinical MTC is rarely observed under 10 years of age; prevalence increases with age, and is 25% at 13 years and about 70% at 70 years. The pentagastrin stimulation test is positive in about 20% of gene carriers at 10 years of age; this increases with age to 50% at 13 years, 65% at 20 years and 95% at 30 years. At present, genetic testing is carried out before 5 years of age in all subjects at risk to establish which individuals are gene carriers. Pheochromocytomas are located in an adrenal gland, and very few cases have been observed in the retroperitoneal region. It is bilateral in 50% of cases, but often after an interval of several years. Pheochromocytoma is almost always benign. Hyperparathyroidism consists of parathyroid hyperplasia, with one or more adenomas in older patients, develops slowly and is usually mild. Clinical and biochemical features do not differ from those seen in sporadic hyperparathyroidism.Cutaneous lichen amyloidosis is a pruritic and hyperpigmented lesion of the skin on the upper portion of the back has been observed in some families with MEN 2A. This lesion may occur early in life and often precedes C-cell disease. Hirschsprung's disease has been observed in a few families with MEN 2A. Patient with multiple endocrine neoplasia type 2A with lichen cutaneous amyloidosis over the interscapular area. The patient reported intense pruritus in this area since 3 years of age.
2. **Multiple Endocrine Neoplasia Type 2B (MEN2B):** MEN2B is a syndrome with MTC, pheochromocytoma, ganglioneuromatosis, marfanoid features and skeletal abnormalities. MTC associated with MEN 2B is the most aggressive form of MTC and occurs early in life, usually before the age of 5 years. It is frequently associated with extension beyond the thyroid capsule, with lymph node and distant metastases at the time of diagnosis. Pheochromocytomas are identified in about one-half of the individuals presenting with the syndrome. Mucosal neuromas are a typical feature of MEN 2B. They occur on the distal portion of the tongue, on the lips, throughout the intestinal tract and eventually in the urinary tract. These patients also have chronic constipation and colonic cramping due to the presence of megacolon disorder. Hypertrophy of corneal nerves is frequent and is evaluated by slit lamp ophthalmic examination. Marfanoid features include long, thin extremities, an altered upper-to-lower body ratio and ligament hyperlaxity. Skeletal abnormalities are frequent, including slipped femoral epiphysis and pectus excavatum.

3. **Familial Medullary Thyroid Carcinoma (FMTC):** FMTC have only hereditary MTC. Clinical presentation of MTC at a later age, 60-70 years old, and a relatively more favourable prognosis respect the others hereditary forms. It is still debated whether FMTC represents a separate syndrome or a variant of MEN 2A in which the genetic component is modified to delay the onset of the array of manifestations typifying the MEN 2A syndrome.

6.4 Genetic alterations

6.4.1 Germline mutations

The predisposing gene for inherited MTC was the RET proto-oncogene localized to centromeric chromosome 10 , identified by genetic linkage analysis in 1987, and germline mutations of were demonstrated in 1993 in MEN 2A, FMTC and MEN 2B. The RET gene is a 21-exon gene that encodes a tyrosine kinase receptor. This membrane-associated receptor is characterised by a cadherin-like region in the extracellular domain, a cysteine-rich region immediately external to the membrane, and an intracellular tyrosine kinase domain. Hereditary MTC is caused by germline autosomal-dominant gain-of-function mutations in the RET proto-oncogene. About 98% of patients with MEN 2 have germline mutations in exons 5, 8, 10, 11, 13, 14, 15 or 16 of the RET gene. Mutations causing MEN 2A affect the cysteine-rich extracellular domain with substitution of a cysteine to another amino acid in exon 10 and, and more commonly (80%), in exon 11. In about 95% of patients with MEN 2B, a single mutation converting methionine to threonine in codon 918 of exon 16 has been identified. It is frequently (>50%) a de-novo mutation in the allele inherited from the patient's father. Other rare intracellular mutations associated with MEN 2B involve exon 15. Rare patients with MEN 2B phenotype have double *RET* mutations. Germline mutations induce different tirosin-kinasi activity. Strong activation of the *RET* proto-oncogene is associated with a more aggressive form of MTC, and mutations providing weaker *RET* activation result in a less aggressive and late-onset form of the disease. On the basis of these findings, the American Thyroid Association (ATA) has recently developed an MTC risk stratification based on genotype (Kloos et al., 2009) (Table 4.)

1. Level D mutations carry the highest risk for MTC. These mutations include codons 883 and 918, and are associated with the youngest age of onset and highest risk of metastases and disease-specific mortality.
2. Level C mutations carry a lower, yet still high, risk of aggressive MTC, and include mutations in codon 634.
3. Level B mutations carry a lower risk for aggressive MTC mutations, and include mutations at *RET* codons 609, 611, 618, 620 and 630.
4. Level A mutations carry the 'least high' risk, and include *RET* gene mutations in codons 768, 790, 791, 804 and 891. This system may be used to individualise the aggressiveness of treatment.

6.4.2 Somatic mutations

Somatic mutations in codon 918 of the *RET* proto-oncogene have been identified in 25–33% of sporadic MTC, and may be associated with a poor outcome compared with sporadic tumours without *RET* mutation (Elisei et al., 2008). Mutations in codons 618, 634, 768, 804 and 883 and partial deletion of the *RET* gene have been identified in a few tumours

Exon	Mutation	Phenotype	ATA risk level*
5	G321R	FMTC/MEN 2A	A
8	C515S	FMTC/MEN 2A	A
	G533C	FMTC/MEN 2A	A
	532 duplication	FMTC	A
	531/9 base pair duplication	FMTC/MEN 2A	A
10	R600Q	FMTC/MEN 2A	A
	K603E	FMTC/MEN 2A	A
	Y606C	FMTC	A
	C609F/R/G/S/Y	FMTC/MEN 2A	B
	C611R/G/F/S/W/Y	FMTC/MEN 2A	B
	C618R/G/F/S/Y	FMTC/MEN 2A	B
	C620R/G/F/S/W/Y	FMTC/MEN 2A	B
11	C630R/F/S/Y	FMTC/MEN 2A	B
	D631Y	FMTC	B
	633/9 base pair duplication	FMTC/MEN 2A	B
	634/12 base pair duplication	FMTC/MEN 2A	B
	C634R	FMTC/MEN 2A	C
	C634G/F/S/W/Y	FMTC/MEN 2A	C
	635/insertion ELCR; T636P	FMTC/MEN 2A	A
	S649L	FMTC/MEN 2A	A
	K666E	FMTC/MEN 2A	A
13	E768D	FMTC/MEN 2A	A
	N776S	FMTC/MEN 2A	A
	L790F	FMTC/MEN 2A	A
	Y791F	FMTC/MEN 2A	A
14	V804L	FMTC/MEN 2A	A
	V804M	FMTC/MEN 2A	A
	V804M+E805K	MEN 2B	D
	V804M+Y806C	MEN 2B	D
	G819K	FMTC	A
	R833C	FMTC	A
	R844Q	FMTC	A
15	R866W	FMTC/MEN 2A	A
	A883F	MEN 2B	D
	S891A	FMTC/MEN 2A	A
16	R912P	FMTC/MEN 2A	A
	M918T	MEN 2B	D
13/14	V804M+V778I	FMTC/MEN 2A	B
14/15	V804M+S904C	MEN 2B/MEN 2A	D

Table 4. MTC risk stratification based on genotype by American Thyroid Association (ATA)

6.5 Therapeutic approach

6.5.1 Initial treatment

Before surgery, all patients with suspicious MTC should undergo a staging work-up. The goal of pre-operative evaluation is to define the extent of disease and to identify the comorbid conditions of hyperparathyroidism, pheochromocytoma or both in the case of hereditary forms. The pre-operative biochemical evaluation should include basal serum Ct, CEA, calcium and 24-h urine collection for metanephrines and normetanephrines determination. Pre-operative imaging, including neck US, should be carried out in all patients; pre-operative chest and neck computed tomography. The primary treatment of both hereditary and sporadic forms of MTC is total thyroidectomy and removal of all neoplastic tissue present in the neck. Several studies have shown that survival in patients with MTC is dependent upon the adequacy of the initial surgical procedure. Multicentric and bilateral MTC is observed in 30% of sporadic cases and in nearly 100% of hereditary cases. The therapeutic option for lymph node surgery should be dictated by the results of presurgical evaluation. Patients with no clinical or imaging evidence of lymph node metastases should undergo prophylactic central compartment (level VI) neck dissection. This strategy will probably include about 30–40% of patients with MTC. In the remaining patients lymph node involvement are documented before surgery. Lymph node metastases may occur in 20–30% of cases with tumours <1 cm in diameter, in 50% of patients with a tumour 1-4 cm in diameter, and in up to 90% in patients with a tumour >4 cm or with a T4 tumour.

6.5.2 Postoperative management

After total thyroidectomy, replacement thyroxine treatment is given to maintain the serum TSH value into the normal range. Measurement of the serum marker Ct and CEA is of paramount importance in the postsurgical follow-up of patients with MTC because this reflects the presence of persistent or recurrent disease. The half-life of serum Ct is reported to be about 30 h. An undetectable basal serum Ct level after surgery is a strong predictor of complete remission. Complete remission may be further confirmed if the serum Ct level remains undetectable after a provocative (pentagastrin or calcium) test. In this situation, no other diagnostic test is indicated. Serum Ct should be repeated every 6 months for the first 2-3 years and annually thereafter. Patients with biochemical remission after initial treatment have only a 3% chance of recurrence during long-term follow-up. On the contrary, if basal serum Ct is detectable or becomes detectable after stimulation, the patient is not cured. Radiological imagines comprise neck US, because frequently recurrence are in locoregional lymph nodes, FNAC with Ct measurement in the washout fluid should typically be carried out to confirm the diagnosis when US demonstrates suspicious lymph nodes enlargement. Chest CT, abdominal MRI, bone scintigraphy, 18 Fluorodeoxyglucose (FDG) positron emission tomography (PET) and 18-F-dihydroxyphenylalanine (DOPA) PET when there is suspicious of diffuse metastasis. These imaging techniques will be positive when Ct levels are high >150 pg/ml. In patients with serum CT <150 pg/ml, clinical evaluation of disease should be limited to neck US and a careful every 6 months follow up with Ct and CEA determinations (Laure Giraudet et al., 2008). Patients with detectable basal serum Ct and no evidence of disease, long-term surveillance is indicated. Pain by bone metastases rapidly improvements with local RT and it can also be useful for brain metastases. In patients with predominant liver involvement, embolisation or chemo-embolisation proved to be efficient for some symptomatic benefit and for partial reduction in tumour mass (Fromigué et al., 2006).

6.5.3 Novel chemotherapy

Traditional chemotherapy is inefficient in metastatic MTC. New strategies to treat metastates of MTC are being evaluated and include radio-immunotherapy and vaccine-based therapies (Kraeber-Bodere et al., 2009). Improved understanding of MTC molecular oncogenesis has resulted in identification of novel molecular targets for treatment, and there has been recent focus on the use of compounds inhibiting receptors of intracellular kinases. These new therapies primarily target RET oncogene and angiogenesis and have entered clinical trials for metastatic MTC. Partial response rates of up to 30% have been reported in single-agent studies, but prolonged disease stabilization is seen more commonly. The most successful agents target the vascular endothelial growth factor receptors (VEGFRs), with focus on tyrosine kinase inhibitors; these compounds include motesanib diphosphate, vandetanib, sorafenib, and sunitinib (Sherman et al., 2009). In a phase I trial, (Kurzrock et al., 2010) treated patients with metastatic MTC with XL184, an oral inhibitor of MET, VEGFR2, and RET that exhibits anti-angiogenic, antiproliferative, and anti-invasive effects. A phase III trial, comparing XL184 with placebo, is now underway. Wells et al. (Wells et al., 2010) describe an open-label, phase III study that assessed the efficacy of vandetanib, a selective inhibitor of RET, VEGFR, and epidermal growth factor receptor. A total of 30 patients with unresectable locally advanced or metastatic hereditary MTC were enrolled. By response evaluation criteria in solid tumors (RECIST), 20% of patients experienced a confirmed partial response and an additional 53% of patients experienced stable disease at 24 weeks; this yielded a disease control rate of 73%. In addition, vandetanib had a tolerable adverse event profile, as well as significant progression-free survival prolongation when compared to placebo.

7. References

ATA Surgery Working Group. (2009).Consensus Statement on the Terminology and Classification of Central Neck Dissection for Thyroid Cancer. *Thyroid*, Vol.19, No.11, pp.1153- 1158.

Bauer, AJ.; Patel, A. & Francis, GL. (2003). Systemic administration of vascular endothelial growth factor monoclonal antibody reduces the growth of papillary thyroid carcinoma in a nude mouse model. *Ann Clin Lab Sci*, Vol.33, No.2 , pp.192–199, ISSN.

Besic, N.; Hocevar, M. & Zgajnar J. (2010). Lower incidence of anaplastic carcinoma after higher iodination of salt in slovenia. *Thyroid*, Vol.20, No.6, pp.623–626, ISSN.

Bilimoria, KY.; Bentrem, DJ. & Sturgeon, C. (2007). Extent of surgery affects survival for papillary thyroid cancer. Ann Surg, Vol.246, No.3, pp.375–381, ISSN.

Boikos, SA. & Stratakis, CA. (2006). Carney complex: pathology and molecular genetics. *Neuroendocrinology*, Vol.83, No.3-4, pp.189–99, ISNN.

Boltze, C.; Roessner, A. & Schneider-Stock, R. (2002). Homozygous proline at codon 72 of p53 as a potential risk factor favoring the development of undifferentiated thyroid carcinoma. *International Journal of Oncology*, Vol.21, No.5 , pp.1151-1154, ISSN.

Cabanillas, ME.; Waguespack, SG. & Busaydi, NL. (2010). Treatment with tyrosine kinase inhibitors for patients with differentiated thyroid cancer. *J Clin Oncol*, Vol.27, N0.6, pp. 6060, ISSN.

Capezzone, M.; Cantara, S. & Pacini, F. (2011). Telomere Length in Neoplastic and Nonneoplastic Tissues of Patients with Familial and Sporadic Papillary Thyroid Cancer. *J Clin Endocrinol Metab,* 2011 Aug 24. (Epub ahead of print)

Castagna, MG.; Brilli, L. & Pacini, F. (2008). Limited value of repeat recombinant thyrotropin (rhTSH)- stimulated thyroglobulin testing in differentiated thyroid carcinoma patients with previous negative rhTSHstimulated thyroglobulin and undetectable basal serumthyroglobulin levels. J Clin Endocrinol Metab, Vol.93, No.1, pp.76-81, ISSN.

Castro, P.; Rebocho, AP. & Sobrinos-Simoes, M. (2006). PAX8-PPARgamma rearrangement is frequently detected in the follicular variant of papillary thyroid carcinoma. *J Clin Endocrinol Metab*, Vol.91, No.1 , pp.213-220, ISSN.

Cetta, F.; Chiappetta, G. & Fusco, A. (1998). The ret/ptc1 oncogene is activated in familial adenomatous polyposis-associated thyroid papillary carcinomas. *J. Clin. Endocrinol. Metab.* Vol.83, No.3, pp.1003-6, ISSN.

Chen, J.; Tward, JD. & Hitchcock, YJ. (2008). Surgery and radiotherapy improves survival in patients with anaplastic thyroid carcinoma: analysis of the surveillance, epidemiology, and end results 1983-2002. *American Journal of Clinical Oncology,* Vol.31, No.5, pp.460-464, ISSN.

Chianelli, M.; Todino, V. & Papini, E. (2009). Low dose (2.0 GBq; 54 mCi) radioiodine postsurgical remnant ablation in thyroid cancer: comparison between hormone withdrawal and use of rhTSH in low risk patients. *Eur J Endocrinol*, Vol.160, No.3, pp.431-436, ISSN.

Cooper, DS.; Doherty, GM. & Tuttle, RM. (2009) Revised American Thyroid Association management guidelines for patients with thyroid nodules and differentiated thyroid cancer. Thyroid, Vol. 19, No. 1167-1214, ISNN.

Davies, H.; Bignel GR & Futreal, PA. (2002).Mutations of the BRAF gene in human cancer. *Nature*, Vol.417, No.6892, pp.949-54, ISSN.

Di Cristofaro, J.; Marcy, M. & De Micco, C. (2006). Molecular genetic study comparing follicular variant versus classic papillary thyroid carcinomas: association of N-ras mutation in codon 61 with follicular variant. Hum. *Pathol,* Vol.37, No.7, pp. 824-30, ISSN.

Dubauskas, Z.; Kunishige, J. & Tannir, N. (2009). Cutaneous squamous cell carcinoma and inflammation of actinic keratoses associated with sorafenib. *Clin Genitourin Cancer,* Vol. 7, No.1 , pp. 20-23, ISSN.

Edwards, B.; Ward, E. & Ries, LAG. (2010). Annual report to the nation on the status of cancer, 1975-2006, featuring colorectal cancer trends and impact of interventions (risk factors, screening, and treatment) to reduce future rates. Cancer, Vol.116, No.3, pp.544-573, ISSN.

Elisei, R.; C. Ugolini, C. & Basolo, F. (2008). BRAF(V600E) mutation and outcome of patients with papillary thyroid carcinoma: a 15-year median follow-up study. *J Clin Endocrinol Metab*, Vol.93, No.10, pp. 3943–3949.

Elisei, R.; Cosci, B. & Pinchera, A. (Mar 2008) Prognostic significance of somatic RET oncogene mutations in sporadic medullary thyroid cancer: a 10-year follow-up study. *J Clin Endocrinol Metab,* Vol. 93, No.3, pp. 682–687, ISSN.

Fadda, G.; Basolo, F. &Palombini, L. (2010). Cytological classification of thyroid nodules. Proposal of the SIAPEC-IAP Italian Consensus Working Group. Phatologyca, Vol.12, No.5, pp.405-408, ISSN.

Farahati, J.; Geling, M. &. Reiners, C. (2004). Changing trends of incidence and prognosis of thyroid carcinoma in lower Franconia, Germany, from 1981–1995. *Thyroid* , Vol.14, No.2, pp. 141-7, ISSN.

Franzius, C.; Dietlein, M. & Schober, O. (2007). Procedure guideline for radioiodine therapy and 131iodine whole-body scintigraphy in paediatric patients with differentiated thyroid cancer. *Nuklearmedizin,* Vol.46, No.5, pp.224–231, ISSN.

Fromigué, J.; De Baere, T. & Schlumberger, M. (2006). Chemoembolization for liver metastases from medullary thyroid carcinoma. *J Clin Endocrinol Metab.* Vol.91, No.7, pp. 2496–2499, ISSN.

Fugazzola, L.; Mannavola, D. & Beck-Peccoz P . (2004). BRAF mutations in an Italian cohort of thyroid cancers, *Clin Endocrinol (Oxf),* Vol.61, No. 2, pp. 239–243, ISSN.

Garcia-Rostan, G.; Zhao, H. & Tallini, G. (2003). ras Mutations Are Associated With Aggressive Tumor Phenotypes and Poor Prognosis in Thyroid Cancer. *Journal of Clinical Oncology,* Vol 21, No.17, pp.3226-3235, ISSN.

Gomez Segovia, I.; Gallowitsch, HJ. & Lind, P. (2004). Descriptive epidemiology of thyroid carcinoma in Carinthia, Austria: 1984–2001. Histopathologic features and tumor classification of 734 cases under elevated general iodination of table salt since 1990: population based age-stratified analysis on thyroid carcinoma incidence. *Thyroid,* Vol.14, No.4, pp.277-86, ISSN.

Hemmings, CT. (2003). Thyroid pathology in four patients with Cowden's disease. *Pathology.* Vol.35, No.4, pp.311–4, ISSN.

Hemminki, K.; Eng, C. & Chen, B. (2005). Familial risks for nonmedullary thyroid cancer. *J. Clin. Endocrinol. Metab,* Vol.90, No.10, pp.5747–53, ISSN.

Hou, P.; Liu, D. & Xing M. (2007). Genetic alterations and their relationship in the phosphatidylinositol 3-kinase/akt pathway in thyroid cancer. *Clin. Cancer Res,* Vol.13,No. 4, pp.1161–70, ISSN.

Hovens, GC.; Stokkel, MP. & Smit, JW. (2007). Association of serum thyrotropin concentration with recurrence and death in differentiated thyroid cancer. J Clin Endocrinol Metab, Vol. 92, No. 7, pp.2610–2615, ISSN.

Kilfoy, BA.; Zheng, T & Zhang, I. (2009). International patterns and trends in thyroid cancer incidence, 1973–2002. *Cancer Causes Control,* Vol.20, No.5, pp. 525–531, ISSN.

Kim, TY.; Kim, KW. & Shong, YK. (2007). Prognostic factors for korean patients with anaplastic thyroid carcinoma. *Head & Neck,* Vol.29, No.8, pp.765–772, ISSN.

Kloos, RT.; Eng, C. & Wells, SA Jr. (Jun 2009). American Thyroid Association Guidelines Task Force, Medullary thyroid cancer: management guidelines of the American Thyroid Association. *Thyroid,* Vol. 19, No. 6, pp. 565–612, ISSN.

Kosary, CL. (2007). Cancer Survival Among Adults: U.S. SEER Program, 1988-2001, Patient and Tumor Characteristics. In: SEER Survival Monograph. LAG Ries, JL Young, GE Keel, MP Eisner, YD Lin and MJ Horner. U.S., National Cancer Institute, SEER Program, NIH No. 07-6215, Bethesda, MD. *http://www.seer.cancer.gov.*

Kraeber-Bodere, F.; Goldenberg, DM. & Barbet, J. (2009). Pretargeted radioimmunotherapy in the treatment of metastatic medullary thyroid cancer. *Curr Oncol,* Vol.116, No.4, pp.16:3–8, ISSN.

Kudo, T.; Miyauchi, A. & Hirokawa, M. (2007). Diagnosis of medullary thyroid carcinoma by calcitonin measurement in fine-needle aspiration biopsy specimens. *Thyroid,* Vol.17, No.7, pp. 635–638, ISSN.

Kurzrock, R. & Cohen, EE. (2010). Long-term results in a cohort of medullary thyroid cancer patients in a phase I study of SL184, an oral inhibitor of MET, VEGFR2, and RET. *J Clin Oncol,* Vol.28, No.15, pp.5502-5505, ISSN.

Leboulleux, S.; Travagli JP. & Baudin, E. (2002). Medullary thyroid carcinoma as part of a multiple endocrine neoplasia type 2B syndrome: influence of the stage on the clinical course. *Cancer,* Vol 94, No.1, pp. 44–50,ISSN.

Lee, J. & Soh, EY. (2010). Differentiated thyroid carcinoma presenting with distant metastasis at initial diagnosis: clinical outcomes and prognostic factors. *Ann Surg ,* Vol.251, No.1, pp. 114–119, ISSN.

Lee, N.; Puri, DR. & Blanco Chao, KS. Intensity-modulated radiation therapy in head and neck cancers: an update. *Head & Neck,* Vol.29, No.4, pp.387–400, ISSN.

Lee, SH.; Lee, SS. & Rho, YS. (2008). Predictive factors for central compartment lymph node metastasis in thyroid papillary microcarcinoma. *Laryngoscope,* Vol.118, No.4, pp. 659–662, ISSN.

Lind, P.; Langsteger, W. & Gomez, I. (1998). Epidemiology of thyroid diseases in iodine sufficiency. *Thyroi* , Vol.8, No.12, pp.1179-83, ISSN.

Machens, A,; Holzhausen, HJ. & Dralle, H. (2005). The prognostic value of primary tumor size in papillary and follicular thyroid carcinoma. *Cancer,* Vol.103, No.11, pp.2269–2273, ISSN.

Maenpaa, HO.; Heikkonen, J. & Joensuu, H. (2008). Low vs. high radioiodine activity to ablate the thyroid after thyroidectomy for cancer: a randomized study. *PLoS One,* Vol.3, No.4, pp.e1885, ISSN.

Mazzaferri, EL. (2007). Management of low-risk differentiated thyroid cancer. *Endocr Pract,* Vol. 13, No.5, pp.498–512, ISSN.

Meinkoth JL. (2004). Biology of Ras in thyroid cells. *Cancer Treat Res,* Vol.122, pp.131-148, ISSN.

Miccoli, P.; Materazzi, G. & Berti, P. (2007). New trends in the treatment of undifferentiated carcinomas of the thyroid. *Langenbecks Arch Surg,* Vol.392, No.4 , pp. 397–404, ISSN.

Moon, WJ.; Jung, SL. & Lee, DH. (2008). Benign and malignant thyroid nodules:US differentiation multicenter retrospective study. *Radiology,* Vol. 247, No.3, pp.762 770, ISSN.

Mrozek, E.; Kloos, RT. & Shaha, MH. (2006). Phase II study of celecoxib in metastatic differentiated thyroid carcinoma. *J Clin Endocrinol Metab*, Vol.91, No.6, pp. 2201–2204, ISSN.

Musholt. TJ.; Musholt, PB. & Klempnauer, J (2000). Prognostic significance of RET and NTRK1 rearrangements in sporadic papillary thyroid carcinoma. *Surgery*, Vol.128, No.6, pp.984-93, ISNN.

Nikiforov, YE. (2002). RET/PTC rearrangement in thyroid tumors. *Endocr Pathol*, Vol.13, No.1, pp.3-16, ISSN.

Nikiforov, YE. (2006). RET/PTC Rearrangement - a link between Hashimoto's thyroiditis and thyroid cancer or not. *J. Clin. Endocrinol. Metab*, Vol. 91, No.6, pp.2040–2, ISNN.

Nikiforova, MN.; Kimura, ET. & Nikiforova, YE. (2003). BRAF mutations in thyroid tumors are restricted to papillary carcinomas and anaplastic or poorly differentiated carcinomas arising from papillary carcinomas. *J. Clin. Endocrinol. Metab*, Vol.88, No.11, pp.5399–404, ISSN.

Pal, T.; Vogl, ED. & Foulkes, WD. (2001). Increased risk for nonmedullary thyroid cancer in the first degree relatives of prevalent cases of nonmedullary thyroid cancer: a hospital-based study. *J. Clin. Endocrinol. Metab*, Vol.86, No.11, pp.5307–12, ISSN.

Papadopoulou, F. & Efthimiou, E. (2009). Thyroid cancer after external or internal ionizing irradiation. *Hell J Nucl Med.* Vol.12, No.3, pp.266-70, ISSN.

Pasqualetti, G.; Ricci, S & Monzani, F. (2011). The emerging role of sunitinib in the treatment of advanced epithelial thyroid cancer: our experience and review of literature. *Mini Rev Med Chem*, Vol.11, No.9, pp.746-52, ISSN.

Rago, T.; Santini, F. & Vitti, P. (2007). Elastography: new developments in ultrasound for predicting malignancy in thyroid nodules. *J Clin Endocrinol Metab*, Vol.92, No.8, pp.2917–2922, ISSN

Robert, C.; Smallridge, SE. & Fatourechi, V. (2007). Monitoring thyreoglobulin in a sensitive Immunoassay has comparable sensitivity to recombinant human TSH-stimulated thyroglobulin in follow-up of thyroid cancer patients. J Clin Endocrinol Metab, Vol.92, No.1, pp.82-87, ISSN.

Roche, B.; Larroumets, G. & Tauveron, I. (2010). Epidemiology, clinical presentation, treatment and prognosis of a regional series of 26 anaplastic thyroid carcinomas (ATC). Comparison with the literature. *Annales d'Endocrinologie*, Vol.71, No.1, pp.38–45, ISSN.

Santoro, M.; Melillo, RM. & Fusco, A. (2006). RET/PTC activation in papillary thyroid carcinoma: European Journal of Endocrinology Prize Lecture. *Eur. J. Endocrinol*, Vol.155, No.5, pp.645–53, ISSN.

Schlumberger, M. & Pacini, F. (2006). Thyroid tumors. *Edition Nucleon*, Vol.18, pp. 313–340, ISSN.

Schlumberger, M.; Berg, G. & Wiersinga, WM. (2004). Follow-up of low risk patients with differentiated thyroid carcinoma: a European perspective. *Eur J Endocrinol*, Vol.150, No.2, pp.105–112, ISSN.

Schoenberger, J.; Grimm, D. & Eilles, C. (2004). Effects of PTK787/ZK222584, a tyrosine kinase inhibitor, on the growth of a poorly differentiated thyroid carcinoma: an animal study. *Endocrinology*, Vol.145, No.3, pp.1031–1038, ISSN.

Sherman SI. (2009). Advances in chemotherapy of differentiated epithelial and medullary thyroid cancers. *J Clin Endocrinol Metab*, Vol.94, No.5, pp.1493–1499, ISSN.

Shimaoka, K.; Schoenfeld, DA. & De Conti, R. (1985). A randomized trial of doxorubicin versus doxorubicin plus cisplatin in patients with advanced thyroid carcinoma. *Cancer*, Vol.56, No.9, pp.2155–2160, ISSN.

Sobrinho-Simoes, M.; Sambade, C. & (2002). Poorly differentiated carcinomas of the thyroid gland: a review of the clinicopathologic features of a series of 28 cases of a heterogeneous, clinically aggressive group of thyroid tumors. Int J Surg Pathol, Vol.10, No.2, pp.123-131, ISSN.

Spencer, CA. (2004). Challenges of serum thyroglobulin (thyroglobulin) measurement in the presence of thyroglobulin autoantibodies. J Clin Endocrinol Metab, Vol.89, No.8, pp.3702–3704, ISSN.

Stulak, JM.; Grant, CS. & Charboneau, JW. (2006). Value of preoperative ultrasonography in the surgical management of initial and reoperative papillary thyroid cancer. *Arch Surg*, Vol.141, No.5, pp.489–494ISSN.

Tuttle, RM.; Brokhin, M. & Robbins, RJ. (2008). Recombinant human TSH-assisted radioactive iodine remnant ablation achieves short-term clinical recurrence rates similar to those of traditional thyroid hormone withdrawal. *J Nucl Med*, Vol.49, No.5, pp.764–770, ISSN.

Tuttle, RM.; Leboeuf, R. & Shaha, AR. (2008). Medical management of thyroid cancer: a risk adapted approach. *J Surg Oncol*, Vol.97, No.8, pp.712-716, ISSN.

Waguespack, SG.; Sherman, SI. & Herzog, CE. (2009). The successful use of sorafenib to treat pediatric papillary thyroid carcinoma. *Thyroid*, Vol.19, No.4, pp. 407–412, ISSN.

Wang, Y.; Hou, P. & Xing, M. (2007). High prevalence and mutual exclusivity of genetic alterations in the phosphatidylinositol-3-kinase/akt pathway in thyroid tumors. *J. Clin. Endocrinol. Metab*, Vol.92, No.6, pp.2387–90, ISSN.

Wells, SA.; Gosnell, JE. & Schlumberger, M. (2010). Vandetanib for the treatment of patients with locally advanced or metastatic hereditary medullary thyroid cancer. *J Clin Oncol*, Vol.28, No.15, pp.767–772, ISSN.

Williams D. (2008). Radiation carcinogenesis: lessons from Chernobyl. *Oncogene.* Vol.27, No.2, pp.S9-18, ISSN.

Wong, CS.; Van Dyk, J. & Simpson WJ. (1991). Myelopathy following hyperfractionated accelerated radiotherapy for anaplastic thyroid carcinoma. *Radiotherapy and Oncology*, Vol.20, No.1, pp.3–9, ISSN.

Xing M. (2005). BRAF mutation in thyroid cancer. *Endocr Relat Cancer*, Vol.12, No.2, pp.245-262, ISSN.

Xing, M.; Westra, WH & Ladenson, PW. (2005). BRAF mutation predicts a poorer clinical prognosis for papillary thyroid cancer. *J. Clin. Endocrinol. Metab*, Vol.90, No.12, pp.6373–9, ISSN.

Yau, T.; Lo, CY. & Lang, BH. (2008). Treatment outcomes in anaplastic thyroid carcinoma: survival improvement in young patients with localized disease treated by combination of surgery and radiotherapy. *Ann Surg Oncol*, Vol.15, No.9, pp.2500-2505, ISSN.

Ying, H.; Suzuki, H. & Cheng, SE. (2003). Mutant thyroid hormone receptor beta represses the expression and transcriptional activity of peroxisome proliferator- activated receptor gamma during thyroid carcinogenesis. *Cancer Res*, Vol.63, No.17, pp.5274-5280, ISSN.

Zaydfudim, V.; Feurer, ID. & Phay, JE. (2008). The impact of lymph node involvement on survival in patients with papillary and follicular thyroid carcinoma. *Surgery*, Vol.144, No.6, pp.1070–1077, ISSN.

5

Thyroid Growth Factors

Aleksander Konturek and Marcin Barczynski
Department of Endocrine Surgery
Jagiellonian University College of Medicine
Kraków
Poland

1. Introduction

The effect of exogenous and endogenous factors on the thyroid is manifested as stimulation or inhibition of the gland's excretory activity and growth regulation of the thyroid tissue itself. External factors affecting thyroid enlargement were known as early as approximately 2000 years B.C. in ancient China, where marine products were administered to inhabitants of the central part of the country. This specific supplementation of iodine-rich products prevented goiter development. [1,2] In modern times, the first country to introduce iodine prophylaxis was Switzerland, followed by the United States. Poland has been implementing a program of common salt iodization since 1986, albeit with an interruption of less than a score of years. We presently know than apart from iodine, there are numerous factors that affect regulation of thyroid secretion and growth. Thyroid homeostasis is thus controlled by several different substances acting on various levels: directly and indirectly by thyrotropin TSH (thyroid stimulating hormone); locally by other growth stimulators, such as the epidermal growth factor (EGF), transforming growth factor alpha (TGF-α), insulin growth factors (IGFs), fibroblast growth factors (FGFs), hepatocyte growth factor (HGF), platelet-derived growth factor (PDGF) and transforming growth factor beta (TGF-β), as well as through programmed cell death in the mechanism of apoptosis. Hence, changes in thyroid size and hormone demand occur mostly through TSH and complex interactions of local growth factors with expression of specific receptors. It has been also observed recently that para- and autocrine effects of growth factors are also associated with expression of particular oncogenes. Except the embryonal and adolescent periods, the volume of a normal thyroid gland does not increase. Each thyroid follicular cell is programmed to undergo five mitotic cycles during adult life and the final population of thyrocytes demonstrates specific differentiation, manifested by hormone secretion in response to thyrotropin via the mechanism of negative feedback. Thus, participation of the thyroid gland in hemostasis is regulated via hormonal, neural and immune pathways. The first level of thyroid growth and function control occurs via the effect of thyrotropin (TSH). The second level of tissue hemostasis is controlled by local factors. The third level consists of interactions between thyroid cells and connective tissue stroma, while the fourth level includes genetic factors with programmed death cell (apoptosis).

2. Regulation of growth and hormonal secretion – Mitogenic pathways

2.1 Role of TSH

Mechanism of activation via a receptor (types of receptors)

Thyrotropin (TSH) is traditionally believed to be the principal stimulator of growth, differentiation and maturation of thyroid follicular cells and connective tissue stroma. It is a 28 kD glycoprotein. Its level is among major parameters describing thyroid function and playing a decisive role in the clinical status of a patient. As early as in mid-thirties (1935 Kippen; Loeb; 1937 Dunhill), observations were made on the effect of TSH on thyroid follicular cells. Both a stimulatory and inhibitory effect of thyrotropin on thyroid follicular cells was described in cells cultured *in vitro*; attempts were undertaken at explaining the role of suppression therapy in preventing thyroid cancer development. For decades, particular research teams obtained contrary results of investigations on the proliferogenic effect on growth and differentiation of thyroid follicular cells. The effect on thyroid function and hormonal secretion has remained unquestioned [3,4]. In the last decade, numerous reports were published that discussed the complex regulation system of thyroid cell growth and proliferation, where thyrotropin alone may play an important role, but is not a prerequisite. Thus, TSH administration to rats resulted in thyroid enlargement both via cell hypertrophy and hyperplasia [5]. TSH-induced thyreocyte proliferation was triggered by human thyroid tissue implantation to mice (thymus-deficient nu/nu mice). In another study, thyrotropin was not necessary for compensatory thyroid growth following hemithyroidectomies, what suggested the effect of other factors that also play a role in the gland's growth [6,7]. Recently, attention has been also focused on the role of cAMP in thyroid growth-associated processes. Numerous reports on the proliferogenic effect of cAMP on thyroid follicular cells point to three pathways of activating growth and proliferation of thyroid cells:

1. first - activation of the adenyl cyclase-cAMP system, stimulated by TSH;
2. second - the phosphatidylinositol-Ca ion system,
3. third - most likely independent of cAMP - protein phosphorylation of tyrosine.

An increase of cAMP level in the majority of differentiated thyroid tumors (in contrast to normal tissue collected from the same patient) was interpreted as a result of an increased response to TSH stimulation. In numerous differentiated thyroid cancers, the functional TSH-cAMP-thyroid follicular cell growth system was noted; nevertheless, the question on intercorrelations of the above factors continue to remain open (Table 1.). Numerous authors have also pointed to a double effect of TSH depending on activation of other transmitters. Thus, 1) thyroid follicular cell growth is stimulated via activation of phosphatidylinositol and protein kinase C, while 2) the function of thyroid follicular cells is regulated by cAMP and protein kinase A (Figure 1). The two alternative pathways may explain diversified effects of thyrotropin in cancerous thyroid tissue [2]. The turning point in explaining many growth-associated phenomena within the thyroid gland was determination of the receptor structure on the molecular level and demonstration of intracellular interactions via activation of other transmitters. The thyrotropin receptor itself belongs to the family of G protein-coupled receptors (similarly as FSH, LH, estrogens, hCG or other steroid receptors). The predominant property of all the above receptors is the presence of a transmembrane domain that crosses the lipid layer (Figure 2.). The N-terminal region of the receptors is the so-called ectodomain situated on cell surface. The C-terminal region, situated within the cell, is much shorter. The TSH receptor, in contrast to other receptors from this family, is modified post-translationally. Approximately 75% of the monomeric, membrane receptor is proteolized. In consequence of proteolysis, the so-called peptide C is released, while the generated subunits A and B are linked by disulfide bridges. Both forms of the receptor - monomeric and dimeric - actively bind TSH. In the cell membrane of thyrocytes, the TSH receptor is found in two forms: active, which binds Gs protein, and inactive, which is prevalent. Both TSH and stimulating autoantibodies bind to the active form of the receptor and stabilize it. In turn, inhibiting antibodies stabilize the inactive ("closed") form of the receptor and thus, the genuine receptor agonist seems to be the active ("open") form of the receptor rather than the thyrotropin (TSH) molecule itself [8,9,10,11].

3. Vascular endothelial growth factor (VEGF), epidermal growth factors (EGFs) and transforming growth factor alpha (TGF-α)

Neoangiogenesis is a process consisting of numerous paracrine and endocrine interactions between cancer cells and vascular endothelial cells, connective tissue stromal cells and some morphotic blood elements, such as macrophages or mastocytes. The result of such interactions is a change in the microenvironment of a tumor that allows for its further uncontrollable growth and progression. A prerequisite for initiation of angiogenic phenomena is disturbance of balance between the system of pro- and anti-angiogenic factors. Not each of the proangiogenic factors that have been described to date (VEGF; bFGF; aFGF; PDGF; TGF-α; TGF-β; EGF; IGF-1) meets all the three characteristic criteria: exerting a specific effect on endothelium, possessing a system of specific cell receptors and manifesting fluctuations that inhibit or induce angiogenesis. Many of such factors, acting in conjunction with mediators secreted by other cells (e.g. macrophages - TNF), induce and promote development of cancer. In keeping with the presently accepted assumptions, angiogenesis is initiated via hypoxia of cancer cells that are situated at the highest distance from the lumen of a blood vessel, as well as via a defect of the genetic apparatus, the consequence of which is formation of the so-called angiogenic phenotype. This term denotes a state of permanent, constitutive activation of growth factors-encoding genes. An additional loss of function of suppressor genes (e.g. the p53 gene) favors the process of neoangiogenesis. One of the relatively well-understood epithelial growth factors is VEGF. This specific protein, defined and named in late eighties, is assumed to play a key role in vascularization of solid tumors, including thyroid tumors. At present, the VEGF group is believed to include six proteins: VEGF-A, VEGF-B, VEGF-C, VEGF-D, VEGF-E and PIGF (Placenta Growth Factor). They act through binding to receptors: VEGFR1, VEGFR2 – on vascular endothelial cells, and VGFR3 – on lymphatic endothelium cells (Figure 3). The necessary cofactors for the VEGF receptor are neuropilins 1 and 2 (Nrp-1,2), which are indispensable for proper activation of the receptor by a ligand. Synthesis of the vascular growth factor is induced by numerous other substances, such as nitrogen oxide, insulin, fibroblast growth factor (FGF), platelet-derived growth factor (PDGF), epidermal growth factor (EGF), tumor necrotic factor (TNF-α), transforming growth factor (TGF-β), IL-1,2. In keeping with the theory of Folkman, which states that tumor growth is limited by its vascularization, attempts have been made to demonstrated higher VEGF expression in cancer tissues as compared to normal cell populations. Similarly as in the case of cancer of the stomach, colon, uterus, breast and ovary, also in thyroid tumors a key role in neoangiogenesis is played by VEGF. As it has been already mentioned, not only thyroid epithelial cells, but also stromal cells are capable of producing and secreting VEGF. The above described results have allowed for formulating a hypothesis that VEGF participates in initiation of neoangiogenesis, yet further tumor development and progression most likely depend on the effect of other chemokines secreted both by tumor cells, its stroma and macrophages migrating to the neoplastic lesion [12.13,14]. In turn, epidermal growth factor EGF is one of the most potent stimulators of thyroid growth and its multiple effect is determined by its binding to specific EGF receptors. *In vitro*, it is a factor that stimulates proliferation of thyroid follicular cells. A factor that increases EGF binding to receptors is thyrotropin (TSH), which - stimulating the increase of the number of EGF receptors - enhances its effect. Yet, in contrast to the above-mentioned TSH, to reveal its mitogenic effect, EGF does not require the presence of other chemokines. In subsequent studies, investigators attempted to determine the effect of positive EGF receptors expression in thyroid cancer tissue on the clinical course of the disease. A comparison was made between the presence of EGF receptors in various types of thyroid cancer, finding their highest expression in anaplastic and medullary carcinoma of the thyroid. Also adenomas demonstrated considerable expression of EGF receptors, but only in some limited areas within the tumor. EGF-R was also noted to bind not only to EGF -α 1, but also to the transforming growth factor alpha (TGF-α). The autocrine mechanism of activating EGF receptors both by the epidermal growth factor molecule and by TGFα was seen in thyroid cancers (papillary carcinoma and its nodal metastases) [15].

4. Insulin growth factors and their receptors (IGFs)

Growth hormone (GH) affects growth processes in tissues and organs through specific substances called the insulin growth factors (IGF-I; IGF-II). IGF-I, termed somatomedin C, and IGF-II affect growth regulation of thyroid endothelial cells. In turn, thyroid follicular cells show high expression of specialized IGF-I and IGF-II receptors. The IGF-I receptor, as a member of the family of receptors that act via tyrosine kinase, is a mediator of the effect of IGF-I on stimulation and growth of thyroid follicular cells. IGF-I has been proven to strongly stimulate growth of the FRTL-5 line cells and to synergistically enhance the mitogenic effect of thyrotropin (TSH). In turn, the IGF-II receptor plays no significant role in thyroid growth stimulation. Autocrine secretion of IGF-I, IGF-II and expression of the IGF-I-Rs receptor were demonstrated in primary cultures of thyroid follicular cells, as well as in adenomas and thyroid papillary carcinoma cell lines [16,17,18].

5. Fibroblast growth factor (FGFs), hepatocyte growth factor (HGF), platelet-derived growth factor (PDGF)

To date, nine subtypes of the fibroblast growth factor belonging to a single family (the "FGF family") have been determined. The FGF factor itself is known as a stimulator of proliferation, differentiation and functioning of various diverse cells of human body. FGF also plays a significant role in neoangiogenesis. The cell response to FGF effect is mediated by its four receptors (FGF-R 1-4) that belong to the family of tyrosine kinases. Thyroid endothelial cells show expression of FGF-R receptors, while the basement membrane of thyroid follicular cells is capable of producing the factor itself. Based on numerous observations in vitro and in vivo in rat thyroid follicular cells, an autocrine, stimulatory effect of FGF-2 ("basic FGF") on thyroid growth processes has been demonstrated. In turn, a paracrine effect has been manifested in neovascularization seen in nodular goiter. Similarly as EGF, FGF has an inhibitory effect on thyroid function. The effect of FGF consists in inhibition of cAMP activation and weakening of TSH activity. FGF-1 administration to rats leads to development of colloid goiter, most likely through inhibition of TSH-dependent colloid transport from the lumen of thyroid follicles (Figure 4.).

The hepatocyte growth factor (HGF) is also a potent myogen for numerous diversified cell types in human body, especially these of epithelial origin. It operates through its receptor that is encoded by the c-met proto-oncogene and belongs to the family of tyrosine kinase receptors. HGF-R expression has been noted both in normal and cancer tissue, with the factor being present in papillary and follicular carcinoma, but absent in anaplastic carcinoma tissue. Some importance in neoplastic proliferation is also ascribed to the platelet-derived growth factor PDGF), the presence of which has been noted in the papillary carcinoma cell line.

6. Interactions between stimulatory growth factors and their inhibitors

A group of factors that inhibit thyroid growth is the family of the thyroid growth inhibiting factor – β (TGF- β). Through their receptors TGF- β-R I to TGF- β-R III, the factors TGF- β1 to TGF- β3 affect inhibition of thyroid follicular cell growth in vitro; their role has also been implicated in development of benign lesions. A drop in TGF production has been observed in thyroid follicular cells of patients with non-toxic goiter.

Stimulation of thyroid tissue growth occurs through an increased frequency of signals reaching the gland from the surrounding structures, resulting in sensitization of follicular cells to normal external stimuli. Such stimuli may be the afore-mentioned growth factors or antibodies or else dietary iodine deficit. A notion of the so-called "grey zone" has become popular in thyreology, to denote a population of cells with a high internal growth potential, which, in consequence of single or multiple genetic damage, change their growth potential (in hyperplastic tumors) towards cancer, yet without obvious neoplastic transformation. The effect on cell cycle, manifested as for example the shortened G0 phase or limitation of apoptosis may lead to an increase in the number of cell divisions prior to programmed cell death.

Within the past decade, development of modern research methods, molecular biology and genetics has allowed for gradual understanding of molecular foundations of thyroid cancers. It is presently known that activation of certain oncogenes and inactivation of suppressor genes may lead to tumor development. Of 35 proto-oncogenes determined in neoplastic transformation of thyroid follicular cells, the following have their effect proven:

1. c-erb encodes the EGF (endothelial growth factor) receptor;
2. flg, bek encodes the FGF receptor type 1 and 2 (fibroblast growth factor);
3. c-met encodes the HGF (hepatocyte growth factor) receptor;
4. c-sis encodes the PDGF (platelet-derived growth factor) receptor;
5. Ras is characteristic of follicular carcinoma, adenoma, anaplastic carcinoma;
6. PTC/ret, TPC – characteristic of papillary carcinoma;
7. Trk encodes NGF (nerve growth factor) characteristic of papillary carcinoma and detected in nodular goiter.

As it follows from the presented data, they play a key role in encoding growth factors and/or their receptors production

Summing up, it should be stressed that the theories presented in the chapter constitute only a very narrow fragment of the bulk of knowledge on the subject. An extensive presentation of the topic is possible only in a monograph, yet the above provided examples help in understanding the foundations of contemporary knowledge on the effect of external factors on cancer development.

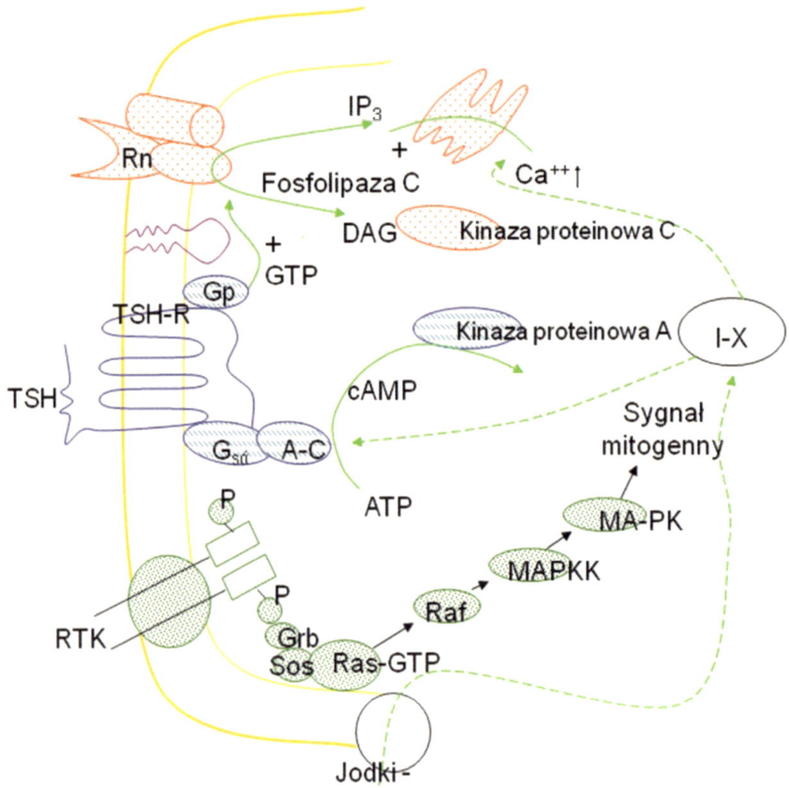

Fig. 1. Mitogenic pathways in regulation of thyroid function and growth. The scheme present the main pathways that participate in regulation of thyroid function and growth.

1. The AC/cAMP/PKA pathway: The main factor that stimulates the pathway in thyrocytes is thyrotropic hormone (TSH), which interacts with the TSH receptor (TSH-R). Stimulation of the TSH-R receptor leads to activations that bind guanosine triphosphate (GTP) of regulatory proteins; Ga protein in the plasma membrane activates adenyl cyclase (AC) that synthesizes cyclic adenosine monophosphate (cAMP), which activates protein kinase A (PKA), and phospholipase C (PLC)-associated Gp protein, which stimulates phosphatidylinositol (PI) metabolism.
2. The PI-PKC-Ca2+ pathway: In addition to TSH-R, the cascade of signal transmission is activated through numerous diversified receptors (marked as Rn in the scheme). Stimulation of TSH and other receptors leads to an increased PLC activity; in consequence, 1,4,5,-inositol triphosphate (IP3) and diacylglycerol (DAG) are formed with

a resultant increase of intracellular level of calcium (Ca2+) and PKC activity. Both PKA and PKC are serine-threonine kinases and they phosphorylate several different proteins.

3. The receptor tyrosine kinase pathway (RTK): Binding of a ligand to RTK leads to phosphorylation of tyrosine residues in the receptor molecule. The stimulated phosphorylated receptors connect to numerous different signaling pathways (the scheme does not show all the pathways) through direct binding of signaling proteins that contain a homology domain with Src proteins (SH2). Nevertheless, the main mitogenic pathway of numerous receptors tyrosine kinase (RTK) includes activation of a chain of events on the *ras* pathway (see the scheme). In brief, phosphorylated RTK interacts with Grb2 adaptor protein. Grb2 binds to a protein called Sos ("son of sevenless"), resulting in activation of the *ras* pathway. The activated form of *ras* GTP protein triggers increased activity of raf protein, with a resultant sequential activation of MAPK cascade proteins (mitogen-activated kinases), what ultimately leads to an increased transcriptional activity (MAPKK kinase, MAPK). The scheme also shows a negative effect of organic forms of iodine (I-X) on various pathways. ATP = adenosine triphosphate.

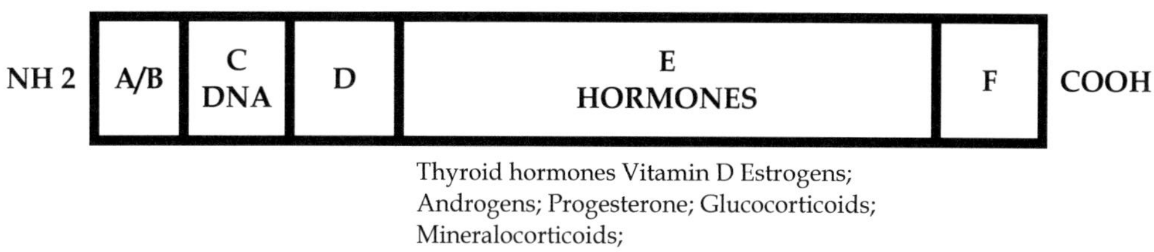

Fig. 2. The family of steroid/thyroid receptors. The marked receptors have similar structure. The C domain consists of DBD domains.

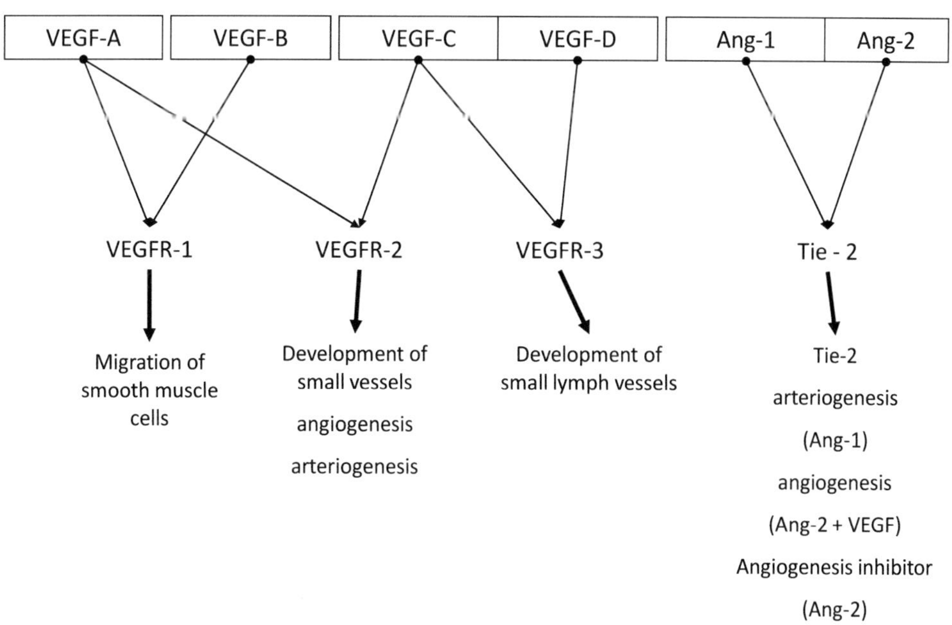

Fig. 3. Vascular growth factors and the effects of their acting through receptors.

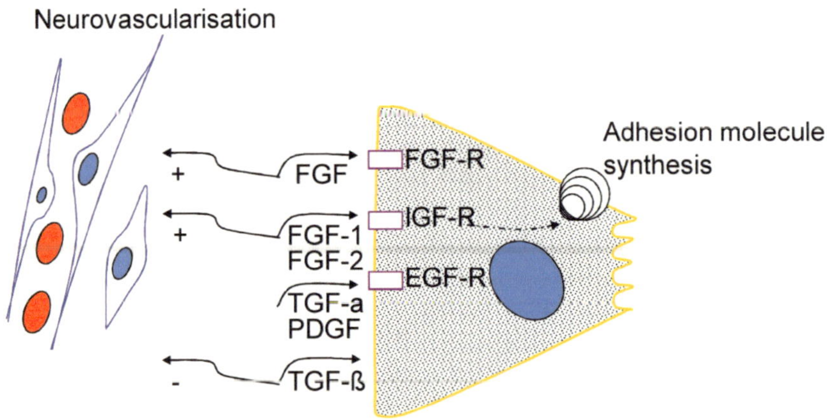

Fig. 4. Autocrine and paracrine regulation of growth and inhibition of thyrocytes via growth factors and their receptors. The factors may be also secreted by the surrounding stromal tissue, thus giving rise to proliferation of endothelial cells and fibroblasts. IGF-insulin growth factor; TGF – transforming growth factor; EGF – epidermal growth factor; FGF – fibroblast growth factor; PDGF – platelet-derived growth factor.

Activation pathway (other transmitter)	Factors	Receptor	Effect	"Related" proto-oncogene
AC-cAMP-PKA	TSH	TSH-R	Stimulatory and inhibitory	
	Iodides (inhibition of cAMP		Stimulatory	
	Epinephrine (inhibition of cAMP)		Stimulatory	
Receptor tyrosine kinases	EGF	EGF-R	Stimulatory	*c-erb* B (EGF-R)
	TGF-a	EGF-R	Stimulatory	
	FGFs	FGF-Rs (1-4)	Stimulatory	*flg, bek* (FGF-R-I, FGF-R-2)
	Insulin	(ffi) IGF-I-R	Stimulatory (via IGF-I-R)	
	IGF-I	IGF-I-R	Stimulatory	
	IGF -n	(IGF-n-R) IGF-I-R	Stimulatory (via IGF-I-R)	
	HGF	HGF-R	Stimulatory	c-met (HGF-R)
	PDGFs (AA, AB, BB)	PDGF-Rs *(a,*)	Stimulatory	*c-sis* (PDGF-BB)
Phosphatidylinositol cascade	TSH	TSH-R	Stimulatory	
	Esters	PKC	Stimulatory	
	TGF -β1	TGF--Rs (1-3)	Inhibitory	
	Iodides		Inhibitory	

Table 1. Major factors with stimulatory and inhibitory effect on growth of thyroid follicular cells.

7. References

[1] Cao X-Y., Jiang X-M., Kareem A.: Iodination of irrigation water as a method supplying iodine to a severely iodine deficient population in Xinjiang, China. Lancet. 1994 Jul 9;344(8915):107-10].

[2] Peter E. Goretzki, M.D., Dietmar Simon, M.D., Cornelia Dotzenrath, M.D., Klaus-Martin Schulte, M.D., Hans-Dietrich Roeher, M.D.: Growth Regulation of Thyroid and Thyroid Tumors in Humans. World J. Surg. 24, 913–922, 2000

[3] Werner SC 1991 History of the thyroid. In: Braverman LE, Utiger RD (eds) The Thyroid: A Fundamental and Clinical Text, ed 6. J, B. Lippincott, Philadelphia, pp 3-6

[4] Goretzki PE, Frilling A, Simon D, Roeher HD. Growth regulation of normal thyroids and thyroid tumors in man. Recent Results Cancer Res. 1990;118:48-63.

[5] Wynford Th,D, Stringer BMJ, Williams ED.: Goitrogen-induced thyroid growth in rat: A quantitive morphometric study. J Endocrinol. 1982,94,131-135

[6] Smeds S, Boeryd B, Jortso E, Lennquist S.: normal and stimulated growth of different humman thyroid tissues in nude mice. In: Goretzki PE, Roeher HD . Growth regulation of thyroid gland and thyroid tumors Vol 18. Basel, Switzerland, Karger, 1989, p98.

[7] Lewiński A, Bartke A, Smith NKR.: Compensatory thyroid hyperplasia In hemithyroidectomized Snell dwarf mice. Endocrinology 1983;113:2317-2319.

[8] Adler G.: Posttranslacyjne modyfikacje receptora tyreotropiny a choroby tarczycy Endokrynol Pol 2005; 1(56): 72-77)

[9] Vassart G., Dumont JE.,: The Thyrotropin Receptor and the Regulation of Thyrocyte Function and Growth. Endocrine Reviews 1992 Vol. 13, No. 3, 596-613.

[10] Bernard Rees Smith, Jadwiga Furmaniak, Jane Sanders TSH receptor blocking antibodies. Thyroid. 2008 Nov ;18 (11):1239

[11] Lazar MA. Thyroid Hormone Receptors: Multiple Forms, Multiple Possibilities. Endocrine Reviews, 1993; Vol. 14, N. 2; 184-193.)

[12] Lin SY, Wang YY, Sheu WH (2003) Preoperative plasma concentrations of vascular endothelial growth factor and matrix metalloproteinase 9 are associated with stage progression in papillary thyroid cancer. Clin Endocrinol 58:513-518.

[13] Lennard CM, Patel A, Wilson J, Reinhardt B, Tuman C, Fenton C, Blair E, Francis GL, Tuttle RM (2001) Intensity of vascular endothelial growth factor expression associated with increased risk of recurrence and decreased disease-free survival in papillary thyroid cancer. Surgery 129:552-558.

[14] Huang SM, Lee JC, Wu TJ, Chow NH (2001) Clinical revelance of vascular endothelial growth factor for thyroid neoplasms. World J Surg 25:302-306.

[15] Konturek A, Barczyński M, Cichoń S, Pituch-Noworolska A, Jonkisz J, Cichoń W. Significance of vascular endothelial growth factor and epidermal growth factor in development of papillary thyroid cancer. Langenbecks Arch Surg. 2005 Jun;390(3):216-21

[16] Tode B, Serio M, Rotella CM et All: Insulin-like growth factor-I Autocrine secretion by human thyroid follicular cells In primary culture. J Clin Endocrinol Metab 198969,621-626.

[17] Onoda N, Ohmura E, Tsushima T et All: Autocrine role of insulin-like growth factor (IGF-I) in thyroid cancer cell Line. Eur J Cancer 1992,28A,1904-1908

[18] Pouliaki V,Mitsiades CS, McMullan C et all: Regulation of Vascular Endothelial Growth Factor Expression by Insulin-Like Growth Factor I in Thyroid Carcinomas. The Journal of Clinical Endocrinology & Metabolism 88(11):5392–5398

6

Vascular Endothelial Growth Factor (VEGF) and Epidermal Growth Factor (EGF) in Papillary Thyroid Cancer

Aleksander Konturek and Marcin Barczynski
Department of Endocrine Surgery
Jagiellonian University College of Medicine, Kraków
Poland

1. Introduction

Early diagnosis and radical management of thyroid cancer do not always result in curing the patient. Long-term analyses of deaths due to thyroid cancer have allowed for establishing systems for distinguishing increased risk groups, such as AMES or AGES. These commonly employed prognostic systems recognize the role of four basic factors only (age, stage, extent of the tumor, its size [AGES] and metastases [AMES]), which constitute the foundation for establishing the low and high-risk groups. Despite the progress in oncology and oncological surgery, a major problem still lies in early cancer detection, when the tumor is still at a stage that allows for curing the patient, as well as in identifying individuals, in whom - despite radical treatment - the prognosis of a complete cure is poor and there is an increased risk of a local recurrence and death due to the cancer.

2. Epidemoilogy of papillary thyroid carcinoma

Papillary thyroid carcinoma accounts for the majority of thyroid cancers and is commonly believed to be the least malignant type. In Europe and the United States, it presently constitutes approximately 75-80% of all diagnosed thyroid cancers [1]. It is characterized by a mild clinical course and a slow growth rate. The tumor is detected in young individuals (usually before they turn 40 years of age) and is 2-3 times more common in females. As a rule, it is a multifocal disease (in 60% of patients) involving one thyroid lobe, although in 50% of cases microscopic neoplastic lesions are present in the contralateral lobe. One should be also aware of the possible presence of a small, 2-10 mm focus of papillary thyroid carcinoma termed „microcarcinoma", which is asymptomatic and detected by chance in the course of histopathology of the thyroid gland resected in a patient with goiter or in serial autopsies of the thyroid (such post-mortem examinations detected 35.6% microcarcinoma foci). Approximately 50% of patients demonstrate the presence of metastases in the lymph nodes. Papillary carcinoma of the thyroid is a hormonally dependent tumor (TSH). The 5-year survival rate is approximately 95% [2, 3]. [Fig. 1,2,3,4]

3. Oncogenesis

The presently prevalent opinion states that genetic factors play an ever-increasing role in the development of neoplastic lesions. In view of the present knowledge, a prerequisite for neoplastic transformation to occur is a mutation involving two basic groups of genes - proto-oncogenes and suppressor genes, also called anti-oncogenes. Proto-oncogenes function as positive proliferation regulators. Under the effect of various external and internal factors, they may be converted into oncogenes. In turn, oncogene products may be divided into two groups of proteins, which are responsible for encoding the production of growth factors and affect the expression of surface receptors, either cytoplasmic or nuclear, thus indirectly participating in transcription inhibition or activation. Early neoplastic lesions usually involve a single cell line and appear as a consequence of a single or several serial mutations. Such mutations result in an increased capability of the cells to undergo mitotic divisions with a simultaneous decrease of their apoptotic capability as compared to the adjacent cells. Thus, a cell line develops that may give origin to for example hyperplasia of the thyroid tissue associated with neoplastic growth, since the borderline separating neoplastic transformation and hyperplastic proliferation is very thin [4,5].

In view of the high metabolism of cells undergoing division, the growth of a non-vascularized tumor is low. The clinical presentation of this growth phase is most commonly carcinoma in situ. The subsequent phase of tumor growth depends on the formation of new blood vessels (neoangiogenesis). Neoangiogenesis is a process composed of numerous interactions occurring in the paracrine and endocrine path between neoplastic cells and cells forming the vascular endothelium, connective tissue interstitium and some morphotic blood elements, such as macrophages or mastocytes. In consequence of these interactions, the microenvironment in the area surrounding the tumor changes, thus providing the neoplastic lesion with an opportunity for further uncontrollable growth and progression. A prerequisite for the initiation of angiogenic phenomena is a disturbed balance between the systems of pro- and anti-angiogenic factors. Of the identified to date proangiogenic factors (VEGF; bFGF; aFGF; PDGF; TGF-α; TGF-β; EGF; IGF-1), not all meet the three defining criteria: exerting a specific effect on the endothelium, possessing the system of specific cell receptors and inhibiting or inducing angiogenesis through changes in their levels. Some of these factors co-act with mediators secreted by other cells (e.g. macrophages - TNF) in triggering and promoting the development of neoplastic disease. In accordance with currently accepted theories, the initiation of angiogenesis occurs through hypoxia of neoplastic cells that are situated the most distally from the lumen of a blood vessel, as well as through a defect of the genetic apparatus, in consequence of which the so-called angiogenic phenotype emerges. The term denotes the condition characterized by a permanent, constitutional activation of genes that encode growth factors. An additional loss of function by suppressor genes (e.g. the p53 gene) facilitates neoangiogenesis [8,19,20]. [Figure 5]

Endocrine glands constitute typical, richly vascularized organs; the circulating blood is the basis of their normal functioning and provides a close control of the feedback systems. As early as more than 20 years ago, investigators demonstrated that an increase in thyroid vascularization in patients with hyperthyroid goiter was regulated by cytokines secreted by thyreocytes. In subsequent years (reports by Goodman), the concept was confirmed and extended by articles on the paracrine effect of connective tissue interstitial cells of the thyroid gland [17].

The regulation of this process is complex and the contributing factors include both neoplastic cells capable of producing such factors as cytokines and chemokines, as well as immunocompetent cells situated in the vicinity of tumor cells or infiltrating the tumor itself; the latter also produce cytokines, chemokines and growth factors. The interrelation of such factor production, especially in the case of chemokines, significantly intensifies angiogenesis. Chemokines, which contain the repeated sequence of glutamine-leucine-arginine, show an angiogenic activity [6-10].

4. Angiogenesis

The basic process of the formation of new blood vessels originating from the previously existing structures is the branching off of capillary vessels and budding of new vascular limbs that takes place both in fetal life and in mature organisms. The process is short-lived (approximately 5 days on the average), subject to strict regulations, and its sudden termination results from the reduction of stimulatory factors and/or a decrease of inhibitor levels. [1-9]. Angiogenesis is a pathomechanism involved in lesions developing in autoimmune diseases (rheumatoid arthritis, lupus erythematosus, hemangiomas, scleroderma, endometriosis) and in neoplastic diseases. [11-13].

A good part of publications in world literature on the role of angiogenic cytokines and epithelial growth factors in the process of tumor growth concentrate on processes occurring in the gastrointestinal tract [14-16]. Nevertheless, their presence and possible effect on the development and growth of tumors of endocrine origin have been recently recognized [17, 18].

VEGF is among relatively well-known endothelial growth factors. This specific protein is believed to play a key role in vascularization of solid tumors, including thyroid cancers. In keeping with the theory adopted by Folkman that states that tumor growth is limited by its vascularization, attempts were made at demonstrating higher VEGF expression in neoplastic tissues as compared to the population of normal cells. These studies show such an association with respect to cancers involving the stomach, colon, uterus, mammary glands and ovaries [14-16]. Also in the case of thyroid tumors, the key role in neoangiogenesis is played by VEGF, especially in view of the fact that the ability to produce and release this factor is characteristic not only of epithelial thyroid cells, but also of interstitial cells [18].

To date, infrequent reports have dealt with peripheral blood serum VEGF determinations in patients with highly differentiated thyroid cancers, what has prompted us to attempt assessing the clinical relevance of determining the level of vascular endothelial growth factor (VEGF) in patients with papillary thyroid cancers.

EGF is among the most potent stimulators of thyroid gland growth and its multiple activity is determined by its binding with specific EGF receptors. In vitro, EGF is a factor that stimulates the proliferation of follicular thyroid cells. A factor that intensifies EGF binding with receptors is thyreotropin (TSH), which - stimulating an increase in the number of EGF receptors - potentiates its activity [24,25]. In contrast to TSH, however, to reveal its mitogenic activity, EGF does not require the presence of other chemokines. [28]. Subsequent investigators have attempted to determine the importance of positive EGF receptor expression in neoplastic thyroid tissue in the clinical course of the disease. EFG levels have been compared in various types of thyroid carcinomas and the highest expression has been found to be characteristic of anaplastic and medullary thyroid cancers. Also adenomas have been demonstrated to show marked expression of EGF receptors; however, this phenomenon involved solely certain regions of the tumor. The observation may weigh in favor of the possible neoplastic transformation of tumor tissues towards malignant processes [26]. The studies of Akslen et al. provided information on the importance of EGF receptor expression in the cytoplasm of papillary thyroid cancer cells, which was closely associated with extrathyroid growth of the tumor [27].

Summing up the results of studies on the serum concentration values of selected growth factors - VEGF and EGF - in patients with papillary thyroid cancer, one should state that they both participate in the induction and progression of neoplastic processes involving the thyroid gland, most likely acting, however, at various stages of tumor development - VEGF at the stage of neoangiogenesis induction, and EGF at the stage of invasion and possible remote metastases formation. [Figure 6]. To provide a firm and unambiguous confirmation of our observations it is necessary to conduct further investigations of the angiogenic activity, demonstrating a correlation between microvessel density (MVD) in the primary and metastatic tumors, as well as the presence and expression of receptors of these chemokines on the one hand, and the clinical stage of the tumor on the other; and showing whether these growth factors indeed have a prognostic value in identifying patients with a poor prognosis and expected shorter recurrence-free survival.

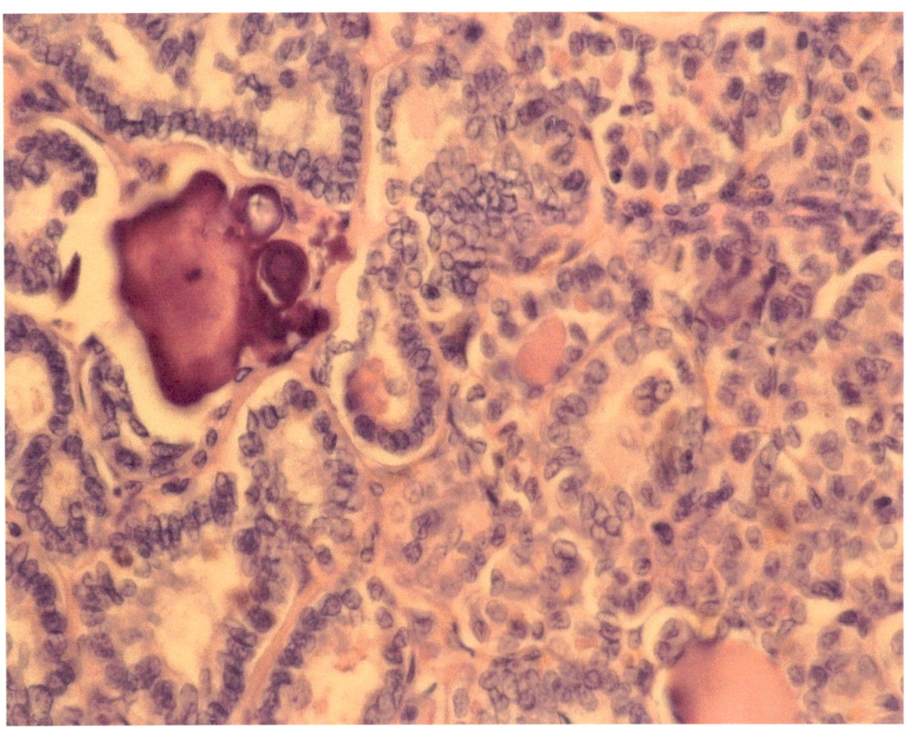

Fig. 1. Papillary thyroid cancer - psammoma body.

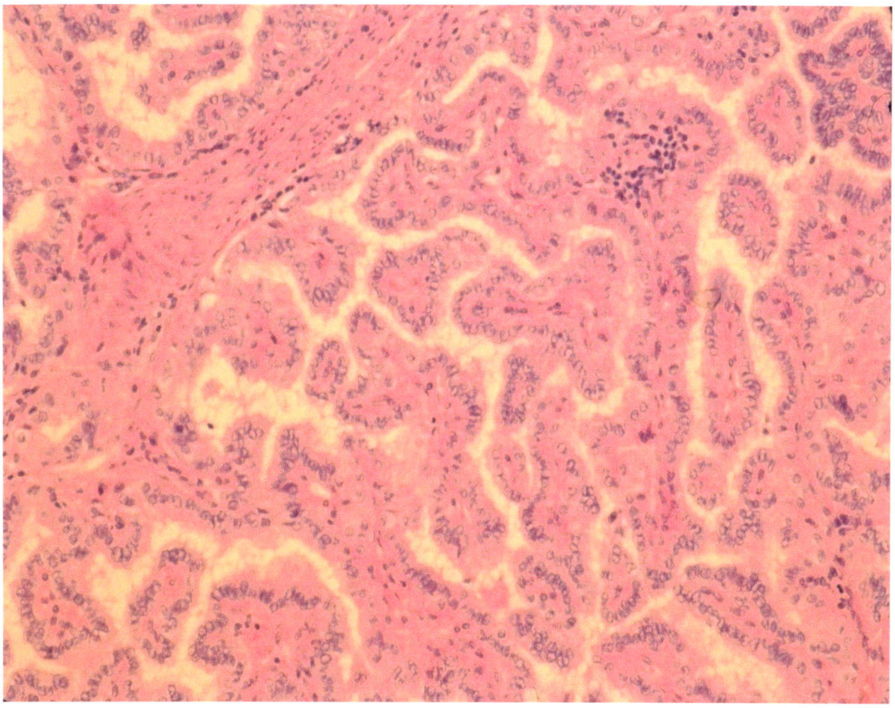

Fig. 2. Papillary thyroid cancer – a typically view

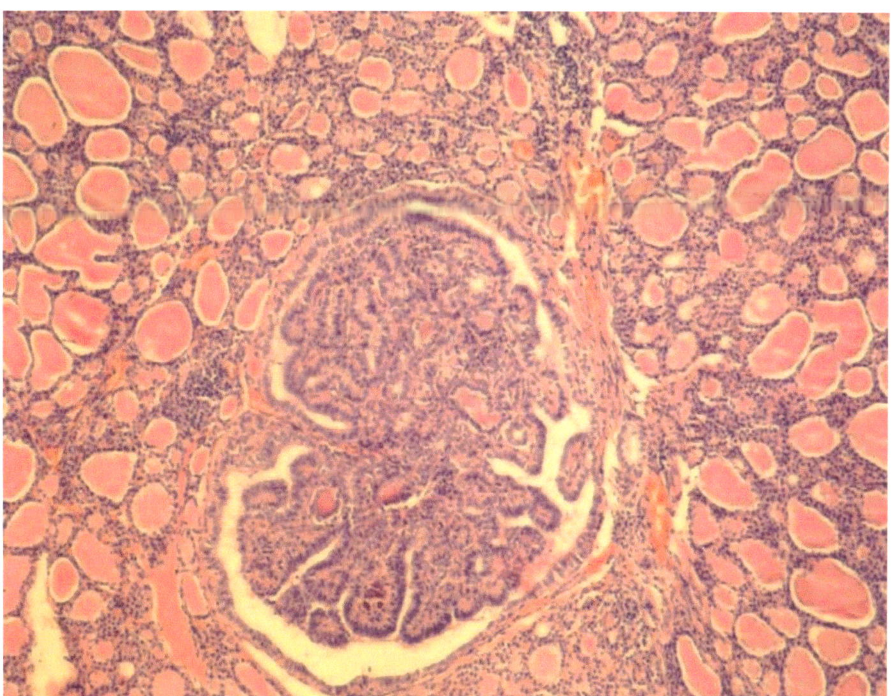

Fig. 3. Papillary thyroid cancer – a microcarcinoma variant

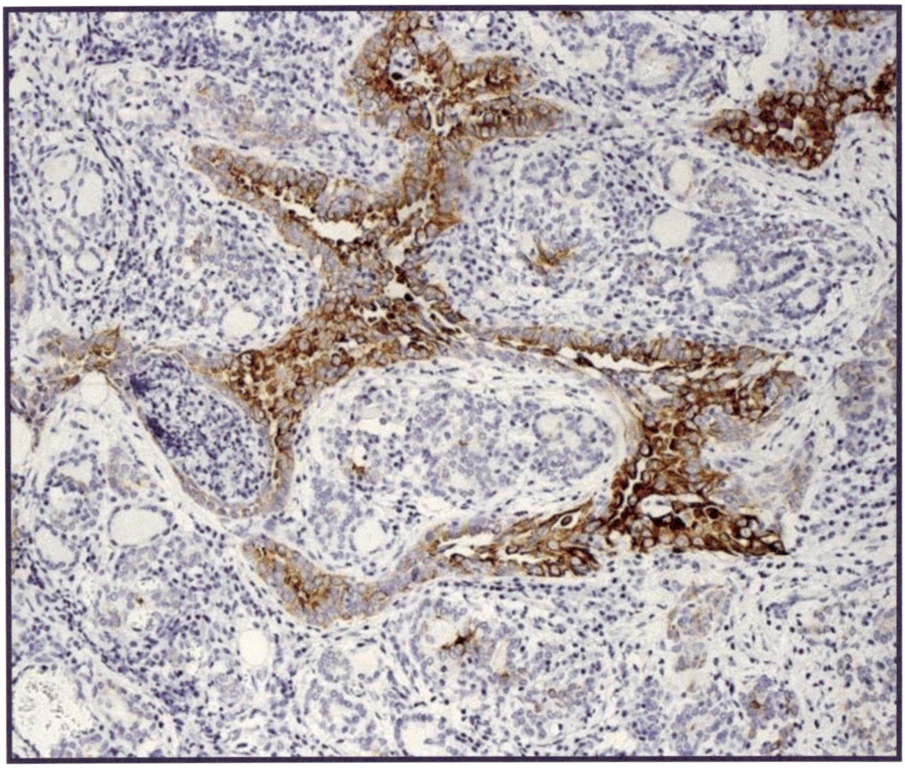

Fig. 4. Papillary thyroid cancer - high positive test of CK - 19

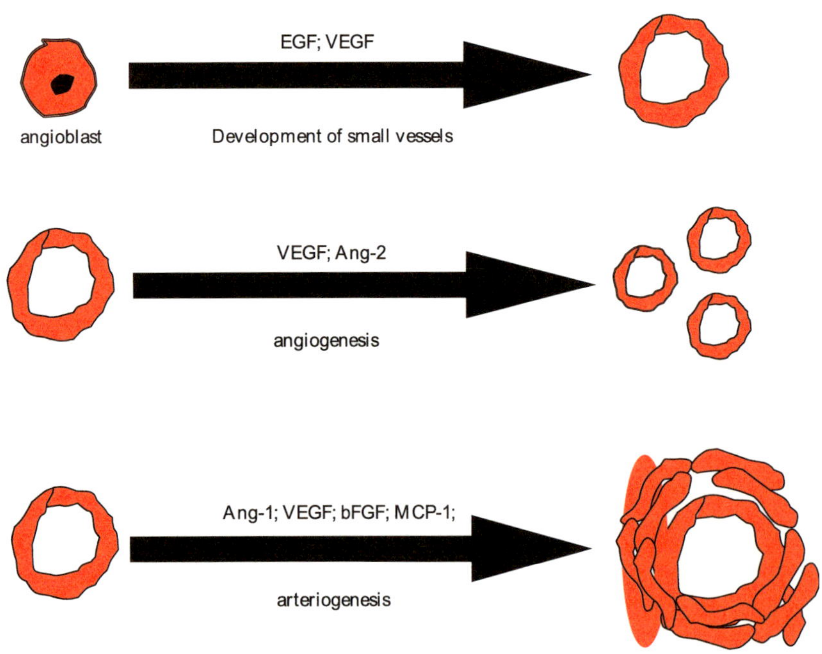

Fig. 5. Vascular growth factors and the effects of their acting.

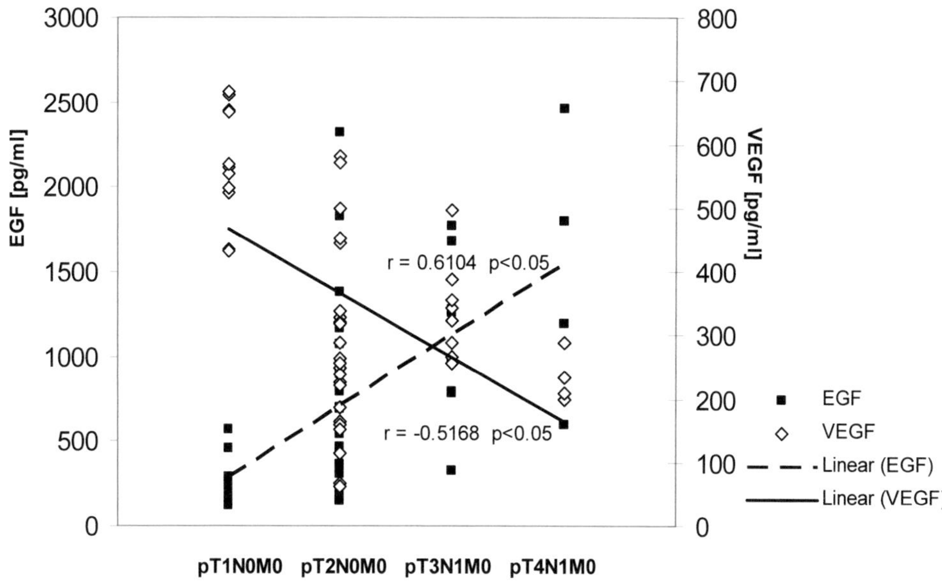

Fig. 6. Correlation between VEGF, EGF and staging of papillary thyroid cancer in pTNM classification (r = Pearson's correlation coefficient). The hypothesis of influence.

5. Keywords

Papillary thyroid cancer, vascular endothelial growth factor, epidermal growth factor, prognostic value

6. References

[1] American Cancer Society (1991) Cancer Statistics 41: 28-29.
[2] DeGroot LJ, Kaplan EL. McCormik M, Straus FH (1990) Natural history, treatment and course of papillary thyroid carcinoma. J Clin Endocrinol Metab 71: 414-424.
[3] Schindler AM, van Melle G, Evequoz B, Scazziga B (1991) Prognostic factors in papillary carcinoma of the thyroid. Cancer 68:324-330.
[4] Goretzki PE, Simon D, Dotzenrath C, Schulte KM, Röher HD (2000) *Growth Regulation of Thyroid and Thyroid Tumors in Humans.* World J Surg 24:913-922.
[5] Falk SA (1997) Thyroid disease: endocrinology, surgery, nuclear medicine and radiotherapy. Lippincott, Williams & Wilkins and Raven Publishers, Philadelphia-New York.
[6] Folkman J, Shing Y (1992) Angiogenesis. J Biol Chem 359:843-848.
[7] Yancopoulos GD, Klagsburn M, Folkman J (1998) Vasculogenesis, angiogenesis and growth factors: ephrins enter the fray at the border. Cell 93:661-664.
[8] Risau W (1997) Mechanism of angiogenesis. Nature 386:671-674.
[9] Carmeliet P (2000) Mechanism of angiogenesis and arteriogenesis. Nature Medicine 6:389-395.

[10] Balkwill F. (2003) :Chemokines biology in cancer. Seminars in Immunology 15: 49-55.

[11] Reichlin M (1998) Systemic lupus erythematosus. In: Rose NR, Mackay IR (eds.) The Autoimmune diseases. Academic Press, Philadelphia, pp 1-37.

[12] Norrby W (1997) Angiogenesis. a new aspects relating to its initiation and control. Acta Pathol Microbiol Immunol Scand 105:417-437.

[13] Eliseenko VI, Skobelkin OK, Chegin VM (1998) Microcirculation and angiogenesis during wound healing by first and second intention. Bull Experiment Biol Med 105:289-292.

[14] Maeda K, Chung YS, Ogawa Y (1996) Prognostic value of vascular endothelial growth factor expression in gastric carcinoma. Caner 77:858-863.

[15] Okada F, Rak J, St.Croix B, Lieubeau B, Kaya M, Roncari L, Shirasawa S, Sasazuki T, Kerbel RS (1998) Impact of oncogenes on tumor angiogenesis: mutant K-ras upregulation of VEGF/VPF is necessary but not sufficient for tumorigenicyity of human colorectal carcinoma cells. Proc Natl Acad Sci 95:3609-3614.

[16] Gasparini G, Toi M, Gion M, Verderio P, Dittadi R, Hanatani M, Matsubara I, Vinante O, Bonoldi E, Boracchi P, Gatti C, Suzuki H, Tominaga T (1997) Prognostic significance of vascular endothelial growth factor protein in node-negativ breast carcinoma. J Natl Cancer Inst 89:139-147.

[17] Goodman AL, Rone JD (1987) Thyroid angiogenesis: endotheliotropic chemoattractant activity from rat thyroid cell in culture. Endocrinology 121:2131-2140.

[18] Turner HE, Harris AL, Melmed SH, Wass JAH (2003) Angiogenesis in endocrine tumors. Endocrine Rev 24:600-632.

[19] Rak J, Mrtsuhashi Y, Bayko L, Filmus J, Sasazuki T, Kerbel RS (1995) Mutant ras oncogenes upregulate VEGF/VPF expression: implications for inducion or inhibition of tumor angiogenesis. Cancer Res 55:4575-4580.

[20] Kerbel RS, Vilona-Petit A, Okada F, Rak J (1998) Establishing a link between oncogenes and tumor angiogenesis. Molecular Medicine 4:286-295.

[21] Lin SY, Wang YY, Sheu WH (2003) Preoperative plasma concentrations of vascular endothelial growth factor and matrix metalloproteinase 9 are associated with stage progression in papillary thyroid cancer. Clin Endocrinol 58:513-518.

[22] Lennard CM, Patel A, Wilson J, Reinhardt B, Tuman C, Fenton C, Blair E, Francis GL, Tuttle RM (2001) Intensity of vascular endothelial growth factor expression associated with increased risk of recurrence and decreased disease-free survival in papillary thyroid cancer. Surgery 129:552-558.

[23] Huang SM, Lee JC, Wu TJ, Chow NH (2001) Clinical revelance of vascular endothelial growth factor for thyroid neoplasms. World J Surg 25:302-306.

[24] Westermark K, Westermark B (1982) Mitogenic effect of epidermal growth factor on sheep thyroid cells in culture. Exp Cell Res 138:47-55.

[25] Westermark K, Karlsson A, Westermark B (1985) Thyrotropin modulates EGF receptor functionin porcine thyroid follicle cells. Mol Cell Endocrinol 40:17-23.

[26] Masuda H, Sugenoya A, Kobayashi S, Kasuga Y, Iida F (1988) Epidermal growth factor receptor on human thyroid neoplasm. World J Surg 12:616-622.

[27] Alslen LA, Myking AO, Salvesen H, Varhaug JE (1993) Prognostic impact of EGF-receptor in papillary thyroid carcinoma. Br J Cancer 68:808-812.

[28] Westermark K, Karlsson FA, Westermark B (1983) Epidermal growth factor modulates thyroid growth and function in culture. Endocrinology 112:1680-1686.

7

Immune Profile and Signal Transduction of T-Cell Receptor in Autoimmune Thyroid Diseases

Adriano Namo Cury
Endocrinology and Metabolism Unit of Santa Casa São Paulo, São Paulo
Brazil

1. Introduction

Autoimmune thyroiditis is of great importance because of its prevalence in global population and represents an organ-specific immune dysfunction whose pathophysiological stages have not yet been fully elucidated. It is well accepted that, as in other autoimmune diseases, there is loss of tolerance to auto-antigens (such as thyroperoxidase or thyroglobulin) with subsequent abnormal lymphocyte activation fostering aggression to thyroid tissue.

From the autoimmune dysfunction, especially in Hashimoto's thyroiditis (HT), the thyrocyte may undergo apoptosis by the FAS-mediated in CD4 + and CD8 + mechanism, or by downregulation of anti-apoptotic protein expression such as Bcl-2 (Mitsiades, Poulaki et al., 1998; Fountoulakis, Vartholomatos et al., 2008). In the HT, lymphocytic infiltrate is intense with formation of germinal centers and destruction of thyroid follicles by chronic inflammation through the natural killer cells (NK) and cytotoxicity induced by auto-antibodies.

In Hashimoto's thyroiditis, chronic inflammation and apoptosis are accepted as a mechanism of the disease and resultant hypothyroidism. It is noteworthy that presence of lymphocytic infiltrate alone does not necessarily induce hypothyroidism (Martin, Colonel et al., 2004) but induces immune dysfunction of T cells response due to genetic and environmental predisposition in different populations and ethnic groups.

T cell and B cell immune dysfunction with production of autoantibodies, cytotoxic cell death, in addition to the previously mentioned apoptosis is the classical model of thyrocytes and thyroid follicle destruction. But recently described as non-classic mechanism and not related to cell death, but to the chronic inflammatory process by inhibiting the thyroid function mediated by inflammatory cytokines TNF-α and INF-γ based upon T cell dysfunction, even without a lymphocytic infiltrate, but by exposure *per se* to inflammatory cytokines (Caturegli, Hejazi et al., 2000; Kimura, Kimura et al., 2005).

Differently, within the group of autoimmune thyroid diseases, Graves' disease (GD) occurs in a unique situation in autoimmunity, with dysfunction in T and B cells, however producing an autoantibody IgG, with great affinity to specific regions of the TSH (TSH-R) receptor that determines hyperfunction, hypertrophy of the thyroid follicle, abnormal dynamics of activation, or even blockade of TSH-R and hyperthyroidism itself (Hadj-Kacem, Rebuffat et al., 2009). Production of TRAb stimulator and sometimes blocker is an expression of the break of tolerance to TSH R specific epitopes with biological effect similar to TSH, yet with longer lasting and slower signaling to thyrocytes.

Exposure of TSH-R subunit-A seems to be responsible for generating the TRAb stimulator, which generates an atypical biological signal to the thyroid cells which respond with activation of the intracellular machinery, hypertrophy, and hypersecretion (Rapoport and McLachlan 2007). In GD the inflammatory infiltrate is less intense when compared to HT, and the phenomenon of apoptosis is less pronounced due to probable protection by soluble FAS (sFas), interfering with the classic mechanism of apoptosis FAS-FASL (Feldkamp, Pascher et al., 2001; Fountoulakis, Vartholomatos et al., 2008) or by upregulation of anti-apoptotic proteins in thyrocytes such as Bcl-2, Bcl-xL and cFLIP (Stassi, Di Liberto et al., 2000).

Comprehension of cell phenotype, dynamics of lymphocyte activation in the break of immune tolerance and its correlation with immunoregulator genes is mandatory to understand the etiology and development mechanism of autoimmune thyroid diseases. Moreover, for the attempt to elucidate the pathways of cellular and humoral dysfunctions that determine the route leading to HT or GD.

2. Immunity and T cells

2.1 Inflammatory response in autoimmune thyroid diseases

Immune behavior of autoimmune thyroid diseases lies in the characterization of the concept of breaking the mechanism of tolerance to self antigens, activation and differentiation of cell clones in charge (T-cell subtypes) of the amplification and execution of inflammatory response in thyroid tissue and dynamics of lymphocyte receptors in HT or GD. Differentiation and amplification of the inflammatory response in different types of T cells plays an essential role in the pathogenesis of the disease.

The understanding of cell phenotype, dynamics of lymphocytes activation in the break of immune tolerance and its correlation with immunoregulator genes is mandatory for the etiology and development mechanism of autoimmune thyroid diseases. Or even for the attempt to elucidate the pathways of cellular and humoral dysfunctions that rule the path leading to HT or GD.

The CD4 + T helper lymphocytes (Th) can be classified into at least three subtypes, Th1, Th2 and Th17 in accordance with a profile of cytokine production (Abbas, Murphy et al., 1996; Mosmann and Sad 1996). In HT the Th1 cell response prevails with predominant production of IFN-γ, IL-2 and TNF-β (Fisfalen, Palmer et al., 1997; Fisfalen, Soltani et al., 1997; Watanabe, Yamamoto et al., 2002). The Th2 humoral response pertains to GD with production of cytokines IL-4, IL-5, IL-6, IL-10 and IL-13 and suppression of INF-γ (Yano, Sone et al., 1995; Abbas Murphy et al., 1996; Fisfalen, Palmer et al., 1997; Fisfalen, Soltani et al., 1997).

Th17 lymphocytes were recently described and specific studies on thyroid autoimmune diseases are scarce. T cells that differentiate to Th17 subtypes secrete IL-17, IL-17F, IL-21 and IL-22 (Wilson, Boniface et al., 2007) playing an important role in chronic inflammatory diseases such as asthma (Traves and Donnelly 2008) or systemic lupus erythematosus (Garrett-Sinha, John et al., 2008). IL-17 has potent proinflammatory action of chemotaxis, with chemokine synthesis and stimulus of cell proliferation (Weaver, Hatton et al., 2007).

Proportion of Th17 lymphocytes in patients with GD was first described by Nanba *et. al.*, whose main finding was a higher rate of Th17, on the peripheral blood of patients with GD without treatment with anti-thyroid drugs when compared to patients with GD in remission (Nanba, Watanabe et al., 2009). Study of the profile of Th17 lymphocytes in Hashimoto's thyroiditis according to Figueroa-Vera *et al.*, (Figueroa-Vega, Alfonso-Perez et al., 2010) discloses a higher expression of the RORC2 gene responsible for differentiation of the Th17 phenotype, in addition to the sheer number of Th17 lymphocytes in peripheral blood and thyroid tissue of patients with HT, however without significant results in those with GD.

2.2 Loss of tolerance and natural regulatory T cells

Autoimmunity occurs mainly by loss of tolerance to auto-antigens from the perpetuation of autoreactive T cells and pathogenic for their cellular targets. Didactically, it can be understood that the stages of loss of tolerance occur in two moments: (1) failure of central tolerance and (2) peripheral. Initially, the correct reading of non-auto-antigens and no formation of autoreactive cells is known as clonal selection theory or negative selection when autoreactive lymphocytes are deleted at the initial stages of cell differentiation in the thymus (Burnet 1959). Evasion of cell clones from the negative central selection, auto-reactive lymphocytes to the periphery may or may not be activated and trigger the process of autoimmune disease, however according to the genetic and environmental interaction. There is a break in the state of anergy or antigenic ignorance, with clonal activation and expansion that will then initiate the autoimmune and inflammatory process (Green, Droin et al., 2003).

This cellular mechanism is known as intrinsic cellular mechanism of peripheral tolerance (Schwartz 2005). The extrinsic cellular mechanism of tolerance is carried out by regulatory T cells CD4 + CD25 + natural (Treg) that exist because of the expression of Forkhead Box Protein 3 (Foxp3), Treg are responsible for suppression of immune response of auto-reactive clones (Sakaguchi, Yamaguchi et al., 2008) and control amplification of the inflammatory response. Failure in negative central and peripheral selection promotes clonal expansion with differentiation of autoreactive cell subtypes, which according to the genetic and environmental triggers differentiate into T cells to produce inflammatory cytokines inducing inflammation and cell destruction.

It is believed that failure of the negative selection process could not per *se* trigger autoimmunity. Perpetuation of pathogenic autoreactive cells associated with a lesser expression and differentiation of Tregs would be another condition for autoimmunity development. It was shown that CD4+ CD25 + cells may experimentally prevent development of autoimmune thyroiditis (Gangi, Vasu et al., 2005; Vergini, Li et al., 2005). As the proportion and function of Tregs seems altered in the ATD when analyzing peripheral and cells of the thyroid ambient itself without the ability to downmodulate the autoimmune response in the thyroid environment (Marazuela, Garcia-Lopez et al., 2006), or even suffer increased apoptosis in the thyroid environment (Nakano, Watanabe et al., 2007) a significant event considering that regulatory action of Treg cells modulates and inhibits inflammatory immune response Th1, Th2 and Th17.

Therefore, the evasion of autoreactive cells, the reduced presence of Tregs, the non- control of inflammatory response, in the genetic context and environmental factor, the predominance of phenotypes Th1, Th2 or even Th17 characterizes autoimmune thyroid disease. Hashimoto's thyroiditis with typical Th1 response and cell infiltrate by thyroid tissue and thyrocyte apoptosis.

In GD, product of a more humoral response Th2, lesser lymphocytic infiltrate and specific failures for TSHR that generate, presumably the only autoimmune condition that promotes hyperplasia, with a lesser degree of apoptosis and IgG by affinity for THSR. The Th17 response might possibly be involved in HT or GD. However studies encompass a limited number of patients and primarily use peripheral blood to isolate lymphocytes, while study of lymphocytes from the thyroid is scarce, since indications for surgery for patients with GD or HT are less frequent nowadays.

3. Immunoregulator genes

The autoimmune thyroid diseases (ATD), such as Hashimoto's thyroiditis and Graves' disease are found in the general population and have an estimated prevalence of 5% (Ban, Davies et al., 2003). Pathogenesis of ATD especially that of GD is brought about by complex interaction between environmental and genetic factors. Genetics of predisposition for ATD involve HLA (human leukocyte antigen) system genes and specific genes that affect any step of the immune response regulation, i.e. activation and suppression of T cells and consequent modulation of B-cells.

Besides genes of the MHC class II system such as HLA-DR3 and DQA1 * 0501 on chromosome 6p21 (Yanagawa, Mangklabruks et al., 1993; Zamani, Spaepen et al., 2000; Maciel, Rodrigues et al., 2001), on chromosome 2q33, we found the *loci* of genes involved in the regulation of T lymphocytes: CD28, CTLA4 and ICOS in which, specifically polymorphisms of the cytotoxic T lymphocyte antigen-4 (CTLA-4) are associated to various autoimmune diseases (Chistiakov and Turakulov 2003; Vaidya and Pearce 2004).

Allelic variants of the CTLA-4 gene with potential effect on functional modulation of the T cell were shown as single-nucleotide polymorphism (SNP) + 49 A> G in exon 1, which seems to modify both the structure and protein expression of CTLA-4 [7]. In 2003, Ueda *et al.,* identified the SNP +6230 G> A in the stop codon of gene CTLA-4 (CT60) associating it to higher risk for GD, HT and type 1 diabetes (DM1) due to expression of different isoforms of mRNA gene CTLA-4 (Ueda, Howson et al., 2003).

In case-control studies during the last decade, polymorphism +49 A> G of CTLA4 gene exon 1 was associated with autoimmune diseases, such as GD, DM1, HT, rheumatoid arthritis, autoimmune Addison's disease, multiple sclerosis (Yanagawa, Hidaka et al., 1995; Nistico, Buzzetti et al., 1996; Kotsa, Watson et al., 1997; Yanagawa, Taniyama et al., 1997; Awata, Kurihara et al., 1998; Fukazawa, Yanagawa et al., 1999; Heward, Allahabadia et al., 1999; Vaidya, Imrie et al., 2000; Ueda, Howson et al., 2003; Blomhoff, Lie et al., 2004; Young-Min and Vaidya 2004; Kavvoura, Akamizu et al., 2007). and in familial studies was associated with GD in Caucasian, Japanese, Chinese and Korean populations (Heward, Allahabadia et al., 1999; Vaidya, Imrie et al., 1999).

Proteins CD28 and CTLA4 are costimulatory molecules found on the surface of T cells that bind to the family of B7 receptors expressed on antigen presenting cells (APC) (Reiser and Stadecker 1996). Immune response relies on the generation of two signals: the first, from the interaction of antigenic peptides with receptors on T cells in the context of MHC and the second signal (costimulatory) that activates, enhances and promotes T cell proliferation by production of cytokines (such as IL-2), where complex CD28/B7 functions as a positive regulator of T cells, and the CTLA4/B7 expressed exclusively in activated T lymphocytes, provides an inhibitory signal, required to limit proliferation of T cells and regulates the autoimmune response (Oosterwegel, Greenwald et al., 1999; Sharpe and Abbas 2006).

4. Polymorphisms, functional impact on the T cell and transduction of TCR

The polymorphism +49 A> G (rs231775) of gene CTLA-4, which promotes the exchange of amino acid threonine for alanine at position 17, has emerged as the natural candidate, among polymorphisms of CTLA-4 gene, because of the ability to promote functional changes of protein CTLA- 4. Kouki *et al.*, (Kouki, Sawai et al., 2000) showed a higher frequency of genotype GG or AG at position 49 of the CTLA-4 gene in GD patients, and lesser control over proliferation and clonal expansion of T cells. Whereas Maurer *et al (Maurer, Loserth et al., 2002)* found differences in the pool of intracellular CTLA-4 protein, prompting imbalance in the expression and competition between CTLA-4 and CD28 on the surface of T cells, possibly modifying the suppression of T cells and generating larger quantities of inflammatory cytokines.

The CT60 polymorphism (rs30807243) seems to determine a distinct expression of mRNA isoforms through alternative splicing, with a lesser expression of soluble CTLA-4 (sCTLA-4) in relation to the total length isoform of CTLA-4 (*fl*CTLA-4) (Ueda, Howson et al., 2003). The correlation between immune-cell genotype and phenotype was demonstrated by presence of susceptibility allele G or allele A of protection, to specific subtypes of T cells in healthy controls, and the quantitative variations of the type CD4 + CD25 + cells called regulatory T cells (Treg) (Atabani, Thio et al., 2005).

Other studies have shown an association between the SNP at exon 2 of CTLA-4 gene in mice, and a new variant of the protein called ligand independent of CTLA-4 (liCTLA-4) (Wicker, Chamberlain et al., 2004), that also has a significant inhibitor function on T cell response when binding and dephosphorilating the T cell receptor (TCR).

Expression of the isoform liCTLA-4 seems to be greater in regulatory and memory T cells (Vijayakrishnan, Slavik et al., 2004), a possible association between the gene CTLA-4 (its isoforms) and immune response after antigen presentation by APC and T cell activation as from the T cell receptor. As such, genetic variations in the CTLA-4 gene region play an important role in T cell signaling and therefore in its function and proliferation of T cells. Different genotypes may determine different phenotypes and probable predisposition to autoimmunity by loss of negative selection mechanisms (central and peripheral immune system dysfunction) and a distinct pattern of CD4 + T cells.

The possibility of analyzing the actions of protein CTLA-4 (and its isoforms) and its correlation with the type of activated T cell (either the memory/effector or naive cell) as well as the profile of tyrosine residues phosphorylation and activity of protein kinases in the intracellular environment (Maier, Anderson et al., 2007) may explain how the genetic profile influences immune response and promotes autoimmune thyroid disease for different clinical or subclinical poles as in HT and GD.

The expression of surface molecules, phenotype, discloses the history of antigenic exposure (Appay, Dunbar et al., 2002) or indicates the functional capacity of each cell subtype (Rufer, Zippelius et al., 2003). Naive or memory / effector cells are pointed out by presence or absence of CD45RA, naive cells are mainly CD4 $^{+}$ CCR7 $^{+}$ CD45RA^{high}, memory cells CD4^{+} CCR7 $^{+}$ CD45RA^{low} and effector cells CD4 $^{+}$ CCR7^{-}CD45RA^{low} (Amyes, McMichael et al., 2005).

During the antigen presentation process, costimulation and clonal expansion of the different populations of T lymphocytes, memory, effector or naive cells use the same pathway on the cell surface by means of the TCR/CD3 complex (Farber 2000), however with different properties in activation of the immune response. Naive cells are hyper-responsive to antigenic and non- antigenic stimuli, with increased susceptibility to apoptosis, while memory cells activated by slower kinetics, and are hyporesponsive to stimulation of the TCR and less susceptible to apoptosis (Hussain, Anderson et al., 2002).

In all T cell lines and their cellular clones, the same mechanism of signal transduction linked to the TCR was identified (Germain and Stefanova 1999), exhibiting phosphorylation of tyrosine residues in the subunits linked to the TCR/CD3 (ζ, ε, δ, γ) by the family proteins tyrosine kinase p56 lck (Iwashima, Irving et al., 1994).

Phosphorylation of the CD3ζ subunit brings about activation and recruitment of other tyrosine kinases such as ZAP-70 that phosphorylate multiple molecules like SLP-76 (Bubeck Wardenburg, Fu et al., 1996) and ligand for activation of the T cell (LAT) (Zhang, Sloan-Lancaster et al., 1998) that associated with Grb2 and GADS (Liu, Fang et al., 1999) activate according to messengers Ras/Erk MAP kinases and activation or suppression of intracytoplasmic events, such as activation of enzymes, modulation of transcription genes, synthesis of inflammatory cytokines, mobilization of intracellular calcium or induction of cell proliferation or cell apoptosis (Wange and Samelson 1996) (figure 1).

Therefore, the antigen-specific response can be well characterized by specific intracellular markers of phosphorylation and development of antibodies for specific epitopes of cytoplasmic proteins (Rosette, Werlen et al., 2001). The phenotypic correlation of T cell subtypes and pattern of TCR/CD3ζ phosphorylation with allelic variants of CTLA-4 (CT60 SNP) gene was recently demonstrated by Maier *et al.*,.(Maier, Anderson et al., 2007), with a different signaling pattern of CD4 + T cells according to presence of allele G.

Polymorphism (rs2476601) of gene PTPN22 (protein tyrosine phosphatase nonreceptor 22) on chromosome 1p13 responsible for the expression of protein tyrosine-specific phosphatase (LYP), with a suppressive and regulatory function of post- TCR phosphorylation are associated with autoimmune diseases such as GD, DM1 and to polyglandular autoimmune conditions (Bottini, Musumeci et al., 2004; Velaga, Wilson et al., 2004; Skorka, Bednarczuk et al., 2005; Dultz, Matheis et al., 2009). The exchange of nucleotide C by T at position 1858

(C1859T) causes at codon 620, the exchange of amino acid arginine by tryptophan and possible changes in signaling and dephosphorylation post- TCR of family kinases through protein LYP (LYP*W620) (Bottini, Musumeci et al., 2004).

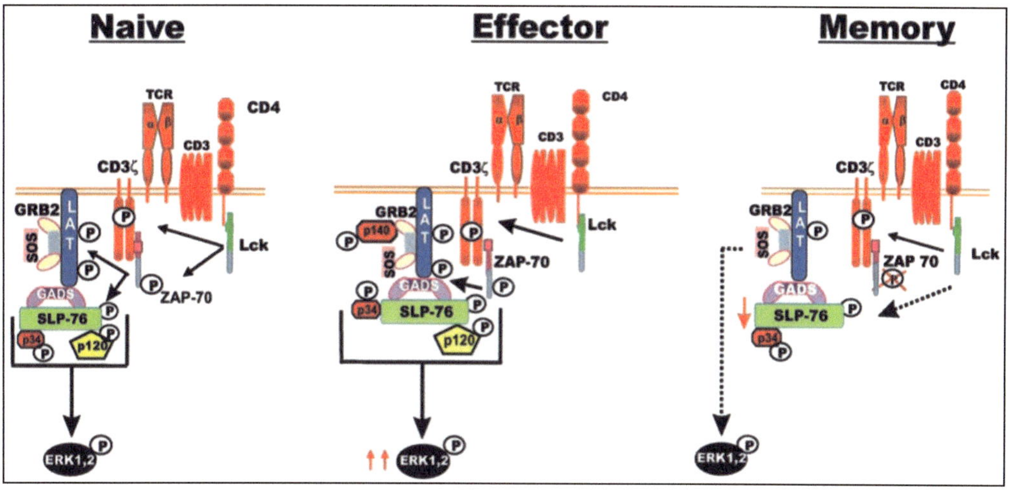

Fig. 1. Representation of T/CD3 cell receptor and signaling pathways and phosphorylation of effector molecules according to the subtype of T lymphocytes (Hussain *et al.*, 2002).

The main function of LYP protein would be to downregulate T cells through TCR signaling, by direct effect on dephosphorylation of the protein kinases Lck and Fyn, from complex TCRζ/CD3 and ZAP70 protein among others (Figure 2) (Cloutier and Veillette 1999; Gjorloff-Wingren, Saxena et al., 1999; Wu, Katrekar et al., 2006). It is noteworthy that, according to the genotype of PTPN22 and the two alleles of LYP (LYP * W620 or LYP * R620), a distinct TCR signaling takes place (Vang, Congia et al., 2005).

The LYP * W620 of "predisposition" (CT or TT genotype of PTPN22) leads to a gain of function, proteins Lck dephosphorylation, TCRζ much more efficiently than LYP * R620 (CC genotype of PTPN22), with less mobilization of intracellular calcium or transactivation of the IL-2 gene (Vang, Congia et al., 2005). That is, predisposition alleles (LYP * W620) activate phosphatases leading to suppression of TCR better than CC homozygotes (LYP * R620 / * R620 LYP), possibly by binding to a larger number of intracellular proteins in TCR signaling than LYP * R620 (Vang, Miletic et al., 2007).

As such LYP * W620 shows gain of function based upon the allelic variation of gene PTPN22 C1859T and possibly predisposes to autoimmune diseases by suppressing the TCR signaling in a much more potent way during thymic development, resulting in loss of negative selection and survival of a greater number of self-reactive cells (Vang, Miletic et al., 2007). Whether they can or not also jeopardize selection of T cells CD4 + CD25 + (Treg), if lineages of T cells are committed in accordance to expression of protein LYP, nevertheless remain scarcely known.

The ATD are a group of autoimmune diseases of poorly understood pathophysiology considering the determinant type of inflammatory response (Th1 or Th2) in the target organ, inducing apoptosis or hyperstimulation and a heterogeneous clinical condition. Thus, different cell phenotypes and immune response may take place when patients with ATD are compared to the population with no autoimmune diseases. There are few studies of autoimmune diseases that have studied the pattern of intracellular signaling of T lymphocytes and possible dysfunctions in T cell activation and immune response, except in rheumatic diseases such as systemic lupus erythematosus (Pang, Setoyama et al., 2002).

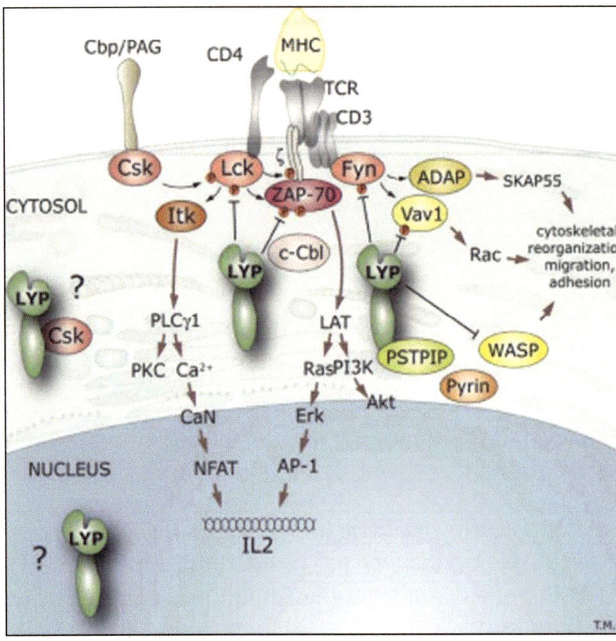

Fig. 2. Possible *loci* of action of protein LYP in signaling of T cell receptor (Vang *et al.*, 2007)

5. Conclusions

Therefore, the main conclusions of this chapter, that is to say correlation of CT60 polymorphism +49 A> G and of the PTPN22 gene with differences in T cell subtypes and intracellular signaling in memory and naive T cells has been established for patients with ATD. But the transduction o TCR activation need to be elucidated in GD a HT. Comparison of immunophenotyping and phosphorylation of TCR, cells in the periphery and of the thyroid environment may answer some questions about genetic profile and predominant phenotype in HT and GD.

Study of CD4 + cell subtypes has extended their association with other thyroid diseases are important, such as the association of Treg and aggressiveness of papillary thyroid carcinoma (French, Weber et al., 2010) was recently published, involving ATD in a different way and impact. Considering that frequency and existence of CD4+CD25+ has already been associated to a worse prognosis in breast adenocarcinoma and lymphomas (Carreras, Lopez-Guillermo et al., 2006; Gobert, Treilleux et al., 2009).

Therefore, study of the microenvironment as well as dynamics of TCR activation and association with specific genotypes might also contribute to a better association between clinical endocrinology and the main genetic and biochemical markers of autoimmune thyroid diseases. As well as the actual evolution of subclinical and clinical phases, therapeutic response in GD and new predictors of remission or relapse, or even the varying presentation of HT, duration of progression to hypothyroidism, and variations on antibodies and different epitopes, glandular volume and texture at ultrasound as well as association with autoimmune polyglandular syndrome or frequency in different ethnic groups.

6. References

Abbas, A. K., K. M. Murphy, et al., (1996). "Functional diversity of helper T lymphocytes." Nature 383(6603): 787-793.

Amyes, E., A. J. McMichael, et al., (2005). "Human CD4+ T cells are predominantly distributed among six phenotypically and functionally distinct subsets." J Immunol 175(9): 5765-5773.

Appay, V., P. R. Dunbar, et al., (2002). "Memory CD8+ T cells vary in differentiation phenotype in different persistent virus infections." Nat Med 8(4): 379-385.

Atabani, S. F., C. L. Thio, et al., (2005). "Association of CTLA4 polymorphism with regulatory T cell frequency." Eur J Immunol 35(7): 2157-2162.

Awata, T., S. Kurihara, et al., (1998). "Association of CTLA-4 gene A-G polymorphism (IDDM12 locus) with acute-onset and insulin-depleted IDDM as well as autoimmune thyroid disease (Graves' disease and Hashimoto's thyroiditis) in the Japanese population." Diabetes 47(1): 128-129.

Ban, Y., T. F. Davies, et al., (2003). "Analysis of the CTLA-4, CD28, and inducible costimulator (ICOS) genes in autoimmune thyroid disease." Genes Immun 4(8): 586-593.

Blomhoff, A., B. A. Lie, et al., (2004). "Polymorphisms in the cytotoxic T lymphocyte antigen-4 gene region confer susceptibility to Addison's disease." J Clin Endocrinol Metab 89(7): 3474-3476.

Bottini, N., L. Musumeci, et al., (2004). "A functional variant of lymphoid tyrosine phosphatase is associated with type I diabetes." Nat Genet 36(4): 337-338.

Bubeck Wardenburg, J., C. Fu, et al., (1996). "Phosphorylation of SLP-76 by the ZAP-70 protein-tyrosine kinase is required for T-cell receptor function." J Biol Chem 271(33): 19641-19644.

Burnet, M. (1959). "Auto-immune disease. I. Modern immunological concepts." British medical journal 2(5153): 645-650.

Carreras, J., A. Lopez-Guillermo, et al., (2006). "High numbers of tumor-infiltrating FOXP3-positive regulatory T cells are associated with improved overall survival in follicular lymphoma." Blood 108(9): 2957-2964.

Caturegli, P., M. Hejazi, et al., (2000). "Hypothyroidism in transgenic mice expressing IFN-gamma in the thyroid." Proceedings of the National Academy of Sciences of the United States of America 97(4): 1719-1724.

Chistiakov, D. A. and R. I. Turakulov (2003). "CTLA-4 and its role in autoimmune thyroid disease." J Mol Endocrinol 31(1): 21-36.

Cloutier, J. F. and A. Veillette (1999). "Cooperative inhibition of T-cell antigen receptor signaling by a complex between a kinase and a phosphatase." J Exp Med 189(1): 111-121.

Dultz, G., N. Matheis, et al., (2009). "The protein tyrosine phosphatase non-receptor type 22 C1858T polymorphism is a joint susceptibility locus for immunthyroiditis and autoimmune diabetes." Thyroid 19(2): 143-148.

Farber, D. L. (2000). "T cell memory: heterogeneity and mechanisms." Clin Immunol 95(3): 173-181.

Feldkamp, J., E. Pascher, et al., (2001). "Soluble Fas is increased in hyperthyroidism independent of the underlying thyroid disease." The Journal of clinical endocrinology and metabolism 86(9): 4250-4253.

Figueroa-Vega, N., M. Alfonso-Perez, et al., (2010). "Increased circulating pro-inflammatory cytokines and Th17 lymphocytes in Hashimoto's thyroiditis." The Journal of clinical endocrinology and metabolism 95(2): 953-962.

Fisfalen, M. E., E. M. Palmer, et al., (1997). "Thyrotropin-receptor and thyroid peroxidase-specific T cell clones and their cytokine profile in autoimmune thyroid disease." The Journal of clinical endocrinology and metabolism 82(11): 3655-3663.

Fisfalen, M. E., K. Soltani, et al., (1997). "Evaluating the role of Th0 and Th1 clones in autoimmune thyroid disease by use of Hu-SCID chimeras." Clinical immunology and immunopathology 85(3): 253-264.

Fountoulakis, S., G. Vartholomatos, et al., (2008). "Differential expression of Fas system apoptotic molecules in peripheral lymphocytes from patients with Graves' disease and Hashimoto's thyroiditis." European journal of endocrinology / European Federation of Endocrine Societies 158(6): 853-859.

French, J. D., Z. J. Weber, et al., (2010). "Tumor-associated lymphocytes and increased FoxP3+ regulatory T cell frequency correlate with more aggressive papillary thyroid cancer." The Journal of clinical endocrinology and metabolism 95(5): 2325-2333.

Fukazawa, T., T. Yanagawa, et al., (1999). "CTLA-4 gene polymorphism may modulate disease in Japanese multiple sclerosis patients." J Neurol Sci 171(1): 49-55.

Gangi, E., C. Vasu, et al., (2005). "IL-10-producing CD4+CD25+ regulatory T cells play a critical role in granulocyte-macrophage colony-stimulating factor-induced suppression of experimental autoimmune thyroiditis." Journal of immunology 174(11): 7006-7013.

Garrett-Sinha, L. A., S. John, et al., (2008). "IL-17 and the Th17 lineage in systemic lupus erythematosus." Current opinion in rheumatology 20(5): 519-525.

Germain, R. N. and I. Stefanova (1999). "The dynamics of T cell receptor signaling: complex orchestration and the key roles of tempo and cooperation." Annu Rev Immunol 17: 467-522.

Gjorloff-Wingren, A., M. Saxena, et al., (1999). "Characterization of TCR-induced receptor-proximal signaling events negatively regulated by the protein tyrosine phosphatase PEP." Eur J Immunol 29(12): 3845-3854.

Gobert, M., I. Treilleux, et al., (2009). "Regulatory T cells recruited through CCL22/CCR4 are selectively activated in lymphoid infiltrates surrounding primary breast tumors and lead to an adverse clinical outcome." Cancer research 69(5): 2000-2009.

Green, D. R., N. Droin, et al., (2003). "Activation-induced cell death in T cells." Immunological reviews 193: 70-81.

Hadj-Kacem, H., S. Rebuffat, et al., (2009). "Autoimmune thyroid diseases: genetic susceptibility of thyroid-specific genes and thyroid autoantigens contributions." International journal of immunogenetics 36(2): 85-96.

Heward, J. M., A. Allahabadia, et al., (1999). "The development of Graves' disease and the CTLA-4 gene on chromosome 2q33." J Clin Endocrinol Metab 84(7): 2398-2401.

Hussain, S. F., C. F. Anderson, et al., (2002). "Differential SLP-76 expression and TCR-mediated signaling in effector and memory CD4 T cells." J Immunol 168(4): 1557-1565.

Iwashima, M., B. A. Irving, et al., (1994). "Sequential interactions of the TCR with two distinct cytoplasmic tyrosine kinases." Science 263(5150): 1136-1139.

Kavvoura, F. K., T. Akamizu, et al., (2007). "Cytotoxic T-lymphocyte associated antigen 4 gene polymorphisms and autoimmune thyroid disease: a meta-analysis." J Clin Endocrinol Metab 92(8): 3162-3170.

Kimura, H., M. Kimura, et al., (2005). "Increased thyroidal fat and goitrous hypothyroidism induced by interferon-gamma." International journal of experimental pathology 86(2): 97-106.

Kotsa, K., P. F. Watson, et al., (1997). "A CTLA-4 gene polymorphism is associated with both Graves disease and autoimmune hypothyroidism." Clin Endocrinol (Oxf) 46(5): 551-554.

Kouki, T., Y. Sawai, et al., (2000). "CTLA-4 gene polymorphism at position 49 in exon 1 reduces the inhibitory function of CTLA-4 and contributes to the pathogenesis of Graves' disease." J Immunol 165(11): 6606-6611.

Liu, S. K., N. Fang, et al., (1999). "The hematopoietic-specific adaptor protein gads functions in T-cell signaling via interactions with the SLP-76 and LAT adaptors." Curr Biol 9(2): 67-75.

Maciel, L. M., S. S. Rodrigues, et al., (2001). "Association of the HLA-DRB1*0301 and HLA-DQA1*0501 alleles with Graves' disease in a population representing the gene contribution from several ethnic backgrounds." Thyroid 11(1): 31-35.

Maier, L. M., D. E. Anderson, et al., (2007). "Allelic variant in CTLA4 alters T cell phosphorylation patterns." Proc Natl Acad Sci U S A 104(47): 18607-18612.

Marazuela, M., M. A. Garcia-Lopez, et al., (2006). "Regulatory T cells in human autoimmune thyroid disease." The Journal of clinical endocrinology and metabolism 91(9): 3639-3646.

Martin, A. P., E. C. Coronel, et al., (2004). "A novel model for lymphocytic infiltration of the thyroid gland generated by transgenic expression of the CC chemokine CCL21." Journal of immunology 173(8): 4791-4798.

Maurer, M., S. Loserth, et al., (2002). "A polymorphism in the human cytotoxic T-lymphocyte antigen 4 (CTLA4) gene (exon 1 +49) alters T-cell activation." Immunogenetics 54(1): 1-8.

Mitsiades, N., V. Poulaki, et al., (1998). "Fas/Fas ligand up-regulation and Bcl-2 down-regulation may be significant in the pathogenesis of Hashimoto's thyroiditis." The Journal of clinical endocrinology and metabolism 83(6): 2199-2203.

Mosmann, T. R. and S. Sad (1996). "The expanding universe of T-cell subsets: Th1, Th2 and more." Immunology today 17(3): 138-146.

Nakano, A., M. Watanabe, et al., (2007). "Apoptosis-induced decrease of intrathyroidal CD4(+)CD25(+) regulatory T cells in autoimmune thyroid diseases." Thyroid : official journal of the American Thyroid Association 17(1): 25-31.

Nanba, T., M. Watanabe, et al., (2009). "Increases of the Th1/Th2 cell ratio in severe Hashimoto's disease and in the proportion of Th17 cells in intractable Graves' disease." Thyroid: official journal of the American Thyroid Association 19(5): 495-501.

Nistico, L., R. Buzzetti, et al., (1996). "The CTLA-4 gene region of chromosome 2q33 is linked to, and associated with, type 1 diabetes. Belgian Diabetes Registry." Hum Mol Genet 5(7): 1075-1080.

Oosterwegel, M. A., R. J. Greenwald, et al., (1999). "CTLA-4 and T cell activation." Curr Opin Immunol 11(3): 294-300.

Pang, M., Y. Setoyama, et al., (2002). "Defective expression and tyrosine phosphorylation of the T cell receptor zeta chain in peripheral blood T cells from systemic lupus erythematosus patients." Clin Exp Immunol 129(1): 160-168.

Rapoport, B. and S. M. McLachlan (2007). "The thyrotropin receptor in Graves' disease." Thyroid: official journal of the American Thyroid Association 17(10): 911-922.

Reiser, H. and M. J. Stadecker (1996). "Costimulatory B7 molecules in the pathogenesis of infectious and autoimmune diseases." N Engl J Med 335(18): 1369-1377.

Rosette, C., G. Werlen, et al., (2001). "The impact of duration versus extent of TCR occupancy on T cell activation: a revision of the kinetic proofreading model." Immunity 15(1): 59-70.

Rufer, N., A. Zippelius, et al., (2003). "Ex vivo characterization of human CD8+ T subsets with distinct replicative history and partial effector functions." Blood 102(5): 1779-1787.

Sakaguchi, S., T. Yamaguchi, et al., (2008). "Regulatory T cells and immune tolerance." Cell 133(5): 775-787.

Schwartz, R. H. (2005). "Natural regulatory T cells and self-tolerance." Nature immunology 6(4): 327-330.

Sharpe, A. H. and A. K. Abbas (2006). "T-cell costimulation--biology, therapeutic potential, and challenges." N Engl J Med 355(10): 973-975.

Skorka, A., T. Bednarczuk, et al., (2005). "Lymphoid tyrosine phosphatase (PTPN22/LYP) variant and Graves' disease in a Polish population: association and gene dose-dependent correlation with age of onset." Clin Endocrinol (Oxf) 62(6): 679-682.

Stassi, G., D. Di Liberto, et al., (2000). "Control of target cell survival in thyroid autoimmunity by T helper cytokines via regulation of apoptotic proteins." Nature immunology 1(6): 483-488.

Traves, S. L. and L. E. Donnelly (2008). "Th17 cells in airway diseases." Current molecular medicine 8(5): 416-426.

Ueda, H., J. M. Howson, et al., (2003). "Association of the T-cell regulatory gene CTLA4 with susceptibility to autoimmune disease." Nature 423(6939): 506-511.

Vaidya, B., H. Imrie, et al., (2000). "Association analysis of the cytotoxic T lymphocyte antigen-4 (CTLA-4) and autoimmune regulator-1 (AIRE-1) genes in sporadic autoimmune Addison's disease." J Clin Endocrinol Metab 85(2): 688-691.

Vaidya, B., H. Imrie, et al., (1999). "The cytotoxic T lymphocyte antigen-4 is a major Graves' disease locus." Hum Mol Genet 8(7): 1195-1199.

Vaidya, B. and S. Pearce (2004). "The emerging role of the CTLA-4 gene in autoimmune endocrinopathies." Eur J Endocrinol 150(5): 619-626.

Vang, T., M. Congia, et al., (2005). "Autoimmune-associated lymphoid tyrosine phosphatase is a gain-of-function variant." Nat Genet 37(12): 1317-1319.

Vang, T., A. V. Miletic, et al., (2007). "Protein tyrosine phosphatase PTPN22 in human autoimmunity." Autoimmunity 40(6): 453-461.

Velaga, M. R., V. Wilson, et al., (2004). "The codon 620 tryptophan allele of the lymphoid tyrosine phosphatase (LYP) gene is a major determinant of Graves' disease." J Clin Endocrinol Metab 89(11): 5862-5865.

Verginis, P., H. S. Li, et al., (2005). "Tolerogenic semimature dendritic cells suppress experimental autoimmune thyroiditis by activation of thyroglobulin-specific CD4+CD25+ T cells." Journal of immunology 174(11): 7433-7439.

Vijayakrishnan, L., J. M. Slavik, et al., (2004). "An autoimmune disease-associated CTLA-4 splice variant lacking the B7 binding domain signals negatively in T cells." Immunity 20(5): 563-575.

Wange, R. L. and L. E. Samelson (1996). "Complex complexes: signaling at the TCR." Immunity 5(3): 197-205.

Watanabe, M., N. Yamamoto, et al., (2002). "Independent involvement of CD8+ CD25+ cells and thyroid autoantibodies in disease severity of Hashimoto's disease." Thyroid : official journal of the American Thyroid Association 12(9): 801-808.

Weaver, C. T., R. D. Hatton, et al., (2007). "IL-17 family cytokines and the expanding diversity of effector T cell lineages." Annual review of immunology 25: 821-852.

Wicker, L. S., G. Chamberlain, et al., (2004). "Fine mapping, gene content, comparative sequencing, and expression analyses support Ctla4 and Nramp1 as candidates for Idd5.1 and Idd5.2 in the nonobese diabetic mouse." J Immunol 173(1): 164-173.

Wilson, N. J., K. Boniface, et al., (2007). "Development, cytokine profile and function of human interleukin 17-producing helper T cells." Nature immunology 8(9): 950-957.

Wu, J., A. Katrekar, et al., (2006). "Identification of substrates of human protein-tyrosine phosphatase PTPN22." J Biol Chem 281(16): 11002-11010.

Yanagawa, T., Y. Hidaka, et al., (1995). "CTLA-4 gene polymorphism associated with Graves' disease in a Caucasian population." J Clin Endocrinol Metab 80(1): 41-45.

Yanagawa, T., A. Mangklabruks, et al., (1993). "Human histocompatibility leukocyte antigen-DQA1*0501 allele associated with genetic susceptibility to Graves' disease in a Caucasian population." J Clin Endocrinol Metab 76(6): 1569-1574.

Yanagawa, T., M. Taniyama, et al., (1997). "CTLA4 gene polymorphism confers susceptibility to Graves' disease in Japanese." Thyroid 7(6): 843-846.

Yano, S., S. Sone, et al., (1995). "Differential effects of anti-inflammatory cytokines (IL-4, IL-10 and IL-13) on tumoricidal and chemotactic properties of human monocytes induced by monocyte chemotactic and activating factor." Journal of leukocyte biology 57(2): 303-309.

Young-Min, S. and B. Vaidya (2004). "CTLA4 exon 1 polymorphism, rheumatoid arthritis and autoimmune endocrinopathy." Clin Rheumatol 23(6): 568-569.

Zamani, M., M. Spaepen, et al., (2000). "Primary role of the HLA class II DRB1*0301 allele in Graves disease." Am J Med Genet 95(5): 432-437.

Zhang, W., J. Sloan-Lancaster, et al., (1998). "LAT: the ZAP-70 tyrosine kinase substrate that links T cell receptor to cellular activation." Cell 92(1): 83-92.

8

Estrogen Signaling and Thyrocyte Proliferation

Valeria Gabriela Antico Arciuch and Antonio Di Cristofano
Department of Developmental and Molecular Biology
Albert Einstein College of Medicine, Bronx
USA

1. Introduction

The development of thyroid cancer is a multifactorial and multistep process. Several factors are thought to predispose people to thyroid cancer, including genetics, environment, and sex hormones. The incidence of thyroid cancer is three to four times higher in women than in men (Libutti, 2005; Machens et al., 2006). This difference in incidence between genders suggests that the growth and outcome of thyroid tumors may be influenced by female sex hormones, particularly E2, which has been widely implicated in the development and progression of several cancers, such as breast, ovarian and prostate cancer (Arnold et al., 2007; Stender et al., 2007). Animal studies support these epidemiological data, and suggest that exogenous estrogen (17β-estradiol, E2) can promote thyroid tumors (Mori et al., 1990; Thiruvengadam et al., 2003).

Several studies have been carried out to address the role of estrogens in the pathogenesis of proliferative and neoplastic disorders. Although the precise mechanism still remains ill-defined, a range of plausible mechanisms explaining their carcinogenic effects has been proposed. On one hand, estrogens may promote cellular proliferation through their receptor-mediated activity (Arnold et al., 2007; Lee et al., 2005). In addition, the natural estrogen E2 or its metabolites 2- hydroxy, 4-hydroxy, and 16-α-hydroxy-estradiol (2-OH-E2, 4-OH-E2, and 16-α-OH E2) can cause neoplastic transformation through a direct genotoxic effect, increasing the spontaneous mutation rate of normal cells (Cavalieri et al., 1997).

In this review, we will analyze the role of estrogen signaling in the proliferation and transformation of the thyroid gland, with a special emphasis on the cross-talk between estrogen signaling and the PI3K pathway.

2. Thyroid cancer

Thyroid carcinoma is the most common and prevalent of all endocrine malignancies, accounting for more than 95% of all endocrine-related cancers (Hodgson et al., 2004; Jemal et al., 2009). Papillary and follicular carcinomas (PTC and FTC respectively) are differentiated tumors arising from thyroid epithelial cells (thyrocytes), while medullary carcinoma originates from parafollicular cells. PTC is by far the most common type of thyroid cancer, representing up to 80% of all thyroid malignancies. Anaplastic carcinomas are undifferentiated tumors deriving from thyroid epithelial cells. They are usually lethal with no effective system therapy. The factors leading to thyroid carcinoma development are not fully understood despite some well-established associations, such as between ionizing radiation and papillary carcinoma, and between iodine deficiency and follicular carcinoma.

From the molecular point of view, papillary and follicular thyroid cancers are completely different diseases. This notion is supported by dissimilar molecular initiating events leading to neoplastic transformation and by differences in DNA ploidy level (PTCs are generally diploid, FTCs aneuploid) (Handkiewicz-Junak et al., 2010).

Follicular Carcinoma	Papillary Carcinoma	Anaplastic Carcinoma
RAS: 20-50%	*BRAF*: 40-45%	*TP53*: 50-80%
PAX8-PPARγ: 20-35%	*RAS*: 10-20%	*BRAF*: 20-40%
PI3K pathway: 20%	*RET-PTC*: 10-30%	*RAS*: 20-40%
		PI3K pathway: 20-50%

Table 1. Most frequent genetic alterations in thyroid cancer

The genetic alterations found in PTC primarily affect two central signalling pathways in thyroid cells: TSH receptor (TSHR)-mediated signalling and mitogen-activated protein kinase (MAPK) pathways (Kim and Zhu, 2009; Lemoine et al., 1998; Nikiforov, 2008). Three important initiating events, *RET/PTC* (rearranged during transfection/ papillary thyroid cancer), *RAS* (resistance to audiogenic seizures) and *BRAF* mutations, are considered mutually exclusive (Fagin, 2004). BRAF mutation and RET/PTC rearrangements differ to some extent in their effects on the shared oncogenic pathway, resulting more frequently in the classic or the solid variant of PTC, respectively, while RAS mutations are more likely to induce the follicular variant of PTC (Xing, 2005).

Follicular carcinomas are often characterized by *RAS* mutations (up to 50%) and *PAX8-PPARγ* rearrangements (20–35%), which lead to a mutant protein incapable of trans-activating a PPARγ signal (Gilfillan, 2010). Phosphatidylinositol 3-kinase (PI3K)/AKT alterations are frequently found in FTC and, even more distinctly, in ATC. In FTC, phosphorylation of AKT, the key player in this pathway, is by far more frequent than that of ERK (Liu et al., 2008).

Anaplastic thyroid carcinomas (ATCs) comprise 2% of thyroid malignancies, and are usually lethal, with no effective therapy (Are and Shaha, 2006). Dedifferentiation, a common hallmark of ATC, is manifested by a loss of specific thyroid cell characteristics and functions, including expression of thyroglobulin, thyroid peroxidase, thyroid stimulating hormone receptor and the Na/I symporter (Neff et al., 2008; Smallridge et al., 2009). Molecular signature events that characterize ATC involve either *BRAF* activation or sustained hyperactivation of the PI3K/AKT cascade, together with *TP53* loss or inactivation (Kouniavsky and Zeiger, 2010).

3. Physiological functions of estrogen and estrogen receptors

3.1 Estrogen production

Estrogens are a group of steroid compounds acting as the primary female sex hormones. Estrogens regulate several physiological processes, including cell growth and development, not only in the reproductive tract but also in other tissues such as bone, brain, liver, cardiovascular system, and endocrine glands.

Although estrogens are present in both men and women, their levels are significantly higher in women of reproductive age. They are mainly produced by the adrenal cortex and ovary. The three major naturally occurring estrogens in women are: estrone, estradiol and estriol (Speroff et al., 1999). In premenopausal women, 17β-estradiol (E2), produced by the ovary, is the estrogen formed in the largest quantity and is the most potent since it has the highest affinity for estrogen receptors. In premenopausal women, the level of circulating E2 varies from 40 to 400 pg/mL during the menstrual cycle (Ruggiero et al., 2002). After menopause, the level of E2 drops to less than 20 pg/mL (Jones, 1992). The second endogenous estrogen is estrone (E1), a less potent metabolite of E2. Estrone is produced from androstenedione in adipose tissue. In postmenopausal women, the ovary ceases to produce E2 while the adrenal gland continues to produce androstenedione, with the result that the level of estrone remains unchanged while the level of E2 falls significantly. The third endogenous estrogen is estriol (E3), also a metabolite of E2. E3 is the main estrogen produced by the placenta during pregnancy, and is found in smaller quantities than E2 and E1 in nonpregnant women (Jones, 1992; Ruggiero et al., 2002).

3.2 Estrogen receptors and their ligands

The actions of estrogens occur through activation of estrogen receptors (ERα, ERβ and GPR30). ERα was initially described in 1973 (Jensen and De Sombre, 1973) while ERβ was identified much later (Kuiper et al., 1996). ERα and ERβ are encoded by separate genes, *ESR1* and *ESR2*, respectively, which share similarities in the DNA-binding domain (97% amino acid similarity) and ligand-binding domain (60% amino acid similarity) (Hall et al., 2001). These two ERs differ in their tissue distributions (Kuiper et al., 1997; Dechering et al., 2000), suggesting that ERα and ERβ might have different physiological functions. It has also been demonstrated that in many systems the activity of ERβ is opposed to that of ERα. For example, in breast cancer cells, ERα is the receptor responsible for E2-induced proliferation, whereas activation of ERβ inhibits this effect (Strom et al., 2004). In the uterus, E2 induces proliferation of both epithelial and stromal cells through ERα, which is the predominant ER in the mature organ, while in the immature uterus, ERα and ERβ are found at similar expression levels in both epithelium and stroma, and ERβ mediates the action of E2 as a suppressor of cell proliferation against activation of ERα by E2 (Weihua et al., 2000).

G protein-coupled receptor 30 (GPR30), a novel transmembrane ER, was identified in different cells by four laboratories between 1996 and 1998 (Takada et al., 1997; Owman et al., 1996; Carmeci et al., 1997; O'Dowd et al., 1998). Since its ligand was unknown at that time, it was named based on its homology to the G protein-coupled receptor (GPCR) super-family. In addition, this receptor was found to be associated with ER expression in breast cancer cell lines (Carmeci et al., 1997). Later in 2000, Filardo et al. demonstrated that estrogen promptly activated ERK1/2 in two breast cancer cell lines, MCF-7 and SKBR3, with the cell line SKBR3 non-expressing ERs. These results demonstrated that estrogen might be a potential ligand for GPR30 (Filardo et al., 2000). This fact was further confirmed by the observation that estrogen did not activate ERK1/2 in the breast cancer cell line MDA-MB-231 without GPR30 expression, whereas ERK1/2 was activated by estrogen after GPR30 transfection into the cells (Filardo et al., 2000). Therefore, GPR30 is necessary for the activation of ERK1/2 by estrogen. So far, GPR30 has been detected in numerous human tissues such as heart, liver, lung, intestine, ovary, brain, breast, uterus, placenta and prostate (He et al., 2009; Filardo et al., 2006; Zhang et al., 2008; Haas et al., 2007; Hugo et al., 2008).

3.3 Genomic and non-genomic actions of estrogen receptors

In the classical, genomic estrogen-signaling pathway, estradiol (E2)-activated ERα translocates to the nucleus, dimerizes, and binds to the 15-bp palindromic estrogen response element (ERE) or interacts with other transcription factors on target genes, recruits coactivators, and stimulates gene transcription thereby promoting cell proliferation (Klinge, 2000). ERα interacts with a number of coactivators and corepressors in a ligand-dependent manner (Klinge, 2000). ERα may also function in a non-traditional manner, interacting with other DNA-binding transcription factors such as activator protein 1 (AP-1) or Sp-1, that in turn bind their cognate DNA elements, leading to remodeling of chromatin, and interactions with components of the basal transcription machinery complex (Ascenzi et al., 2006; Deroo and Korach, 2006).

Another more rapid mechanism of estrogen action is termed 'non-genomic' or 'membrane-initiated' because it involves E2 activation of plasma membrane-associated ERα or ERβ and leads to rapid activation of intracellular signaling pathways, e.g., ERK1/2 and PI3K/AKT (Wong et al., 2002; Watson et al., 2007; He et al., 2009). It can also result in an increase of Ca^{2+} or nitric oxide and the promotion of cell cycle progression. The ERs may be targeted to the plasma membrane by adaptor proteins such as caveolin-1 or Shc (Kim et al., 2008). GPR30 also activates ERK1/2 and PI3K/AKT signaling, although its exact role in estrogen action remains controversial (Pedram et al., 2006). GPR30 ligands, for example, estrogen (Muller et al., 1979), tamoxifen (Dick et al., 2002) and ICI 182780 (Hermenegildo and Cano, 2000) bind to GPR30, and activate heterotrimeric G proteins, which then activate Src and adenylyl cyclase (AC) resulting in intracellular cAMP production. Src is involved in matrix metalloproteinases (MMP) activation, which cleave pro-heparan-bound epidermal growth factor (pro-HB-EGF) and release free HB-EGF. The latter activates EGF receptor (EGFR), leading to multiple downstream events such as activation of phospholipase C (PLC), PI3K, and MAPK. Activated PLC produces inositol triphosphate (IP3), which further binds to IP3 receptor and leads to intracellular calcium mobilization. The activation of MAPK and PI3K results in activation of numerous cytosolic pathways and nuclear proteins, which further regulate transcription factors such as serum response factor and members of the E26 transformation specific (ETS) family by direct phosphorylation (Posern and Treisman, 2006; Gutierrez-Hartmann et al., 2007).

The non-genomic pathway may cross-talk with the genomic pathway, since ERα can be translocated from the membrane into the nucleus both in a E2-dependent or independent manner (Lu et al., 2002). It has also been demonstrated that E2-induced ERK activation stimulates the expression of AP-1-mediated genes via both serum response factor ELK-1 (ER activated in the membrane) and the recruitment of coactivators to AP-1 sites on gene promoters by the nuclear ER (Ascenzi et al., 2006). The intricate relationship between membrane and nuclear effects induced by estrogens has also been observed in the regulation of many other genes including PI3K (Ascenzi et al., 2006).

Therefore, integrative signaling by E2 from several places in the cell can lead to both rapid and sustained actions, which synergize to provide plasticity for cell response.

3.4 Estrogen receptors in the mitochondria

Glucocorticoid and thyroid hormones have been shown to modify the levels of mtDNA-encoded gene transcripts. These effects are mediated through direct interactions of their receptors with mtDNA. It has also been established that thyroid hormone can cause the direct stimulation of mitochondrial RNA synthesis (Casas et al., 1999; Enriquez et al., 1999) and that a variant form of the thyroid hormone receptor is imported in and localized within liver mitochondria (Casas et al., 1999; Wrutniak et al., 1995).

These findings suggest that mitochondria could also be a target site for the action of estrogens. Monje and colleagues (Monje and Boland 2001; Monje et al., 2001) demonstrated the presence of both ERα and ERβ in mitochondria of rabbit uterine and ovarian tissue, and ER translocation into mitochondria suggests the presence of E2 effects on mitochondrial function and protein expression (Chen et al., 2004). The mitochondrial genome contains estrogen response elements (ERE)-like sequences (Demonacos et al., 1996; Sekeris et al., 1990). Furthermore, several studies have detected the presence of estrogen-binding proteins (EBPs) in the organelle (Grossman et al., 1989; Moats and Ramirez 2000). Estrogen treatment increases the transcript levels of several mitochondrial DNA (mtDNA)-encoded genes in rat hepatocytes and human Hep G2 cells (Chen et al., 1996; Chen et al., 1998).

Estrogen response elements have been found in the D-loop, in the master regulatory region, and within the structural genes of the mtDNA (Demonacos et al., 1996). As a consequence, E2 may exert coordinated effects on both nuclear and mitochondrial gene expression. E2 can increase mtDNA transcripts for cytochrome oxidase IV subunits I and II in cultured cancer cells (Chen et al., 2004). E2 profoundly affects mitochondrial function in cerebral blood vessels, enhancing efficiency of energy production and suppressing mitochondrial oxidative stress by increasing protein levels of Mn-SOD and aconitase, and stabilizing mitochondrial membrane (Stirone et al., 2005).

The mechanisms of ER translocation into mitochondria are still quite elusive but recent data in MCF7 cells demonstrated that human ERβ posses a putative internal mitochondrial targeting peptide signal to the organelle (Chen et al., 2004). These authors observed that around 12% of total cellular ERα and 18% of ERβ is present in the mitochondrial fraction in E2-treated MCF7 cells. Furthermore, the localization of both ERα and ERβ to mitochondria in response to E2-treatment is accompanied by a concomitant time- and concentration-dependent increase in the transcript levels of the mtDNA-encoded genes (Chen et al., 2004).

3.5 Target molecules of estrogen receptors in the thyroid gland

Besides the adrenal cortex and ovary, also the human thyroid gland has the ability to synthesize estrogens and such ability seems to be higher in women than men (Dalla Valle et al., 1998). In the thyroid gland, E2 provokes a considerable increase in the thyroid weight, stimulates thyroid iodide uptake, enhances thyroperoxidase activity, and increases the level of T3 (Lima et al., 2006).

ERK1/2 regulate various cellular activities, such as gene expression, mitosis, differentiation, proliferation, and cell survival/apoptosis (Roberts and Der, 2007; Dunn et al., 2005). Zeng and colleagues have demonstrated that E2 can activate ERK1/2 in the thyroid by inducing its phosphorylation (Zeng et al., 2007). ERK1/2 activation by E2 depends on the interaction between estradiol and ERα (Zeng et al., 2007).

Bcl-2 family proteins play a central role in controlling mitochondrial-mediated apoptosis. They include proteins that suppress apoptosis such as Bcl-2 and Bcl-XL, and proteins that promote apoptosis such as Bax, Bad and Bcl-X_S (Antonsson and Martinou, 2000). Bcl-2 proteins localize or translocate to the mitochondrial membrane and modulate apoptosis by permeabilization of the inner and/or outer membrane, leading to the release of citochrome *c* or stabilization of the barrier function. Bcl-2 family members are altered in thyroid cancer (Kossmehl et al., 2003) and their levels are regulated by estrogen in some cell systems (Song and Santen, 2003). The antiapoptotic member Bcl-2 is up-regulated by E2 and by the ERα agonist PPT, but down-regulated by the ERβ agonist DPN in thyroid cancer cells, suggesting that ERα induces Bcl-2 expression whereas ERβ reduces it (Zeng et al., 2007). In addition, it has been shown that ERβ but not ERα promotes the expression of Bax (Lee et al., 2005; Zeng et al., 2007).

Recent work on the WRO thyroid cancer cells revealed that E2 increases cathepsin D transcription and that cathepsin D expression is inhibited upon siRNA-mediated knockdown of ERα and ERβ (Kumar et al., 2010). Cathepsin D is a classical E2 target gene regulated by Sp1-ERα promoter binding (Wang et al., 1997). It is well established that cathepsin D expression is elevated in thyroid tumors and correlates with disease aggressiveness (Leto et al., 2004).

The expression of another classical E2 target gene, cyclin D1 (Pestell et al., 1999), is stimulated by E2 in thyroid cancer cell lines, and co-treatment with siERα and siERβ shows roles for ERα and ERβ in regulating cyclin D1 transcription. E2 regulation of cyclin D1 transcription involves ERα-Sp1 (Castro-Rivera et al., 2001) and AP-1-ERα (Liu et al., 2002) interactions.

In Nthy-ori3-1 and BCPAP cells (derived from thyroid carcinoma), ERα was found to be complexed with Hsp90 and AKT (Rajoria et al., 2010). The complex of Hsp90 and AKT with ERα has major implications for its non-genomic signaling. In the presence of E2, Hsp90 dissociates, allowing ERα to dimerize and induce gene expression. At the same time, AKT is also rendered free to participate in the signal transduction cascade.

Rajoria and colleagues observed that E2 dramatically increases the ability of thyroid cells to adhere (137-140%) and migrate (27-75%). They also found downregulation of β-catenin in the thyroid cells treated with E2 (Rajoria et al., 2010).

4. PI3K-AKT pathway

In 1991, three independent research groups identified the gene that encodes for the serin/threonin kinase AKT/PKB (Jones et al., 1991; Bellacosa et al., 1991; Coffer and Woodgent, 1991). AKT plays a major role in cell proliferation, survival, adhesion, migration, metabolism and tumorigenesis. The effects of AKT activation are determined by the phosphorylation of its downstream effectors located in the cytoplasm, nucleus and mitochondria (Manning and Cantley, 2007; Bijur and Jope, 2003; Antico Arciuch et al., 2009). Mammals have three closely related PKB genes, encoding the isoforms AKT1/PKBα, AKT2/PKBβ and AKT3/PKBγ. Although the AKT isoforms are ubiquitously expressed, evidence suggests that the relative isoform expression levels differ between tissues. AKT1 is the mainly expressed isoform in most tissues, while AKT2 is highly enriched in insulin target tissues. *Akt1* deficient mice show normal glucose tolerance and insulin-stimulated glucose clearance from blood, but display severe growth retardation (Cho et al., 2001). It has also been shown that cells derived from *Akt1* deficient mouse embryos are also more susceptible to pro-apoptotic stimuli (Chen et al., 2001). On the other hand, deficiency of *AKT2* alone is sufficient to cause a diabetic phenotype in mice (Withers et al., 1998; Cho et al., 2001) and a loss-of-function mutation in AKT2 is associated with diabetes in one human family (George et al., 2004).

AKT kinases are typically activated by engagement of receptor tyrosine kinases by growth factors and cytokines, as well as oxidative stress and heat shock. AKT activation relies on phosphatidylinositol 3,4,5-triphosphate (PtdIns-3,4,5-P3) which is produced from phosphatidylinositol 4,5-biphosphate (PtdIns-4,5-P2) by phosphatidylinositol 3-kinase (PI3K) (Franke et al., 1995). The interaction between the Pleckstrin homology (PH) domain of AKT with PtdIns-3,4,5-P3 favors its phosphorylation at two residues, one in the C-terminal tail (Ser^{473}) and the other in the activation loop (Thr^{308}). Phosphorylation at Ser^{473} appears to precede and facilitate phosphorylation at Thr^{308} (Sarbassov et al., 2005). AKT is phosphorylated in Ser^{473} by mTORC2 (Ikenoue et al., 2008), while PI-3K-dependent kinase 1 (PDK1) accounts for the phosphorylation in Thr^{308} (Chan et al., 1999).

The proliferative effects of AKT result from phosphorylation of several substrates. For example, GSK3β once phosphorylated is inactivated and this prevents degradation of cyclin D1 (Diehl et al., 1998). Furthermore, AKT activation leads to increased translation of cyclin D1 and D3 transcripts via mTOR (Muise-Helmericks et al., 1998). AKT phosphorylates the cell cycle inhibitors $p21^{WAF1}$ and $p27^{Kip1}$ inducing their cytoplasmic retention (Testa and Bellacosa, 2001).

AKT activity prevents apoptosis through the phosphorylation and inhibition of pro-apoptotic mediators such as Bad, FOXO family members, and IκB kinase-β (IKK-β) (Datta et al., 1999). AKT activity also attenuates the response of cells to the release of cytochrome *c* into the cytoplasm (Kennedy et al., 1999).

AKT can also antagonize p53-mediated cell cycle checkpoints by modulating the subcellular localization of Mdm2. Phosphorylation of Mdm2 by AKT triggers its localization to the nucleus, where Mdm2 can complex with p53 to promote its ubiquitin/proteasome-mediated degradation (Mayo and Donner, 2001).

The crucial role of the PI3K signaling cascade in the pathogenesis of thyroid neoplastic disorders has been recently confirmed by the development and study of a relevant mouse model (Yeager et al., 2007, 2008; Miller et al., 2009), as well as by solid clinicopathological data (Garcia-Rostan et al., 2005; Hou et al., 2007, 2008; Vasko and Saji, 2007; Wang et al., 2007). Thyrocyte-specific deletion of the *Pten* tumor suppressor constitutively activates the PI3K signaling cascade, leading to hyperplastic thyroid glands at birth, and to the development of thyroid nodules and follicular adenomas by 6-8 months of age (Yeager et al., 2007) and thyroid carcinomas by one year of age (Antico Arciuch et al., 2010).

5. PI3K-estrogen cooperation during proliferation

The *Pten* mouse model of thyroid disease displays a unique and remarkable characteristic: the higher proliferative index of female mutant thyrocytes, compared with males. This difference leads to increased cellularity in the thyroids of female mutants at a young age, to an increased incidence of thyroid adenomas in mutant females at 8 months of age (Yeager et al., 2007), and to an increased incidence of thyroid carcinomas in mutant females at one year of age (Antico Arciuch et al., 2010). The direct role of estrogen signaling in determining this difference in proliferative response to PI3K activation is underlined by the fact that these effects could be completely reversed by estrogen depletion in the females, and by slow-release estrogen pellet implantation in the males.

Several groups had anticipated a role for estrogen in thyroid proliferation, based on the effects of estradiol on thyroid carcinoma cells in culture (Manole et al., 2001; Vivacqua et al., 2006; Chen et al., 2008; Kumar et al., 2010; Rajoria et al., 2010). The *Pten* mouse model represents the first *in vivo* validation of the direct role played by estrogen in establishing the increased prevalence of thyroid disorders in the female.

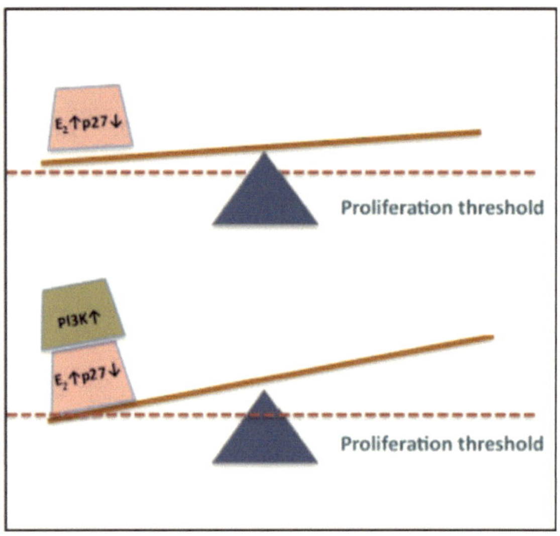

Fig. 1. Schematic model of the cooperation between estrogen signaling and PI3K activation.

The analysis of *Pten* mutant mice also shed some light on the molecular basis of the differential thyrocyte proliferative index and risk of adenoma and carcinoma development between male and female mutant mice. Genetic approaches, by crossing *Pten* mutant mice and *p27* mutant mice, and cell culture-based experiments have provided evidence that these gender-based differences in this mouse model are due, at least in part, to the ability of estrogens to down-regulate p27 levels through mechanisms that include transcriptional regulation, in addition to the known effects on p27 protein degradation through regulation of Skp2 (Antico Arciuch et al., 2010; Foster et al., 2003).

Thus it is conceivable that, in thyroids harboring mutations that confer elevated proliferative signals and thus a low cell cycle progression threshold, E2-mediated p27 depletion further increases the thyrocyte proliferative index (Figure 1).

Additional mechanisms, including E2-mediated mitochondrial effects, are also likely to contribute to this phenotype. Maintenance of a normal intracellular redox status plays an important role in such processes as DNA synthesis, gene expression, enzymatic activity, and others. Signaling cascades involving protein tyrosine kinases can be enhanced by oxidative inhibition of protein tyrosine phosphatases, and pathways involving NF-kB, JNK, p38 MAPK, and AP-1 are strongly responsive to redox regulation (Droge, 2002). Recent data have suggested that physiological concentrations of E2 trigger a rapid production of intracellular reactive oxygen species (ROS) in endothelial and epithelial cells, and that E2-induced DNA synthesis is at least in part mediated by ROS signaling in these cells (Felty et al., 2005; Felty, 2006). This notion is particularly intriguing, since E2-mediated ROS production in thyroid follicular cells would have two effects: an immediate stimulation of cell proliferation, and a long-term accumulation of oxidative DNA damage. Furthermore, these effects would be further enhanced if PI3K activation resulted in an alteration of the thyrocyte antioxidant and detoxification system. Strikingly, in an ongoing proteomic effort (manuscript in preparation), we have recently identified Glutathione S-transferase Mu 1 (GSTM1), an enzyme important for the reduction (detoxification) of hydrogen peroxide, as one of the most significantly down-regulated proteins in mutant thyroids, suggesting that, indeed, PI3K-mediated GSTM1 reduction might indeed further amplify the effects of ROS in the thyroid.

Finally, the increased expression level of *Tpo*, *Duox1* and *Slc5a5* genes in female mice, irrespective of their genotype, strongly suggests that estrogen has a significant role in their transcriptional regulation, providing additional targets for future studies on the role of estrogen in the pathophysiology of the thyroid gland.

6. Conclusion

A role for estrogen in thyroid proliferation has been proposed for several years, based on the analysis of the effects of estrogen on thyroid cells in culture. Now, for the first time, our hormone manipulation experiments in a relevant mouse model of thyroid proliferative disorders and neoplastic transformation have provided *in vivo* evidence that circulating estrogens increase thyroid follicular cells proliferation. It is tempting to suggest that the relatively mild effect of estrogens on thyroid cells is uncovered and amplified by oncogenic events lowering the thyrocyte proliferation threshold. Further studies will validate this hypothesis in the context of different oncogenic mutations.

7. References

Antico Arciuch VG, Dima M, Liao XH, Refetoff S and Di Cristofano A. (2010) Cross-talk between PI3K and estrogen in the mouse thyroid predisposes to the development of follicular carcinomas with a higher incidence in females. *Oncogene*. 29:5678-86.

Antico Arciuch VG, Galli S, Franco MC, Lam PY, Cadenas E, Carreras MC, and Poderoso JJ. (2009) AKT1 intramitochondrial cycling is a crucial step in the redox modulation of cell cycle progression. *PLoS One* 4: e7523.

Antonsson B and Martinou JC. (2000) The Bcl-2 protein family. Exp Cell Res. 256:50-7.

Are C and Shaha AR. (2006) Anaplastic thyroid carcinoma: biology, pathogenesis, prognostic factors, and treatment approaches. *Ann Surg Oncol*. 13:453-64.

Arnold JT, Liu X, Allen JD, Le H, McFann KK and Blackman MR. (2007) Androgen receptor or estrogen receptor-beta blockade alters DHEA-, DHT-, and E(2)-induced proliferation and PSA production in human prostate cancer cells. *Prostate*. 67:1152-62.

Ascenzi P, Bocedi A, Marino M. (2006) Structure-function relationship of estrogen receptor alpha and beta: impact on human health. *Mol Aspects Med*. 27:299-402.

Bellacosa A, Testa JR, Staal SP and Tsichlis PN. (1991) A retroviral oncogene, akt, encoding a serine-threonine kinase containing an SH2-like region. *Science.* 254:274-277.

Bijur GN, Jope RS. Rapid accumulation of AKT in mitochondria following phosphatidylinositol 3-kinase activation. (2003) *J Neurochem* 87:1427 35.

Carmeci C, Thompson DA, Ring HZ, Francke U and Weigel RJ. (1997) Identification of a gene (GPR30) with homology to the G-protein-coupled receptor superfamily associated with estrogen receptor expression in breast cancer. *Genomics.* 45:607-617.

Casas F, Rochard P, Rodier A, Cassar-Malek I, Marchal-Victorion S, Wiesner RJ, Cabello G, and Wrutniak C. (1999) A variant form of the nuclear triiodothyronine receptor c-ErbAalpha1 plays a direct role in regulation of mitochondrial RNA synthesis. *Mol Cell Biol.* 19:7913-7924.

Castro-Rivera E, Samudio I and Safe S. (2001) Estrogen regulation of cyclin D1 gene expression in ZR-75 breast cancer cells involves multiple enhancer elements. *J Biol Chem.* 276:30853-30861.

Cavalieri EL and Rogan EG. (2001) Evidence that a burst of DNA depurination in SENCAR mouse skin induces error-prone repair and forms mutations in the H-ras gene. *Oncogene* 20:7945-7953.

Cavalieri EL, Stack DE, Devanesan PD, Todorovic R, Dwivedy I, Higginbotham S, Johansson SL, Patil KD, Gross ML, Gooden JK, Ramanathan R, Cerny RL and Rogan EG. (1997) Molecular origin of cancer: catechol estrogen-3,4-quinones as endogenous tumor initiators. *Proc Natl Acad Sci U S A.* 94:10937-42.

Chan TO, Rittenhouse SE and Tsichlis PN. AKT/PKB and other D3 phosphoinositideregulated kinases: kinase activation by phosphoinositide-dependent phosphorylation. (1999) *Annu Rev Biochem* 68: 965-1014.

Chen GG, Liu ZM, Vlantis AC, Tse GM, Leung BC and van Hasselt CA. (2004) Heme oxygenase-1 protects against apoptosis induced by tumor necrosis factor-alpha and cycloheximide in papillary thyroid carcinoma cells. *J Cell Biochem.* 92:1246-56.

Chen GG, Vlantis AC, Zeng Q and van Hasselt CA. (2008) Regulation of cell growth by estrogen signaling and potential targets in thyroid cancer. *Curr Cancer Drug Targets.* 8:367-377.

Chen J, Gokhale M, Li Y, Trush MA, and Yager JD. (1998) Enhanced levels of several mitochondrial mRNA transcripts and mitochondrial superoxide production during ethinyl estradiol-induced hepatocarcinogenesis and after estrogen treatment of HepG2 cells. *Carcinogenesis.* 19:2187-2193.

Chen J, Schwartz DA, Young TA, Norris JS, and Yager JD. (1996) Identification of genes whose expression is altered during mitosuppression in livers of ethinyl estradiol-treated female rats. *Carcinogenesis.* 17:2783-2786.

Chen JQ, Delannoy M, Cooke C and Yager JD. (2004) Mitochondrial localization of ERalpha and ERbeta in human MCF7 cells. *Am J Physiol.* 286:E1011-E1022.

Chen WS, Xu PZ, Gottlob K, Chen ML, Sokol K, Shiyanova T, Roninson I, Weng W, Suzuki R, Tobe K, Kadowaki T and Hay N. Growth retardation and increased apoptosis in mice with homozygous disruption of the AKT1 gene. (2001) *Genes Dev* 15:2203-8.

Cho H, Mu J, Kim JK, Thorvaldsen JL, Chu Q, Crenshaw EB 3rd, Kaestner KH, Bartolomei MS, Shulman GI and Birnbaum MJ. Insulin resistance and a diabetes mellitus-like syndrome in mice lacking the protein kinase AKT2 (PKB beta). (2001) *Science* 292:1728-1731.

Cho H, Thorvaldsen JL, Chu Q, Feng F and Birnbaum MJ. (2001) AKT1/pkbalpha is required for normal growth but dispensable for maintenance of glucose homeostasis in mice. *J Biol Chem* 276:38349-52.

Coffer PJ and Woodgett JR. (1991) Molecular cloning and characterisation of a novel putative protein-serine kinase related to the cAMP-dependent and protein kinase C families. *Eur J Biochem.* 201:475-481.

Dalla Valle L, Ramina A, Vianello S, Fassina A, Belvedere P and Colombo L. (1998) Potential for estrogen synthesis and action in human normal and neoplastic thyroid tissues. *J. Clin. Endocrinol. Metab.* 83:3702-3709.

Datta SR, Brunet A and Greenberg ME. Cellular survival: a play in three AKTs. (1999) *Genes Dev.* 13:2905-27.

Dechering K, Boersma and Mosselman S. (2000) Estrogen receptors alpha and beta: two receptors of a kind? *Curr. Med. Chem.* 7:561-576.

Demonacos CV, Karayanni N, Hatzoglou E, Tsiriyiotis C, Spandidos DA and Sekeris CE. (1996) Mitochondrial genes as sites of primary action of steroid hormones. *Steroids.* 61:226-232.

Deroo BJ, Korach KS. (2006) Estrogen receptors and human disease. *J Clin Invest.* 116:561-70.

Dick GM, Hunter AC and Sanders KM. (2002) Ethylbromide tamoxifen, a membrane-impermeant antiestrogen, activates smooth muscle calcium-activated large-conductance potassium channels from the extracellular side. *Mol Pharmacol.* 61(5):1105-13.

Diehl JA, Cheng M, Roussel MF and Sherr CJ. (1998) Glycogen synthase kinase-3beta regulates cyclin D1 proteolysis and subcellular localization. *Genes Dev.* 12:3499-3511.

Droge W. (2002) Free radicals in the physiological control of cell function. *Physiol Rev* 82, 47-95.

Dunn KL, Espino PS, Drobic B, He S and Davie JR. (2005) The Ras-MAPK signal transduction pathway, cancer and chromatin remodeling. *Biochem Cell Biol.* 83:1-14.

Enriquez JA, Fernandez-Silva P, Garrido-Perez N, Lopez-Perez MJ, Perez-Martos A, and Montoya J. (1999) Direct regulation of mitochondrial RNA synthesis by thyroid hormone. *Mol Cell Biol.* 19:657-670.

Fagin JA. (2004) How thyroid tumors start and why it matters: kinase mutants as targets for solid cancer pharmacotherapy. *J Endocrinol.* 183:249-56.

Felty Q. (2006) Estrogen-induced DNA synthesis in vascular endothelial cells is mediated by ROS signaling. *BMC Cardiovasc Disord* 6, 16-22.

Felty Q., Singh K.P. and Roy, D. (2005) Estrogen-induced G1/S transition of G0-arrested estrogen-dependent breast cancer cells is regulated by mitochondrial oxidant signaling. *Oncogene* 24, 4883-93.

Filardo EJ, Quinn JA, Bland KI, Frackelton AR Jr. (2000) Estrogen-induced activation of Erk-1 and Erk-2 requires the G protein-coupled receptor homolog, GPR30, and occurs via trans-activation of the epidermal growth factor receptor through release of HB-EGF. *Mol. Endocrinol.* 14:1649-1660.

Filardo EJ, Graeber CT, Quinn JA, Resnick MB, Giri D, DeLellis RA, Steinhoff MM and Sabo E. (2006) Distribution of GPR30, a seven membrane-spanning estrogen receptor, in primary breast cancer and its association with clinicopathologic determinants of tumor progression. *Clin. Cancer Res.* 12:6359-6366.

Franke TF, Yang SI, Chan TO, Datta K, Kazlauskas A, Morrison DK, Kaplan DR and Tsichlis PN. The protein kinase encoded by the AKT proto-oncogene is a target of the PDGF-activated phosphatidylinositol 3-kinase. (1995) *Cell* 2:727-36.

Foster JS, Fernando RI, Ishida N, Nakayama KI and Wimalasena J. (2003) Estrogens down-regulate p27Kip1 in breast cancer cells through Skp2 and through nuclear export mediated by the ERK pathway. *J Biol Chem.* 278:41355-41366.

Garcia-Rostan G, Costa AM, Pereira-Castro I, Salvatore G, Hernandez R, Hermsem MJ et al. (2005) Mutation of the PIK3CA gene in anaplastic thyroid cancer. *Cancer Res.* 65:10199-10207.

George S, Rochford JJ, Wolfrum C, Gray SL, Schinner S, Wilson JC, Soos MA, Murgatroyd PR, Williams RM, Acerini CL, Dunger DB, Barford D, Umpleby AM, Wareham NJ, Davies HA, Schafer AJ, Stoffel M, O'Rahilly S and Barroso I. A family with severe insulin resistance and diabetes due to a mutation in AKT2. (2004) *Science* 304:1325-1328.

Gilfillan, CP. (2010) Review of the genetics of thyroid tumours: diagnostic and prognostic implications. *ANZ Journal of Surgery.* 80:33-40.-

Grossman A, Oppenheim J, Grondin G, St. Jean P and Beaudoin AR. (1989) Immunocytochemical localization of the [3H]estradiol-binding protein in rat pancreatic acinar cells. *Endocrinology.* 124:2857-2866.

Gutierrez-Hartmann A, Duval DL and Bradford AP. (2007) ETS transcription factors in endocrine systems. *Trends Endocrinol Metab.* 18(4):150-8.

Haas E, Meyer MR, Schurr U, Bhattacharya I, Minotti R, Nguyen HH, Heigl A, Lachat M, Genoni M and Barton M. (2007) Differential effects of 17beta-estradiol on function and expression of estrogen receptor alpha, estrogen receptor beta, and GPR30 in arteries and veins of patients with atherosclerosis. *Hypertension.* 49:1358-1363.

Hall JM, Couse JF and Korach KS. (2001) The multifaceted mechanisms of estradiol and estrogen receptor signaling. *J. Biol. Chem.* 276:36869-36872.

Handkiewicz-Junak D, Czarniecka A and Jarzab B. (2010) Molecular prognostic markers in papillary and follicular thyroid cancer: Current status and future directions. *Mol Cell Endocrinol.* 322:8-28.

He YY, Cai B, Yang YX, Liu XL and Wan XP. (2009) Estrogenic G protein-coupled receptor 30 signaling is involved in regulation of endometrial carcinoma by promoting proliferation, invasion potential, and interleukin-6 secretion via the MEK/ERK mitogen-activated protein kinase pathway. *Cancer Sci.* 100:1051-1061.

Hermenegildo C and Cano A. (2000) Pure anti-oestrogens. *Hum Reprod Update.* 6(3):237-43.

Herrmann BL, Saller B, Janssen OE, Gocke P, Bockisch A. Sperling H, Mann K and Broecker M. (2002) Impact of estrogen replacement therapy in a male with congenital aromatase deficiency caused by a novel mutation in the CYP19 gene. *J. Clin. Endocrinol. Metab.* 8:5476-5484.

Hodgson NC, Button J and Solorzano CC. (2004) Thyroid cancer: is the incidence still increasing? *Ann Surg Oncol.* 11:1093-7.

Hou P, Ji M and Xing M. (2008) Association of PTEN gene methylation with genetic alterations in the phosphatidylinositol 3-kinase/AKT signaling pathway in thyroid tumors. *Cancer.* 113:2440-2447.

Hou P, Liu D, Shan Y, Hu S, Studeman K, Condouris S et al. (2007) Genetic alterations and their relationship in the phosphatidylinositol 3-kinase/AKT pathway in thyroid cancer. *Clin Cancer Res.* 13:1161-1170.

Hugo ER, Brandebourg TD, Woo JG Loftus J, Alexander JW, Ben-Jonathan N. (2008) Bisphenol A at environmentally relevant doses inhibits adiponectin release from human adipose tissue explants and adipocytes. *Environ. Health Perspect.* 116:1642-1647.

Ikenoue T, Inoki K, Yang Q, Zhou X and Guan KL. Essential function of TORC2 in PKC and AKT turn motif phosphorylation, maturation and signaling. (2008) *EMBO J* 23:1919-31.

Jemal A, Siegel R, Ward E, Hao Y, Xu J and Thun MJ. (2009) Cancer statistics, 2009. *CA Cancer J Clin.* 59:225-49.

Jensen EV, DeSombre ER. (1973) Estrogen-receptor interaction. *Science.* 182:126-134.

Jones KP (1992). Estrogens and progestins: what to use and how to use it. *Clin. Obstet. Gynecol.* 32:871-883.

Jones PF, Jakubowicz T, Pitossi FJ, Maurer F and Hemmings BA. (1991) Molecular cloning and identification of a serine/threonine protein kinase of the second-messenger subfamily. *Proc Natl Acad Sci U S A.* 88:4171-4175.

Kennedy SG, Kandel ES, Cross TK and Hay N. (1999) AKT/Protein kinase B inhibits cell death by preventing the release of cytochrome c from mitochondria. *Mol Cell Biol* 19:5800-5810.

Kim CS and Zhu X. (2009) Lessons from mouse models of thyroid cancer. *Thyroid.* 19:1317-31.

Kim KH, Moriarty K and Bender JR. (2008) Vascular cell signaling by membrane estrogen receptors. *Steroids.* 73(9-10):864-9.

Klinge CM. (2000) Estrogen receptor interaction with co-activators and co-repressors. *Steroids* 65: 227-25.

Kossmehl P, Shakibaei M, Cogoli A, Infanger M, Curcio F, Schönberger J, Eilles C, Bauer J, Pickenhahn H, Schulze-Tanzil G, Paul M and Grimm D. (2003) Weightlessness induced apoptosis in normal thyroid cells and papillary thyroid carcinoma cells via extrinsic and intrinsic pathways. *Endocrinology.* 144:4172-9.

Kouniavsky G and Zeiger MA. (2010) Thyroid tumorigenesis and molecular markers in thyroid cancer. *Curr Opin Oncol.* 22:23-9.

Kuiper GG, Enmark E, Pelto-Huikko M, Nilsson S and Gustafsson JA. (1996) Cloning of a novel receptor expressed in rat prostate and ovary. *Proc Natl Acad Sci USA.* 93:5925-5930.

Kuiper GG, Carlsson B, Grandien K, Enmark E, Häggblad J, Nilsson S and Gustafsson JA. (1997) Comparison of the ligand binding specificity and transcript tissue distribution of estrogen receptors alpha and beta. *Endocrinology.* 138:863-870.

Kumar A, Klinge CM and Goldstein RE. (2010) Estradiol-induced proliferation of papillary and follicular thyroid cancer cells is mediated by estrogen receptors alpha and beta. *Int J Oncol.* 36:1067-1080.

Lee ML, Chen GG, Vlantis A C, Tse GM, Leung BC and van Hasselt CA. (2005) Induction of thyroid papillary carcinoma cell proliferation by estrogen is associated with an altered expression of Bcl-xL. *Cancer J.* 11:113-121.

Lemoine NR, Mayall ES, Wyllie FS, Farr CJ, Hughes D, Padua RA, Thurston V, Williams ED and Wynford-Thomas D. (1988) Activated ras oncogenes in human thyroid cancers. *Cancer Res.* 48:4459-4463.

Leto G, Tumminello FM, Crescimanno M, Flandina C and Gebbia N. (2004) Cathepsin D expression levels in non-gynecological solid tumors: clinical and therapeutic implications. *Clin Exp Metastasis.* 21:91-106.

Libutti SK. (2005) Understanding the role of gender in the incidence of thyroid cancer. *Cancer J.* 11:104-105.

Lima LP, Barros IA, Lisbôa PC, Araújo RL, Silva AC, Rosenthal D, Ferreira AC and Carvalho DP. (2006) Estrogen effects on thyroid iodide uptake and thyroperoxidase activity in normal and ovariectomized rats. *Steroids.* 71:653-9.

Liu MM, Albanese C, Anderson CM, Hilty K, Webb P, Uht RM, Price RH Jr, Pestell RG and Kushner PJ. (2002) Opposing action of estrogen receptors alpha and beta on cyclin D1 gene expression. *J Biol Chem.* 277:24353-24360.

Liu Z, Hou P, Ji M, Guan H, Studeman K, Jensen K, Vasko V, El-Naggar AK and Xing M. (2008) Highly prevalent genetic alterations in receptor tyrosine kinases and phosphatidylinositol 3-kinase/akt and mitogen-activated protein kinase pathways in anaplastic and follicular thyroid cancers. *J. Clin. Endocrinol. Metab.* 93:3106-3116.

Lu Q, Ebling H, Mittler J, Baur WE and Karas RH. (2002) MAP kinase mediates growth factor-induced nuclear translocation of estrogen receptor alpha. *FEBS Lett.* 516(1-3):1-8.Manning BD, and Cantley LC. (2007) AKT/PKB signaling: navigating downstream. *Cell* 129:1261-74.

Machens A, Hauptmann S and Dralle H. (2006) Disparities between male and female patients with thyroid cancers: sex difference or gender divide? *Clin Endocrinol (Oxf).* 65:500-5.

Manole D, Schildknecht B, Gosnell B, Adams E and Derwahl M. (2001) Estrogen promotes growth of human thyroid tumor cells by different molecular mechanisms. *J Clin Endocrinol Metab.* 86:1072-1077.

Mayo LD and Donner DB. (2001) A phosphatidylinositol 3-kinase/AKT pathway promotes translocation of Mdm2 from the cytoplasm to the nucleus. *Proc Natl Acad Sci U S A.* 98:11598-603.

Miller KA, Yeager N, Baker K, Liao XH, Refetoff S and Di Cristofano A. (2009) Oncogenic Kras requires simultaneous PI3K signaling to induce ERK activation and transform thyroid epithelial cells in vivo. *Cancer Res.* 69:3689-3694.

Moats RK II and Ramirez VD. (2000) Electron microscopic visualization of membrane-mediated uptake and translocation of estrogen-BSA:colloidal gold by hep G2 cells. *J Endocrinol.* 166:631-647.

Monje P and Boland R. (2001) Subcellular distribution of native estrogen receptor alpha and beta isoforms in rabbit uterus and ovary. *J Cell Biochem.* 82:467-479.

Monje P, Zanello S, Holick M and Boland R. (2001) Differential cellular localization of estrogen receptor alpha in uterine and mammary cells. *Mol Cell Endocrinol.* 181:117-129.

Mori M, Naito M, Watanabe H, Takeichi N, Dohi K and Ito A. (1990) Effects of sex difference, gonadectomy, and estrogen on N-methyl-N-nitrosourea induced rat thyroid tumors. *Cancer Res.* 50:7662-7.

Muise-Helmericks RC, Grimes HL, Bellacosa A, Malstrom SE, Tsichlis PN and Rosen N. (1998) Cyclin D expression is controlled post-transcriptionally via a phosphatidylinositol 3-kinase/AKT-dependent pathway. *J. Biol. Chem.* 273:29864-29872.

Müller RE, Johnston TC and Wotiz HH. (1979) Binding of estradiol to purified uterine plasma membranes. *J Biol Chem.* 254(16):7895-900.

Neff RL, Farrar WB, Kloos RT and Burman KD. (2008) Anaplastic thyroid cancer. *Endocrinol Metab Clin North Am.* 37:525-38.

Nikiforov YE. (2008) Thyroid carcinoma: molecular pathways and therapeutic targets. *Mod Pathol.* 2:S37-S43.

O'Dowd BF, Nguyen T, Marchese A, Cheng R, Lynch KR, Heng HH, Kolakowski LF Jr and George SR. (1998) Discovery of three novel G-protein-coupled receptor genes. *Genomics.* 47:310-313.

Owman C, Blay P, Nilsson C and Lolait SJ. (1996) Cloning of human cDNA encoding a novel heptahelix receptor expressed in Burkitt's lymphoma and widely distributed in brain and peripheral tissues. *Biochem. Biophys. Res. Commun.* 228:285-292.

Pedram A, Razandi M and Levin ER. (2006) Nature of functional estrogen receptors at the plasma membrane. *Mol Endocrinol* 20:1996-2009.

Pestell RG, Albanese C, Reutens AT, Segall JE, Lee RJ and Arnold A. (1999) The cyclins and cyclin-dependent kinase inhibitors in hormonal regulation of proliferation and differentiation. *Endocr Rev.* 20:501-534.

Posern G and Treisman R. (2006) Actin' together: serum response factor, its cofactors and the link to signal transduction. *Trends Cell Biol.* 16(11):588-96.

Rajoria S, Suriano R, Shanmugam A, Wilson YL, Schantz SP, Geliebter J and Tiwari RK. (2010) Metastatic phenotype is regulated by estrogen in thyroid cells. *Thyroid.* 20:33-41.

Roberts PJ and Der CJ. (2007) Targeting the Raf-MEK-ERK mitogen-activated protein kinase cascade for the treatment of cancer. *Oncogene.* 26:3291-310.

Ruggiero RJ and Likis FE. (2002) Estrogen: physiology, pharmacology, and formulations for replacement therapy. *J. Midwifery Womens Health.* 47:130-138.

Sarbassov DD, Guertin DA, Ali SM and Sabatini DM. Phosphorylation and regulation of AKT/PKB by the rictor-mTOR complex. (2005) *Science* 18:1098-1101.

Sekeris CE. (1990) The mitochondrial genome: a possible primary site of action of steroid hormones. *In Vivo.* 4:317-320.

Smallridge RC, Marlow LA and Copland JA. (2009) Anaplastic thyroid cancer: molecular pathogenesis and emerging therapies. *Endocr Relat Cancer.* 16:17-44.

Song RX and Santen RJ. (2003) Apoptotic action of estrogen. *Apoptosis.* 8:55-60

Speroff L, Glass RH and Kase NG. (1999) *Clin. Gynecol. Endocrinol. Infert. (6th ed).* Lippincott Williams & Wilkins: Philadelphia.

Stender JD, Frasor J, Komm B, Chang KC, Kraus WL and Katzenellenbogen BS. (2007) Estrogen-regulated gene networks in human breast cancer cells: involvement of E2F1 in the regulation of cell proliferation. *Mol Endocrinol.* 21:2112-23.

Stirone C, Duckles SP, Krause DN and Procaccio V. (2005) Estrogen increases mitochondrial efficiency and reduces oxidative stress in cerebral blood vessels. *Mol Pharmacol.* 68:959-965.

Strom A, Hartman J, Foster JS, Kietz S, Wimalasena J and Gustafsson JA. (2004) Estrogen receptor beta inhibits 17beta-estradiol-stimulated proliferation of the breast cancer cell line T47D. *Proc. Natl. Acad. Sci. USA.* 101:1566-1571.

Takada Y, Kato C, Kondo S, Korenaga R and Ando J. (1997) Cloning of cDNAs encoding G protein-coupled receptor expressed in human endothelial cells exposed to fluid shear stress. *Biochem. Biophys. Res. Commun.* 240:737-741.

Testa JR and Bellacosa A. AKT plays a central role in tumorigenesis. (2001) *Proc. Natl. Acad. Sci. USA* 98:10983-10985.

Thiruvengadam A, Govindarajulu P and Aruldhas MM. (2003) Modulatory effect of estradiol and testosterone on the development of N-nitrosodiisopropanolamine induced thyroid tumors in female rats. *Endocr Res.* 29:43-51.

Vasko VV and Saji M. (2007) Molecular mechanisms involved in differentiated thyroid cancer invasion and metastasis. *Curr Opin Oncol.* 19:11-17.

Vivacqua A, Bonofiglio D, Albanito L, Madeo A, Rago V, Carpino A et al. (2006) 17beta-estradiol, genistein, and 4-hydroxytamoxifen induce the proliferation of thyroid cancer cells through the G protein-coupled receptor GPR30. *Mol Pharmacol.* 70:1414-1423.

Wang F, Porter W, Xing W, Archer TK and Safe S. (1997) Identification of a functional imperfect estrogen-responsive element in the 5'- promoter region of the human cathepsin D gene. *Biochemistry.* 36:7793-7801.

Wang Y, Hou P, Yu H, Wang W, Ji M, Zhao S et al. (2007) High prevalence and mutual exclusivity of genetic alterations in the phosphatidylinositol-3-kinase/akt pathway in thyroid tumors. *J Clin Endocrinol Metab.* 92:2387-2390.

Watson CS, Alyea RA, Jeng YJ and Kochukov MY. (2007) Nongenomic actions of low concentration estrogens and xenoestrogens on multiple tissues. *Mol Cell Endocrinol* 274:1-7.

Weihua Z, Saji S, Makinen S, Cheng G, Jensen EV, Warner M and Gustafsson JA. Estrogen receptor (ER) beta, a modulator of ERalpha in the uterus. *Proc. Natl. Acad. Sci. USA.* 97:5936-5941.

Withers DJ, Gutierrez JS, Towery H, Burks DJ, Ren JM, Previs S, Zhang Y, Bernal D, Pons S, Shulman GI, Bonner-Weir S and White MF. (1998) Disruption of IRS-2 causes type 2 diabetes in mice. *Nature* 391:900-904.

Wong CW, McNally C, Nickbarg E, Komm BS and Cheskis BJ. (2002) Estrogen receptor-interacting protein that modulates its nongenomic activity-crosstalk with Src/Erk phosphorylation cascade. *Proc Natl Acad Sci U S A.* 99:14783-14788.

Wrutniak C, Cassar-Malek I, Marchal S, Rascle A, Heusser S, Keller JM, Flechon J, Dauca M, Samarut J, Ghysdael J and Cabello G. (1995) A 43-kDa protein related to c-Erb A alpha 1 is located in the mitochondrial matrix of rat liver. *J Biol Chem.* 270:16347-16354.

Xing M. (2005) BRAF mutation in thyroid cancer. *Endocr. Relat. Cancer.* 12:245-262.

Yeager N, Brewer C, Cai KQ, Xu XX and Di Cristofano A. (2008) mTOR is the key effector of PI3K-initiated proliferative signals in the thyroid follicular epithelium. *Cancer Res.* 68:444-449.

Yeager N, Klein-Szanto A, Kimura S and Di Cristofano A. (2007) Pten loss in the mouse thyroid causes goiter and follicular adenomas: insights into thyroid function and Cowden disease pathogenesis. *Cancer Res.* 67:959-66.

Zeng Q, Chen GG, Vlantis AC and van Hasselt CA. (2007) Oestrogen mediates the growth of human thyroid carcinoma cells via an oestrogen receptor-ERK pathway. *Cell Prolif.* 40:921-35.

Zhang Z, Duan L, Du X, Ma H, Park I, Lee C, Zhang J and Shi J. (2008) The proliferative effect of estradiol on human prostate stromal cells is mediated through activation of ERK. *Prostate.* 68:508-516.

9

Suspicious Thyroid Fine Needle Aspiration Aspiration Biopsy: TSH as a Malignancy Marker?

Renata Boldrin de Araujo, Célia Regina Nogueira, Jose Vicente Tagliarini, Emanuel Celice Castilho, Mariângela de Alencar Marques, Yoshio Kiy, Lidia R. Carvalho and Gláucia M. F. S. Mazeto
Botucatu Medical School, Sao Paulo State University, Unesp
Brazil

1. Introduction

Thyroid nodules are common, affecting from 5 to 15% of the population (Tunbridge et al., 1977; Vander et al., 1968). Thyroid cancer, on the other hand, is uncommon and represents only 5% of all nodules, with an incidence in the United States of 1/10,000 inhabitants (Davies & Welch, 2006). Among thyroid neoplasms, the differentiated carcinomas (DTC) are the most frequent, and are responsible for about 75% of the malignant nodules of this gland (Schlumberger & Pacini, 1997).

Despite the fact that the great majority of thyroid lesions are benign and the mortality rate due to thyroid cancer is low (Schlumberger & Pacini, 1997), the incidence of thyroid cancer is increasing at a rate of greater than 5% per year (Davies & Welch, 2006). Thus, it is important to identify the nodules which are malignant and require surgical treatment.

The method of choice for the diagnostic evaluation of thyroid nodules is fine needle aspiration biopsy (FNAB) (Bennedbaek et al., 1999; Bennedbaek & Hegedus, 2000; Cooper et al., 2006; Schlumberger, 1998). FNAB is both highly sensitive (65 - 98%) and highly specific (72 - 100%) (Gharib & Goellner, 1993; Mazzaferri, 1993; Sherman, 2003), and provides satisfactory diagnostic results in 80% of cases, with an increase of this percentage after a new FNAB (Gharib & Goellner, 1993). In cases of DTC, FNAB has been shown to be particularly useful in the diagnosis of papillary carcinoma (PC). However, in cases of follicular (FC) and Hürthle carcinoma (HC), as in the case of the follicular variant of PC (FVPC), FNAB is useful only as a screening test. In these cases FNAB indicates the corresponding cytological pattern (follicular or Hürthle), but is not able to differentiate benign tumors from the malignant tumors. In these cases, the patients undergo surgery for histological analysis and definitive diagnosis (Faquin & Baloch, 2010; Tuttle et al., 1998).

Faced with the uncertainty of the diagnostic evaluation of thyroid nodules, several clinical risk factors (Kimura et al., 2009; Tuttle et al., 1998), imaging tests (Wiest, 1998; Frates, 2006) and molecular markers (Melck & Yip, 2011) have been proposed as malignancy indicators. Recently, some studies have reported an association between increased serum levels of thyroid stimulating hormone (TSH) and thyroid cancer (Boelaert et al., 2006; Gul et al., 2010; Jonklaas et al., 2008). However, this relationship has not yet been established for the more doubtful cases, such as those with an inconclusive cytological diagnosis for FC or HC.

The objective of this study was to evaluate whether the TSH serum levels can help to differentiate benign cases from the malignant cases in patients with an FNAB that shows a follicular or Hürthle pattern.

2. Material and methods

This retrospective study was approved by the Committee of Ethics in Research of Botucatu Medical School (FMB) of the Sao Paulo State University - UNESP (protocol number 3626-2010).

We analyzed the cytological reports from patients carrying thyroid nodules that were submitted for thyroid FNAB at the Clinics Hospital FMB–Unesp between the years of 2003 and 2008. Of these, 59 cases with suspicious or inconclusive cytological diagnosis for FC or HC were selected. We included those nodules that presented a follicular or Hürthle pattern with the following reported descriptions: "follicular lesion," "follicular tumor," "follicular neoplasia," "Hürthle follicular lesion," "Hürthle tumor" or "Hürthle neoplasia." The medical data of these patients were evaluated, and we found 31 cases that were submitted to surgery and with histological diagnosis. The effective study sample consisted of 28 women and three men, with an average age of 52.1 years.

The patients were divided into two groups according to the presence (group M) or absence (group WM) of a histological diagnosis of malignancy. Pre-operative TSH serum levels were compared between group M and group WM. The two groups were also compared in regards to gender, age, smoking history, previous exposure to radiation and free thyroxine (FT4) serum levels. These same comparisons were performed after the exclusion of the cases which presented hypo- or hyperthyroidism.

The histological diagnosis of malignancy was based on the criteria set by the World Health Organization (WHO). Reports of PC, FC, HC and FVPC were considered to be malignant, and reports of follicular adenoma, Hürthle adenoma, colloid goiter and Hashimoto's thyroiditis were considered to be benign (DeLellis et al., 2004).

The serum levels of TSH and FT4 were obtained from the medical records. The average pre-operative hormone levels of each patient were determined by the average of three separate test results for these hormones, which were collected at different times up to one year prior to surgery. TSH and FT4 were measured by chemiluminescence, with a normal range of 0.8-1.9 ng/dL and 0.4-4.0 mUI/mL, respectively (DPC, Los Angeles, CA). Thyroid function was considered normal when TSH and FT4 were within normal reference ranges; hypothyroid, when TSH was elevated; and hyperthyroid, when TSH was suppressed.

2.1 Statistical analysis

The collected data were charted in a Microsoft Excel® worksheet (Microsoft Corporation, EUA) and submitted to statistical analysis through the computer program SPSS/Windows (version 10.0.7). To study the association between the qualitative variables, we used the Chi-square test. For the quantitative variables, we used the Student's T test. The significance level was of 5% (Zar, 1999).

3. Results

Of the 31 cases submitted to surgery, 14 showed malignancy upon histopathological analysis (group M). The malignancies included nine PCs, three FCs (one case with both PC and FC), one HC, one Hürthle tumor and one follicular tumor of uncertain malignant meaning. Thus, the concordance of suspicious or inconclusive FNAB for FC or HC with malignancy was 45.2% and the concordance with FC or HC was 12.9%. 17 patients (54.8%) had benign histological reports (group WM).

The M and WM groups did not differ significantly as to serum levels of TSH and FT4 ($p>0.05$). There were no significant differences in age or gender distribution ($p>0.05$). There were two smokers in the WM group and no smokers in the M group. In addition one patient in the WM group had previous exposure to radiation (Table 1).

Seven patients (22.6%) presented hypo- or hyperthyroidism and were under treatment with thyroid medication. These included two (28.6%) patients from the M group and five (71.4%) patients from the WM group. After excluding such cases, the M and WM groups still did not differ in regards to the analyzed parameters (Table 2).

Data	Group		P
	M	WM	
Female Gender n (%)**	12 (85.7)	16 (94.1)	0.43
Age (years)*	48.8 ± 12.5	54.8 ± 13.9	0.21
Smoking n (%)***	0 (0.0)	2 (100.0)	-
Previous exporsure to radiation ***	0 (0.0)	1 (100.0)	-
TSH (mUI/L)*	2.04 ± 1.74	3.08 ± 2.67	0.22
FT4 (ng/dL)*	1.56 ± 0.59	1.35 ± 0.19	0.17

* Average ± standard deviation (Student's T test); ** Chi-square test; ***not submitted to statistical analysis due to small sample number. M: presence of malignancy; WM: absence of malignancy; TSH: thyroid stimulating hormone; FT4: free thyroxine.

Table 1. General data from 31 patients, with fine needle aspiration biopsies (FNAB) with suspicious or inconclusive cytological diagnosis for FC or HC, submitted to thyroidectomy, according to the final histological diagnosis of presence (group M) or absence (group WM) of malignancy.

Data	Group		P
	M	WM	
Female Gender n (%)**	10 (83.3)	11 (91.7)	0.54
Age (years)*	50.4 ± 11.3	52.3 ± 15.8	0.74
Smoking n (%)***	0 (0.0)	2 (100.0)	-
TSH (mUI/L)*	1.79 ± 1.03	1.81 ± 1.16	0.96
FT4 (ng/dL)*	1.59 ± 0.64	1.33 ± 0.18	0.19

* Average ± standard deviation (Student's T test); ** Chi-square test; ***not submitted to statistical analysis due to small sample number. M: presence of malignancy; WM: absence of malignancy; TSH: thyroid stimulating hormone; FT4: free thyroxine.

Table 2. General data from 24 patients, without hypo- or hyperthyroidism, with fine needle aspiration biopsies (FNAB) with suspicious or inconclusive cytological diagnosis for FC or HC, submitted to thyroidectomy, according to the final histological diagnosis of presence (group M) or absence (group WM) of malignancy.

4. Discussion

Considering that in DTC the follicular cell physiologic characteristic of TSH responsiveness is preserved (Biondi et al., 2005; Carayon et al., 1980; Ichikawa et al., 1976), it is presumable that a greater stimulation provided by this hormone might be a contributing factor to the tumor genesis. In fact, some studies have reported an association between increased TSH serum levels and thyroid malignancy. Boelaert et al. have observed that the malignancy risk of a thyroid nodule rises along with the TSH serum levels, indicating that these levels are an independent prognostic factor for malignancy and may be used in conjunction with FNAB in detecting such tumors (Boelaert et al., 2006). Gul et al. have reported that low serum levels of FT4, associated with high levels of TSH (still within the normal patterns), are associated with a greater probability of thyroid cancer, independent of gender and goiter type (Gul et al., 2010). This study also suggests that hormone levels may be used in conjunction with FNAB in diagnosing thyroid cancer, as do gender, age and goiter type (Boelaert et al., 2006; Kumar et al., 1999; Tuttle et al., 1998).

Although FNAB is the method of choice for the evaluation of thyroid nodules, the technique presents limitations in the investigation of lesions of follicular or Hürthle patterns (Faquin & Baloch, 2010). Thus, the TSH serum levels might be used as a malignancy marker in such lesions. However, few studies have evaluated the relationship between thyroid malignancy and levels of this hormone specifically in follicular or Hürthle lesions (Tuttle et al., 1998). In the present study we have evaluated such relationship, and observed no association between TSH serum levels and malignancy in follicular or Hürthle lesions: the average serum levels of TSH and FT4 were not significantly different between the benign and the malignant cases.

One possible reason for such discordance in comparison with the majority of previous studies may be that, in this study, only the cases with suspicious or inconclusive aspiration for FC or HC were analyzed. Others have evaluated the presence of malignancy by studying DTC in general, including PC (Gul et al., 2010; Haymart et al., 2008; Jonklaas et al., 2008), or several types of carcinomas, including those independent from TSH (Boelaert et al., 2006; Polyzos et al., 2008). When evaluating only the FNABs with a diagnosis of follicular neoplasia, Tuttle et al. also did not find any differences in the results of thyroid function tests between benign and malignant cases (Tuttle et al., 1998).

Another reason for the distinct findings in this study may be that we have evaluated only the cases with histological confirmation of the diagnosis. Others have included non-thyroidectomized patients, who had "diagnostic confirmation" only through the evolutionary evaluation during a two year follow-up period (Boelaert et al., 2006; Polyzos et al., 2008; Fiore et al., 2009), a time that might be considered insufficient in the DTC cases.

Another divergence between this study and others (Gul et al., 2010; Jonklaas et al., 2008) is that this study excluded the cases with cytological diagnosis of malignancy and those without recent TSH level measurements. At first, the cases with radiation exposure were not excluded. However, only one patient had been submitted to previous external radiotherapy, presenting a final histological diagnosis of benignity. Although those with thyroid dysfunction were also not excluded at first, when these patients were withdrawn from the analysis, there was still no statistically significant difference between the hormone levels in benign and malignant cases.

In regards to the remaining clinical aspects examined in this study, there was also divergence between the present study and previous reports mentioned. We did not find any significant differences regarding age and gender that might predict nodular malignancy. In fact, the influence of such aspects is controversial and, similar to TSH evaluation, many of the previous studies did not restrict their evaluation only to cases with suspicion of FC or HC. Boelaert et al. showed an association of the male sex or the age extremes with a greater malignancy risk (Boelaert et al., 2006). Haymart et al. has also reported an association of greater risk of malignancy with the male sex and younger age groups, although they found no association with older age (Haymart et al., 2008). On the other hand, Gul et al. associated age of greater than 60 years to a greater risk of malignancy, but did not find an association with gender (Gul et al., 2010). Considering the lesions of follicular pattern, Raber et al., when evaluating cases with diagnostic FNAB for follicular neoplasia, also did not associate the age extremes or the male gender to a greater risk of malignancy (Raber et al., 2000). Tuttle et al. did not find an association between age and the occurrence of malignant tumors, although they did associate the male gender to a greater risk of malignancy (Tuttle et al., 1998). Schlinkert et al. also studied cases with diagnostic FNAB for follicular neoplasia and associated younger ages, but not older ages, with a greater risk of malignancy (Schlinkert et al., 1997). However, other authors have found an association between older ages and greater probability of malignant tumor (Cooper et al., 2006; Tuttle et al., 1998). Thus, there is a great divergence even among findings of studies that are restricted to the cytological diagnosis of follicular neoplasia. Moreover, the criteria for surgery submission were different in each study, which complicates the comparison between studies.

Another characteristic examined in this study was smoking history, which also could not be associated with a greater risk of malignancy. This finding is in agreement with other case-control studies (Kreiger & Parkes, 2000; Mack et al., 2003). In contrast to these studies, Sokic et al. found an association between smoking and a greater risk of thyroid cancer. However, the Sokic study was carried out in a population of hospitalized patients (Sokic et al., 1994), for whom tobacco exposure was modified due to the hospital condition.

We must highlight that the present study presents important limitations. One of the most relevant limitations is the small number of cases evaluated (31 patients). The retrospective nature of the study contributed to that small number by presenting problems such as irregular follow-up, non-submission to thyroidectomy and therefore absence of a histopathological report, and the absence of TSH measurements close in time to the surgical procedure. However, independent of the limitations of this and similar studies, it is a fact that the reports investigating nodular malignancy criteria in follicular tumors cases are not in unanimous agreement.

Therefore, there is still much controversy surrounding the pre-operative diagnosis of thyroid nodules with FNAB compatible with a follicular or Hürthle pattern. Recently, the *National Cancer Institute Thyroid Fine-needle Aspiration State of the Science Conference* (Bethesda, Maryland, USA) attempted to minimize such divergences by reclassifying many of these lesions as benign, follicular lesions of uncertain meaning or follicular neoplasia, presenting a malignancy risk lower than 1%, between 5 and 10% and between 20 and 30%, respectively (Baloch et al., 2008). However, many services have not yet adhered to this new cytological classification and, even when this classification is used, there is still a significant percentage of thyroid nodules for which diagnostic doubt will only be clarified after surgical approach.

5. Conclusion

In conclusion, in this study the serum levels of TSH and FT4, in addition to gender, age and smoking habits, were not useful in differentiating FC or HC from benign lesions of similar cytological patterns. Considering the controversy surrounding this area and the absence of significant evidence, there is a need for more studies examining the correlation between the cytological diagnoses in cases of follicular tumors with the pre-operative TSH serum levels. Future studies should have an adequate study design and a greater study population, in order to improve the diagnosis of these lesions.

6. References

Baloch Z.W., LiVolsi V.A., Asa S.L., Rosai J., Merino M.J., Randolph G., Vielh P., DeMay R.M., Sidawy M.K., & Frable W.J. (2008). Diagnostic Terminology and Morphologic Criteria for Cytologic Diagnosis of Thyroid Lesions: A Synopsis of the National Cancer Institute Thyroid Fine-Needle Aspiration State of the Science Conference. Diagn Cytopathol., 36:425–437.

Bennedbaek F.N., Perrild H., & Hegedus L. (1999). Diagnosis and treatment of the solitary thyroid nodule. Results of a European survey. *Clin Endocrinol* (Oxf), 50:357–363

Bennedbaek F.N. & Hegedus L. (2000). Management of the solitary thyroid nodule: results of a North American survey. *J Clin Endocrinol Metab* 85:2493–2498.

Biondi B., Filetti S. & Schlumberger M. (2005). Thyroidhormone herapy and thyroid cancer: a reassessment. Nature Clinical Practice. *Endocrinology & Metabolism,* 1(1): 32–40.

Boelaert K., Horacek J., Holder R. L., Watkinson J. C., Sheppard M. C., & Franklyn J. A. (2006). Serum Thyrotropin Concentration as a Novel Predictor of Malignancy in Thyroid Nodules Investigated by Fine-Needle Aspiration. *J Clin Endocrinol Metab,* 91(11):4295-4301.

Carayon P., Thomas-Morvan C., Castanas E., & Tubiana M. (1980). Human thyroid cancer: membrane thyrotropin binding and adenylate cyclase activity. *J Clin Endocrinol Metab,* 51:915–920.

Cooper D.S., Doherty G.M., Haugen B.R., Kloos R.T., Lee S.L., Mandel S.J., Mazzaferri E.L., McIver B., Sherman S.I., & Tuttle R.M. (2006). Management guidelines for patients with thyroid nodules and differentiated thyroid cancer. *Thyroid,* 16:1–33

Davies L. & Welch H.G. (2006). Increasing incidence of thyroid cancer in the United States, 1973–2002. *Journal of the American Medical Association,* 295 2164–2167.

DeLellis R.A., Lloyd R.D., Heitz P.U., Eng C. (editors). (2004) WHO: Pathology and Genetics, In: *Tumours of Endocrine Organs,* IARC Press, Lyon, France.

Faquin W.C., Baloch Z.W. (2010). Fine-Needle Aspiration of Follicular Patterned Lesions of the Thyroid: Diagnosis, Management, and Follow-Up According to National Cancer Institute (NCI) Recommendations. Diagn Cytopathol, 38(10):731-739.

Fiore E., Rago T., Provenzale M.A., Scutari M., Ugolini C., Basolo F., Di Coscio G., Berti P., Grasso L., Elisei R., Pinchera A., Vitti P. (2009). *Endocr. Relat. Cancer,* 16, 1251–1260.

Frates M.C., Benson C.B., Doubilet P.M., Kunreuther E., Contreras M., & Cibas E.S. (2006). Prevalence and distribution of carcinoma in patients with solitary and multiple thyroid nodules on sonography. *J Clin Endocrinol Metab,* 91:3411-7.

Gharib H. & Goellner J.R. (1993). Fine-needle aspiration biopsy of the thyroid: an appraisal. *Ann Intern Med,* 118:282–289

Gul K., Ozdemir D., Dirikoc A., Oguz A., Tuzun D., Baser H., Ersoy R., & Cakir B. (2010). Are endogenously lower serum thyroid hormones new predictors for thyroid malignancy in addition to higher serum thyrotropin? *Endocrine.* 37(2):253-260.

Haymart M.R., Repplinger D.J., Leverson G.E, Elson D.F, Sippel R.S., Jaume J.C., & Chen H. (2008). *J. Clin. Endocrinol. Metab.*, 93, 809–814.

Ichikawa Y., Saito E., Abe Y., Homma M., & Muraki T. (1976). Presence of TSH receptor in thyroid neoplasms. *J Clin Endocrinol Metab,* 42:395–398.

Jonklaas J, Nsouli-Maktabi H, & Soldin SJ. (2008). Endogenous thyrotropin and triiodothyronine concentrations in individuals with thyroid cancer. *Thyroid,* 18(9):943-52.

Kimura ET, Tincani AJ, Ward LS, Nogueira CR, Carvalho GA, Maia AL, Tavares MR, Teixeira G, Kulcsar MAV, Biscolla RPM, Cavalcanti CEO, Correa LAC, del Negro A, Friguglieti CUM, Hojaij F, Abrahão M, & Andrada NC. (2009). Doença nodular da tireóide: Diagnóstico, In: *Diretrizes Clínicas na Saúde Suplementar,* Sociedade Brasileira de Endocrinologia e Metabolismo, Sociedade Brasileira de Cirurgia de Cabeça e Pescoço, pp. 1-14, Associação Médica Brasileira e Agência Nacional de Saúde Suplementar, retrieved from http://www.projetodiretrizes.org.br/ans/diretrizes/29.pdf.

Kreiger N. & Parkes R. (2000). Cigarrete smoking and the risk of thyroid cancer. *European Journal of Cancer,* 36, 1969-1973.

Kumar H., Daykin J., Holder R., Watkinson J. C., Sheppard M. C., & Franklin J. A. (1999) Gender, Clinical Findings, and Serum Thyrotropin Measurements in the Prediction of Thyroid Neoplasia in 1005 Patients Presenting with Thyroid Enlargement and Investigated by Fine-Needle Aspiration Cytology. *Thyroid,* 9(11):1105-1109.

Mack, W.J., Martin, S.P., Dal Maso, L., Galanti, R., Xiang M., Franceschi S., Hallquist A., Jin F., Kolonel L., La Vecchia C., Levi F., Linos A., Lund E., McTiernan A., Mabuchi K., Negri E., Wingren G., & Ron E. (2003). A pooled analysis of case–control studies of thyroid cancer: cigarette smoking and consumption of alcohol, coffee, and tea. *Cancer Causes and Control,* 14: 773–785.

Mazzaferri E.L. (1993). Management of a solitary thyroid nodule. *N Engl J Med,* 328:553–559.

Melck AL, Yip L. (2011). Predicting malignancy in thyroid nodules: Molecular advances. *Head Neck.* Aug 4. doi: 10.1002/hed.21818. [Epub ahead of print].

Polyzos S.A., Kita M., Efstathiadou Z., Poulakos P., Slavakis A., Sofianou D., Flaris N., Leontsini M., Kourtis A., & Avramidis A. (2008). *J. Cancer Res. Clin. Oncol.,* 134, 953–960.

Raber W., Kaserer K., Niederle B., & Vierhapper H. (2000). Risk factors for malignancy of thyroid nodules initially identified as follicular neoplasia by fine-needle aspiration: results of a prospective study of one hundred twenty patients. *Thyroid,* Aug;10(8):709-712.

Schlinkert, R.T., van Heerden, J.A., Goellner, J.R., Gharib, H., Smith, S.L., Rosales, R.F., & Weaver, A.L. (1997). Factors that predict malignant thyroid lesions when Fine-Needle Aspiration is "Suspicious for Follicular Neoplasm". *Mayo Clin Proc,* 72:913-916.

Schlumberger M.J. (1998). Papillary and follicular thyroid carcinoma. *N Engl J Med,* 338:297–306.

Schlumberger M. & Pacini F. (1997). *Tumeurs de la thyroïde,* Nucléon. Sherman S.I. (2003). *Thyroid carcinoma,* Lancet, 361:501–511.

Sherman SI. (2003). Thyroid carcinoma. *Lancet* 361:501–511.

Sokic, S.I., Adanja, B.J., Vlajinac, H.D., Jankovic, R.R., Marinkovic, J.P., Zivaljevic, V.R. (1994). Risk factors for thyroid cancer. *Neoplasma*, 41, 371-374.

Tunbridge W.M., Evered D.C., Hall R., Appleton D., Brewis M., Clark F., Evans J.G., Young E., Bird T., & Smith P.A. (1977). The spectrum of thyroid disease in a community: the Whickham survey. *Clin Endocrinol* (Oxf), 7:481–493.

Tuttle R.M., Lemar H., & Burch H.B. (1998). Clinical Features Associated with an Increased Risk of Thyroid Malignancy in Patients with Follicular Neoplasia by Fine-Needle Aspiration. *Thyroid*, 8(5):377-383.

Vander J.B., Gaston E.A., & Dawber T.R. (1968). The significance of nontoxic thyroid nodules. Final report of a 15-year study of the incidence of thyroid malignancy. *Ann Intern Med*, 69:537–540

Wiest P.W., Hartshorne M.F., Inskip P.D., Crooks L.A., Vela B.S., & Telepak R.J. (1998). Thyroid palpation versus high-resolution thyroid ultrasonography in the detection of nodules. *J Ultrasound Med*;17:487-96.

Zar J. (1999). *Biostatistical analysis*, 4th ed. New Jersey: Prebtice-Hall.

Part 2

Treatment of Thyroid and Parathyroid Diseases

10

Minimally-Invasive Parathyroid Surgery

David Rosen, Joseph Sciarrino and Edmund A. Pribitkin
Thomas Jefferson University, Philadelphia, PA
USA

1. Introduction

Parathyroid surgery was first performed to correct primary hyperparathyroidism less than 100 years ago, and surgical treatment remains the only successful and durable cure for the disorder. [1,2] Techniques have evolved over the past century and continue to change and develop to this day. The conventional technique of bilateral neck exploration, though effective, has the disadvantage of being an invasive procedure, resulting in greater pain, poorer cosmesis, longer operative time, and longer hospitalization. More recently, developments in adjunctive technologies have allowed the development of less invasive techniques to achieve the same end result. This chapter will briefly discuss the conventional surgical treatment of primary hyperparathyroidism followed by a look at the minimally invasive techniques that are being developed and used today.

2. Anatomy and embryology

Knowledge of the anatomy and embryology of the parathyroid glands is paramount to the success of surgery, regardless of the techniques employed. The variability in gland position can make localization difficult both pre-operatively and intra-operatively. The parathyroids are endocrine glands that develop from the endoderm of the 3rd and 4th pharyngeal pouches beginning in the 5th week of gestation. They migrate from this position inferiorly, reaching their final locations by the 7th week. The 3rd pharyngeal pouch develops into both the thymus and the inferior parathyroids, while the 4th arch becomes the superior glands.[1-3] Parathyroid glands are usually about 5 x 3 x 1 mm in size with an average weight of 35 mg, although adenomatous glands may be much larger.[3]

Normally, each set of glands is paired, resulting in 2 superior and 2 inferior glands. This is the case in 84% of patients. About 3% of patients will have only 3 glands, and 13% of patients may have 5 or more glands. The superior parathyroid glands normally reside postero-medial to the superior thyroid lobes, near the cricothyroid junction, while the inferior glands tend to be on the postero-lateral side of the inferior thyroid lobe, inferior to where the recurrent laryngeal nerve and inferior thyroid artery cross. The inferior parathyroids are usually found within 2 cm of the lower pole of the thyroid. This anatomic arrangement of glands is true in about 80% of patients. However, aberrant migration is common, and the glands can be found in ectopic locations in many cases. Ectopic superior parathyroid glands may be retroesophageal, intrathyroidal, or in the posterior mediastinum. Inferior parathyroid glands have more variable ectopic sites as a result of their longer migration. These sites include the thyrothymic tissue, thyroid, thymus, anterior mediastinum, and within the carotid sheath. Understanding of this anatomic variability is important in interpreting preoperative imaging and directing operative exploration [1-3]

3. Pathophysiology

Overproduction of parathyroid hormone (PTH) is the defining feature of hyperparathyroidism. Hyperparathyroidism may be caused by a single parathyroid adenoma, multi-gland hyperplasia, double adenomas, or parathyroid carcinoma. Single adenoma accounts for about 81-96% of hyperparathyroidism, depending on the series. Multigland hyperplasia accounts for 4-14%, double adenomas 2-11%, and parathyroid carcinoma <1%.[1,2,4] Traditional bilateral neck exploration remains the standard of care for parathyroid carcinoma[1] so the focus of this chapter on minimally invasive techniques will be on benign disease.

Single adenoma	81-96%
Multi gland hyperplasia	4-14%
Double adenoma	2-11%
Carcinoma	<1%

Table 1. Causes of Primary Hyperparathyroidism

4. Traditional bilateral neck exploration

Traditional bilateral neck exploration (BNE) was the primary approach used by parathyroid surgeons until this past decade when minimally invasive techniques became more prevalent. Even as recently as 1998 nearly ¾ of parathyroid surgeons were still performing bilateral cervical exploration as the primary surgical technique.[3] In the absence of other significant contraindications, all patients with diagnosed primary hyperparathyroidism, tertiary hyperparathyroidism, or select cases of secondary hyperparathyroidisim are candidates for this operation, and no preoperative localization studies are required, as all glands should be visualized intraoperatively. [1,2,5]

BNE requires general anesthesia, typically with endotracheal intubation and often with a nerve integrity monitoring tube. A midline, transverse 3-5 cm cervical incision is made and carried through platysma, subplatysmal flaps elevated, the strap muscles divided in midline, and dissection and exploration continued until all parathyroid glands are visualized. This typically entails anteromedial retraction of the thyroid lobe to reveal the parathyroids posteriorly. Care is taken to safeguard the recurrent laryngeal nerve. Glands that are abnormal in appearance are resected. Those that are questionable may be biopsied and sent for frozen section pathology to guide decision of whether or not to resect. If all glands appear abnormal as is the case with multi-gland hyperplasia, the surgeon may perform a subtotal or total resection with autotransplantation. A subtotal resection, also known as a 3.5 gland resection is accomplished by resecting 3 abnormal glands, and approximately ½ of the most normal-appearing gland, leaving approximately 50 mg of parathyroid tissue. This approach removes the majority, but not all of the PTH secreting tissue in an attempt to allow the patient to become normocalcemic without needing chronic vitamin D and calcium supplementation. A total resection with autotransplantation involves resecting all found glands and then implanting small sections of the gland into a distant site; typically 12-24 sites within the subcutaneous tissue or the brachioradialis of the non-dominant forearm. Again, this maintains functioning parathyroid tissue to reduce the risk of lifetime supplementation and permits titration of hormone level by future selective removal of auto-transplanted parathyroid tissue. [1,2,5]

Intraoperative PTH monitoring is frequently used to determine completeness of resection of abnormal tissue. If PTH does not drop to <50% of the pre-operative level, then the exploration is continued in the neck and mediastinum to look for ectopic tissue. If all ectopic sites have been explored and the Miami criterion has not been met, the operation is concluded and further work-up postoperatively with imaging must be done.[1-3,6,7]

Cure rates have been reported at >95% with a single operation, and complications at <4%. [1,2,5] Complications include recurrent laryngeal nerve (RLN) paresis, persistent hypocalcemia, and hematoma. Postoperatively patients are admitted at least overnight, and postoperative calcium levels are followed to screen for hypocalcemia. Patients are typically placed on vitamin D and calcium postoperatively and go home on this supplementation.[1]

Despite the decrease in its incidence (10% of endocrine surgeons surveyed in 2008 used BNE as their primary technique, as opposed to 74% in 1998[3]), bilateral exploration is still the preferred primary technique in cases of MEN, non-MEN familial isolated hyperparathyroidism (both of which carry an increased risk of multi-gland disease), and non-localizing pre-op imaging.[2] Additionally, a minimally invasive technique failure may need to be converted to a bilateral neck exploration to achieve a cure.

5. Minimally invasive techniques

The term "minimally invasive" is applied to several different techniques. These techniques share the objectives of reduced dissection, operative time, and duration of hospitalization as well as an improvements in patient comfort and cosmesis through smaller or more discretely located incisions. Technological advancements in imaging, laboratory, and operative techniques have made these approaches possible. These adjuncts will be discussed, followed by an explanation of the techniques themselves.

6. Preoperative localization studies

6.1 Parathyroid scintigraphy

This imaging technique uses a radiotracer (usually ^{99m}Tc-sestamibi) injected intravenously to locate the parathyroid glands. ^{99m}Tc-sestamibi preferentially distributes to cells with high concentrations of mitochondria, resulting in greater concentration in cells of thyroid, heart, liver, salivary gland, and parathyroid tissue. Parathyroid glands that are hyperplastic or adenomatous tend to concentrate sestamibi to levels significant for detection, while normal glands are not typically seen. This is likely due to increased mitochondria as well as increased blood flow to these glands. Due to their anatomic relationship and shared affinity for the radiotracer, signal from the thyroid and parathyroids may overlap, obscuring the definition of an abnormal parathyroid gland. Fortunately, the retention of the radiotracer over time is greater in parathyroid than thyroid tissue. Combining early and delayed (2-3 hours) imaging permits better identification of abnormal parathyroid tissue. Additionally, an abnormal signal contour or a signal clearly separate from the thyroid bed raises suspicion of abnormal parathyroid tissue on either early or late images.[3,8] Sestamibi scanning may be done with planar imaging, or with 3-dimensional imaging using single-photon emission computed tomography (SPECT). SPECT has been reported to allow better differentiation of parathyroid tissue from the thyroid gland, and thus better detection and localization.[1-3]

This technology does have limitations, however. Uptake and retention of the radiotracer by abnormal parathyroid tissue may be variable. If washout from an adenoma is rapid, no discrete signal will be seen on the delayed images, despite the presence of a diseased gland (false negative). False negatives are also more commonly seen in patients with multi-gland disease, such as double adenomas or multi-gland hyperplasia. Additionally, multiple factors may cause false positive results, such as adenomas of thyroid origin, lymph nodes, or multinodular goiter, all of which have affinity for ^{99m}Tc-sestamibi and can be located in the same region as an abnormal gland.[2,3] Arguably, the greatest utility of sestamibi scanning is in the identification of ectopically located parathyroid tissue.

6.2 Ultrasonography

This relatively low-cost modality has the advantages of the absence of radiation and providing anatomic information in the area of intended surgery. Moreover, ultrasonography enables excellent visualization of the thyroid gland and can diagnose concurrent thyroid disease, limiting re-operation rates. Normal parathyroid glands are typically not seen on ultrasound due to their small size and location. Adenomatous glands tend to appear homogenous on ultrasound and are usually hypoechoic to the thyroid gland signal. The use of Doppler imaging can provide information regarding parathyroid galnd vascularity and can identify an artery feeding an adenomatous gland, which greatly increases the accuracy of diagnosis.[3]

Shortcomings of ultrasound include poor sensitivity for some ectopic glands such as retrotracheal or mediastinal glands. Glands in these locations are shadowed by the tracheal air column and bones of the sternum and clavicle, respectively. Large adenomas may also complicate diagnosis, because their imaging characteristics may be atypical. They can appear heterogeneous and/or hyperechoic to thyroid tissue. Disease of the thyroid such as mulitinodular goiter or posterior thyroid nodules may also increase the difficulty of detection of parathyroid adenomas. Enlarged lymph nodes associated with anthracotic pigment, thyroiditis and malignant thyroid disease can also confound parathyroid localization. However, as previously mentioned, even a study that fails to reveal a parathyroid adenoma may be useful by identifying thyroid disease in a patient that is being considered for surgery for hyperparathyroidism. Incidence of concurrent thyroid disease has been reported as high as 51% in patients being considered for parathyroid surgery, and the incidence of thyroid malignancy as 2-6%.[2,3]

6.3 Combined scintigraphy and ultrasonography

Radiotracer imaging and ultrasound alone show similar sensitivities. Sensitivity for sestamibi scanning has been reported in the range of 68-95% for single adenomas, with one meta-analysis putting it at 88%. Sensitivity is far less for multi-gland disease and has been reported at 44% for hyperplasia and 30% for double parathyroid adenomas.[1-4,6,8,10] Sensitivity of ultrasound alone has been reported at 72-89% for patients with single adenomas. Again, sensitivity drops for multi-gland disease and has been reported at 16% for parathyroid hyperplasia and 35% in double adenomas. [1-4,6,8,10]

Ultrasonography and Radio-guided imaging complement each other and increase diagnostic accuracy when used together. The surgeon may use both the functional information from scintigraphy along with the anatomic information from ultrasound. Additionally, ectopic glands that are missed by ultrasonography may be detected with scintigraphy, while ultrasonography may detect thyroid abnormalities helping to interpret scintigraphy findings. Combining these techniques results in a sensitivity of 74-95% for single gland disease. However, the sensitivity for double adenomas is 60%, and multi-gland disease is only accurately predicted 30% of the time by these techniques. When the two imaging studies are concordant (which occurs in 50-60% of cases) the sensitivity is in the range of 94-99%.[1,3] In fact, some surgeons suggest that intraoperative PTH monitoring not be used in cases of concordant ultrasound and sestamibi scan, and simply terminate the procedure after excising the gland indicated on the imaging studies. Combined ultrasonography and sestamibi is the preferred imaging method of most parathyroid surgeons.[1]

6.4 Other imaging techniques

Computed tomography [CT] and magnetic resonance imaging [MRI] scans may provide additional anatomical information, but are not first-line studies. CT offers the advantage of scanning the entire neck and mediastinum to help with localization of ectopic glands. Sensitivity of CT scanning alone ranges from 46-87%. When combined with ultrasonography, it results in only slightly increased sensitivity compared with ultrasonography alone. CT tends to be used only in patients undergoing reoperation or in patients with an ectopic gland detected on sestamibi.[1,3-5,8]

CT can also be combined with SPECT to give images that contain a combination of anatomic and functional information. This allows better localization and sensitivities ranging from 88-93%. Benefits may be greater in the subset of patients with multi-gland disease or goiter, but such combination scans require further investigation. [3]

MRI has sensitivities rivaling other modalities, but its high cost and other options for imaging have limited its use to select cases. [1,3-5,8]

7. Introperative adjunctive techniques

7.1 Intraoperative parathyroid hormone monitoring

The serum half-life of parathyroid hormone (PTH) is 3-5 minutes. This short turn-over time along with the availability of rapid assays that take from 8-20 minutes for results allow the operative team to monitor and predict the success of surgery based on the amount of circulating PTH. Typically, pre-operative and pre-incision blood samples are taken for baseline measurements. After excision of all of the suspected diseased tissue, samples are usually sent at 0, 5, and 10 minutes. The criteria used for a successful operation at most centers is a drop of the PTH level to 50% or less of the pre-incision level. If this occurs at 5 or 10 minutes, the operation is deemed complete. If it does not occur, further cervical exploration is performed to identify additional parathyroid tissue that may be causing the patient's hyperparathyroidism, and the suspicion for multi-gland disease increases. If the 50% criterion is met, surgical success rates (as measured by postoperative normocalcemia) are in the range of 97-98%. This technique may be used in both minimally invasive and bilateral neck exploration techniques. Additionally, rapid PTH assay may be performed on excised tissue, allowing rapid identification of parathyroid tissue if there is any doubt.[1,2,4-7]

7.2 Gamma probe

The radioactivity of ^{99m}Tc-sestamibi may also be detected by a hand-held probe. This adjunctive technology can help direct dissection as well as provide information regarding completeness of excision. This will be further discussed in the section regarding radio-guided parathyroid surgery.

8. Minimally invasive operative techniques

8.1 Focused parathyroidectomy

Focused parathyroid surgery is possible and effective because of the availability of pre-operative localization studies and the fact that about 75-90% of hyperparathyroidism is due to single adenomas. These factors allow for limited dissection in the area of the diseased gland, decreasing the invasiveness of bilateral neck dissection.

Candidates for this surgery are patients who meet the guidelines for surgical treatment of hyperparathyroidism, have positive pre-operative localization imaging, and do not have a condition that would predispose them to multi-gland disease, such as MEN or non-MEN familial isolated hyperparathyroidism. Patients with such conditions or non-localizing preoperative imaging should undergo traditional or minimally invasive bilateral neck exploration instead.[1,2]

This technique involves making a small (2-4 cm) transverse incision in a skin crease in the midline or on the side indicated by pre-operative imaging. The incision is carried down to the strap muscles, which are dissected and lateralized. The thyroid is mobilized and retracted medially for access. Directed dissection based on preoperative imaging allows identification of the offending gland, while care is taken not to injure the recurrent laryngeal nerve. Since the other parathyroid glands are not visualized in this technique, intraoperative parathyroid hormone monitoring is employed to determine completeness of the operation. If the 50% criterion is not met, explorative dissection to visualize the other glands is employed.[1,2,5,6,11]

Given the limited amount of dissection, this procedure may be performed under sedation with local and regional anesthesia instead of general anesthesia.[1,2] This helps reduce the risk of anesthesia in these cases. Whether general or local anesthesia is used, the majority of cases can be performed on an outpatient basis. Postoperative calcium levels do not typically have to be checked because the remaining parathyroid glands remain undisturbed. For this same reason, patients do not typically require postoperative supplementation with calcium and vitamin D. Hungry bone syndrome may still occur, however, and inpatient hospitalization and calcium testing should be performed when the concern of postoperative hypocalcemia is high.[1,2,5]

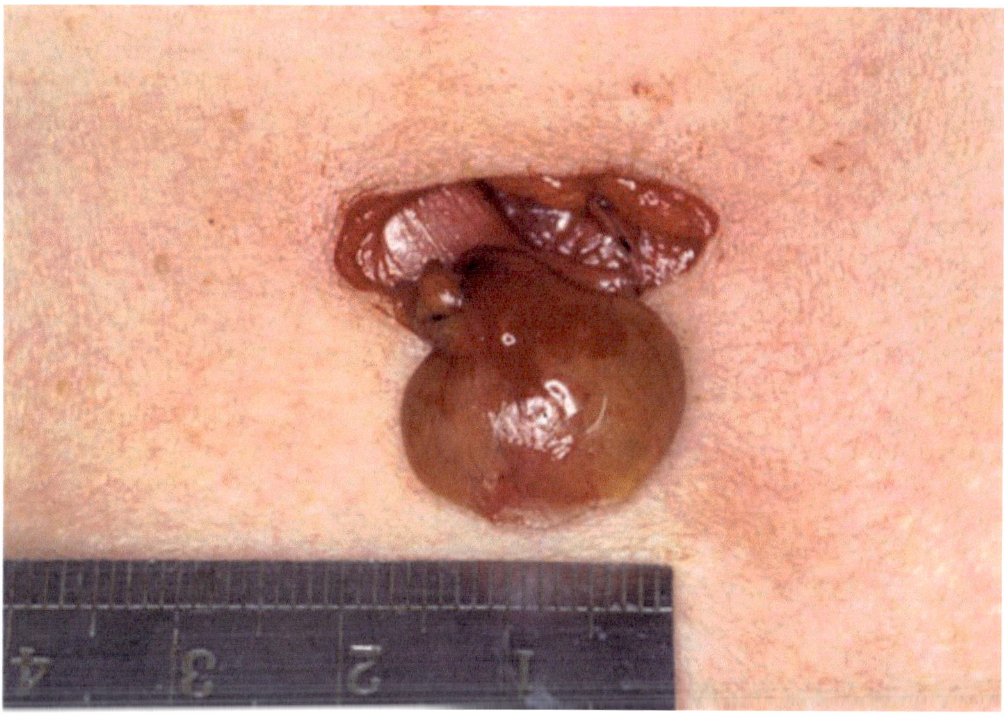

Fig. 1. An example of a 2 cm incision possible with minimally invasive techniques.

- Failure of pre-operative localization
- Known multigland disease
- MEN
- Non-MEN familial isolated hyperparathyroidism
- Lithium-associated hyperpathyroidism
- Parathyroid carcinoma

Table 2. Contraindications to Focused Exploration Techniques for Parathyroidectomy

Benefits of this approach over bilateral neck exploration include shorter operative time, shorter hospitalization, and the avoidance of general anesthesia.[1,2,5] These factors contribute to a decreased overall cost of the procedure. One surgeon compared 613 BNE operations to 1037 focused parathyroidectomies under local and regional anesthesia, and found the average cost savings in his institution to be $1471 per case.[5] Additionally, cosmesis is typically improved with this technique due to a smaller incision.[1,2,5,11] One disadvantage of this technique is the failure to visualize all parathyroids resulting in the potential risk of missing an abnormal gland which may occur in 10-25% of cases. However, the use of IPM helps to decrease this risk.

Outcomes using this technique are generally comparable to the traditional approach, with relatively high cure (95-99%) and low complication (1-4%) rates. Many studies have confirmed that this is a viable alternative to the traditional bilateral neck exploration.[1,2,5,11]

8.2 Radio-guided surgery

^{99m}Tc-sestamibi radioactivity can be detected by a handheld gamma probe which can be used intraoperatively to help locate the hyperfunctioning parathyroid tissue. This technique involves intravenous injection of the radiotracer 2 hours prior to surgery. In the operating room, the gamma probe can be used to determine on which side of the neck to place the incision. As in focused parathyroidectomy, efforts are made to keep the incision as short as possible (2-4 cm) without limiting the exposure. After the skin and platysma are incised, the probe can be inserted into the wound and the dissection directed in the area of highest radioactivity. Dissection is continued until the hyperfunctioning parathyroid gland is encountered and excised.[2,4,8] The excised tissue can be placed directly against the probe to measure its radioactivity relative to a background level that is found by placing the probe over the thyroid isthmus. If the ex-vivo count of the excised tissue is >20% of the background radiation at the thyroid isthmus, it is strong evidence that the excised tissue is indeed parathyroid adenoma. Hyperplastic parathyroid glands tend to exhibit <16% of background radiation, and normal parathyroids, fat, and lymph nodes are usually around 2%.[4,8] Much like the focused parathyroidectomy technique previously described, this technique benefits from the ability to use local and regional anesthesia with sedation. Also, it too is often used in conjunction with IPM.

Like the focused parathyroidectomy technique, this approach benefits from a small incision, limited dissection, and potential for avoidance of general anesthesia and inpatient hospitalization. Use of the gamma probe was found to have a 93-94% sensitivity and 88% positive predictive value in localization of a parathyroid adenoma.[2,4,8] However, failure of localization does occur, and conversion rates to convential bilateral exploration have been found to be 10% inpatients with single adenomas, and 50% for multi-gland disease and hyperplasia, though similar rates have been observed in focused parathyroidectomy.[2,5] Additionally, logistical concerns over timing of surgery and equipment may be seen as a disadvantage of this technique.

Radio-guided minimally invasive bilateral neck exploration has been advocated by high volume thyroid centers as yielding optimal cure rates while decreasing costs. Norman et al have noted that even highly selected unilateral explorations in patients with a clearly positive, "in focus" sestamibi scan with a solitary localization of radioactivity clearly distinct from a normal thyroid gland can still fail to achieve cure in up to 6% of cases. Following a planar sestamibi scan performed two hours before surgery, through a 2.5 cm incision under general laryngeal masked anesthesia, Norman identifies each of the four parathyroid glands and determines its metabolic activity by removing a portion of the gland and measuring the contained gamma radioactivity against a standard curve of hormone production. This permits classification of each gland as normal (dormant), adenoma, hyperplastic or clinically enlarged non-dormant. By protocol, all glands that are non-dormant are removed with more than 1 gland removed in 24.7% of cases.[12] Norman employs neither frozen section analysis nor intra-operative PTH assay, and operative times average 22.3 minutes per case. One, three and ten year cure rates for radioguided minimally invasive bilateral neck exploration exceed 99% in this case series.

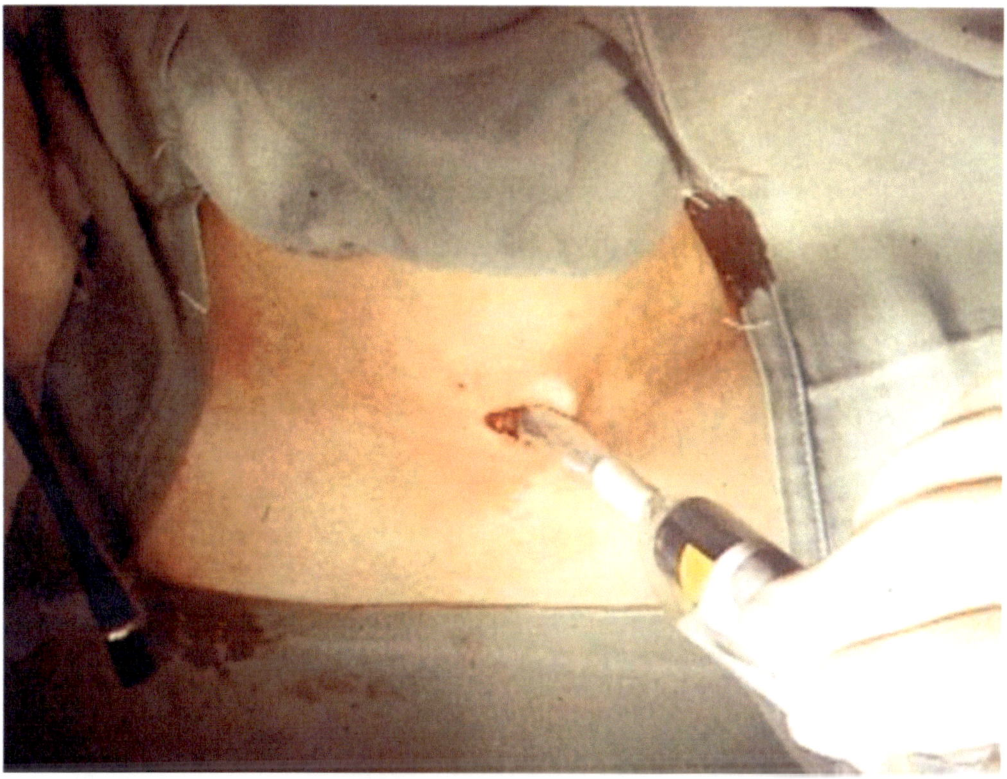

Fig. 2. A gamma probe inserted into the incision to guide dissection.

8.3 Endoscopic parathyroidectomy

Endoscopic parathyroidectomy attempts to take the techniques developed for minimally invasive laparoscopic surgeries and apply them to the neck. This technique was first reported by Gagner in 1996 for a bilateral cervical exploration.[13] It uses several very small incisions (about 5mm) as ports for an endoscope and endoscopic instruments. Generally, a 5mm trocar is inserted superior to the sternal notch in the midline of the neck through which a 30° endoscope is placed. Three additional ports are placed, two in the right neck and one in the left. Working space is created by insufflation of CO_2. The strap muscles are divided at the raphe, and the thyroid is mobilized antero-medially to reveal the parathyroid glands for resection.[1,2,9,13] Other techniques include approaches from the lateral neck, anterior chest wall, and axilla. Some of these techniques change the trocar sites to improve cosmesis. Others, such as the lateral approach, attempt to improve access to superior glands—although the technique described by Gagner provides excellent access to the lower pole of the thyroid, access to the superior poles is limited.[2]

These endoscopic approaches provide the benefit of improved cosmesis by reducing the incisions on the neck to small port sites, which in some cases are covered by clothing. Additionally, focused parathyroidectomy and bilateral cervical exploration both may be carried out with this technique. One important advantage of this method is the ability to visualize and dissect in the mediastinum if ectopic glands are suspected. Some have argued that the magnification of the endoscope allows better visualization of the recurrent laryngeal nerve, while others state that visualization of the never is poorer due to less exposure.[1,2,9,13]

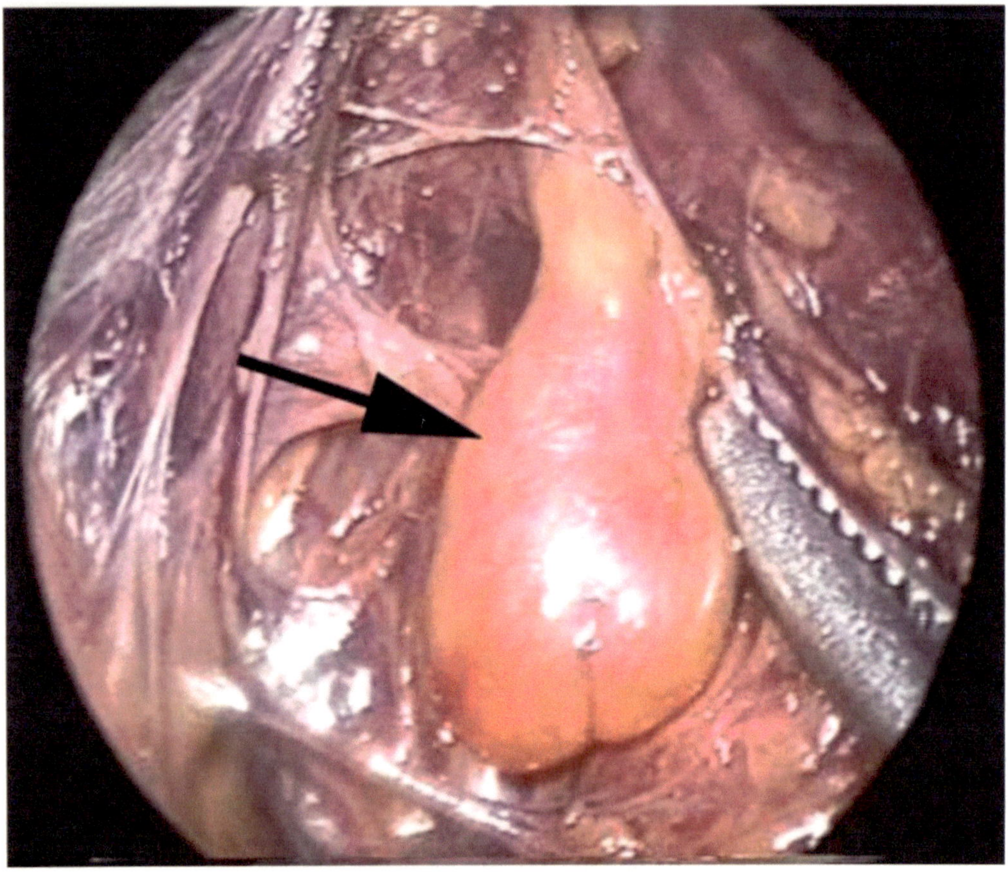

Fig. 3. View of a parathyroid adenoma through an endoscope.

A major disadvantage of this method is the steep learning curve for the surgical team to become proficient with the technique. Dedicated equipment must be purchased and maintained. Most endoscopic approaches to parathyroid surgery tend to have longer overall operative time, particularly in the early part of the learning curve. Some complications specific to this technique include subcutaneous emphysema, hypercapnia, respiratory acidosis, tachycardia, and air embolism.[1,2,9,13] These may be reduced by lower-pressure insufflation used in some approaches.[9] Also, the surgeon loses the tactile assessment that is possible in an open approach, and violation of the parathyroid capsule may be more likely when removing an adenoma from a small port.[2] Despite these disadvantages, cure rates with this technique are comparable to the previous techniques listed.[1,2,9]

8.4 Minimally invasive video-assisted parathyroidectomy

Minimally Invasive Video-Assisted Parathyroidectomy (MIVAP) was first described by Miccoli in 1998. [14] It is considered a gasless endoscopic technique, and, as with focused parathyroidecotmy, relies on preoperative localization studies and IPM. Like the focused technique, MIVAP is not an option for patients with multi-gland disease, conditions predisposing to multi-gland disease, parathyroid carcinoma, or failed preoperative localization. Additionally, patients with large goiters are not candidates for this approach.[2,15]

A 15-20mm incision is made in the midline, and the strap muscles are divided in at the raphe. Blunt dissection on the side of the neck as indicated by localization studies, and the strap muscles are retracted laterally from the thyroid using direct visualization. Then, a 5mm 30° endoscope is inserted into the wound. Working space is created by use of external retractors, so insufflation of CO_2 is not necessary. Specialized 2mm endoscopic instruments are used to complete the dissection of the parathyroid adenoma and excise it from the surrounding tissue. If the adenoma is not found, or if PTH levels do not drop appropriately, the procedure is converted to a conventional bilateral neck exploration.[1,2, 14, 15]

The absence of insufflation in this technique avoids many of the complications of the total endoscopic approach. Also, operative times tend to be shorter than total endoscopic procedures. Miccoli reported an average operative time of 36.2 minutes in a series of 370 operations, and an average time of 25.7 minutes for the last 100 in that series.[15] This procedure also affords the surgeon tactile assessment of the surgical bed, which is not available with total endoscopic approaches. However, the disadvantages of a long learning curve and specialized equipment remain. Also, 2 assistants are required for this technique.[1,2]

Cure rates with MIVAP are comparable to the other procedures described and have been reported at 96-100%. Complication rates are also comparable to the other approaches.[1,2, 15]

9. Conclusion

Although first performed nearly 100 years ago, parathyroid surgery has undergone rapid evolution over the past few decades. Advances in imaging, laboratory assay, and operative technique have made new methods possible. The varied minimally invasive techniques described in this chapter are all capable of producing satisfactory outcomes, and many offer significant advantages over traditional bilateral cervical exploration. Nonetheless, cure rates approaching 100% can only be achieved through evaluation of all four glands[16]. Parathyroid surgeons must be well versed in both traditional and minimally invasive techniques. As cure rates are high among all techniques listed, future refinement and innovation are likely to be directed at reducing complications, lowering overall cost, and improving patient satisfaction.

10. References

[1] M. Augustine, P. Bravo, M. Zeiger. Surgical Treatment of Primary Hyperparathyroidism. Endocrine Practice. Volume 17. Supplement 1 / March-April 2011.

[2] John I. Lew, Carmen C. Solorzano. Surgical Management of Primary Hyperparathyroidism: State of the Art. Surgical Clinics of North America. Volume 89. Issue 5. October 2009: Pages 1205-1225.

[3] N. Johnson, S. Carty, M. Tublin. Parathyroid Imaging. Radiol Clin N Am. Volume 49. Issue 3. May 2011: 489-509.

[4] H. Chen, E. Mack, J.R. Sterling. A Comprehensive Evaluation of Perioperative Adjuncts During Minimally Invasive Parathyroidectomy. Ann Surg September2005. 242(3). 375–383.

[5] R. Udelsman, Z. Lin, P. Donovan. The Superiority of Minimally Invasive Parathyroidectomy Based on 1650 Consecutive Patients With Primary Hyperparathyroidism. Ann Surg. Volume 253. Issue 3. March 2011: 585-591.

[6] H. Takami, Y. Ikeda, N. Wada Surgical management of primary hyperparathyroidixsm. Biomedicine & Pharmacotherapy. Volume 54. Supplement 1. June 2000: Pages 17s-20s

[7] D. Canerio-Pla. Contemporary and Practical Uses of Intraoperative Parathryoid Hormone Monitoring. Endocrine Practice. Vol 17. Suppl 1. March/April 2011: 44-53.

[8] Y. Ikeda, J. Takayama, H. Takami. Minimally Invasive Radioguided Parathyroidectomy for Hyperparathyroidism. Annals of Nuclear Medicine. Volume 24. Number 4. March 2010: 233-240.

[9] Y. Ikeda, H. Takami, G. Tajima, Y. Sasaki, J. Takayama, H. Kurihara, M. Niimi. Section 1. Parathyroid: Total Endoscopic Parathyroidectomy. Biomed Pharmacotherapy. Volume 56. Supplement 1. 2002: 22s-25s.

[10] M. Weiss, R. Schmid, M. Hacker, T. Pfluger. Hyperparathryoidism: How to Optimize Parathyroid Imaging by Means of Tc-99m Sesta-MIBI Scintigraphy and Ultrasound? The Endocrinologist. Volume 17. Number 1. February 2007: 50-56.

[11] Y. Ikeda, H. Takami, G. Tajima, Y, Sasaki, J. Takayama, H. Kurihara, M. Niimi. Section 1: Parathyroid: Direct Mini-Incision Parathyroidectomy. Biomed Pharmacotherapy. Volume 56. Suplement 1. 2002: 14s-17s.

[12] Norman J, Politz D. Measuring individual parathyroid gland hormone production in real time during radio guided parathyroidectomy. Experience in over 8,000 operations. Minerva Endocrinology. Volume 33, Issue 3. September 2008: 147-157.

[13] M. Gagner. Endoscopic subtotal parathyroidectomy in patients with primary hyperparathyroidism. Br J Surg. 83. 1996: 875 [letter].

[14] P. Micoli, C. Bendinelli, E. Vignali, S. Mazzeo, G. Matteo Cecchini, L. Pinchera, C. Marcocci. Endoscopic Parathyroidectomy: Report of an Initial Experience. Surgery. Volume 124. Issue 6. December 1998: 1077-1080.

[15] P. Miccoli, P. Berti, G. Materazzi, M. Massi, A. Picone, M. Minuto. Results of Video-assisted Parathyroidectomy: Single Institution's Six-year Expierence. World J Surg. Volume 28. Number 12. December 2004: 1216-1218.

[16] Norman J. Controversies in Parathyroid Sugery: The Quest of a "mini" unilateral operation seems to have gone too far. J Surg Oncol. 2011. In press.

11

Management of Primary Hyperparathyroidism: 'Past, Present and Future'

Sanoop K. Zachariah
Department of Surgical Disciplines, MOSC Medical College, Kolenchery, Cochin India

1. Introduction

Over the years the disease known as primary hyperparathyroidism has undergone a dramatic change in the clinical spectrum ranging from a symptomatic disease to an asymptomatic disease. In spite of the current understanding of the disease perspective, the mainstay of treatment is still surgical.

The standard treatment advocated and practiced for years could be considered as a source control operation involving routine bilateral exploration of the neck with an attempt to identify and eliminate the offending gland or glands. These surgeries were elaborate, time consuming and the success rates depended on the experience of the surgeon. Of late, certain novel and more patient-friendly techniques such as minimally invasive surgery and targeted selective gland excision are being performed with reportedly excellent outcomes.

This chapter reviews and discusses the surgical aspects of parathyroid surgery including the evolution of surgery from the 'conventional bilateral cervical exploration' to recent advances such as 'minimally invasive surgery' and 'focused parathyroidectomy'. The clinical features of primary hyperparathyroidism and indications for parathyroidectomy are also described, followed by a review of surgical techniques currently being practiced.

2. Anatomy

2.1 The surgical anatomy of the parathyroid glands

A good surgeon should also be an excellent anatomist. The ultimate triumph of the surgical management of primary hyperparathyroidism is often based on the surgeon's knowledge of the normal anatomical relationships and more so about the important embryologic variations of the parathyroid anatomy.

Practically everyone has at least four parathyroid glands, but their number can vary between 2 to 6. [Figure 1]. Thus in about 80% of cases there are symmetrically four (2 on either side) and in 5-13% of the cases they may be supernumerary (Hooghe et al., 1992). For example, in an autopsy study of 503 cases, in 84% there were four glands, 3% of the cases had only three glands, and in 13% there were supernumerary glands. The supernumerary gland was often a fifth gland tucked away in the thymus (Akerström et al., 1984).

The parathyroid glands are oval shaped, well encapsulated and smooth, often the size of a split pea, and yellow, pink or tan in colour weighing around 20-40 mg each. Normal parathyroid glands measure approximately 6 mm in length, 3–4 mm in transverse diameter, and 1–2 mm in anteroposterior diameter. In addition to the yellowish tinge, these small glands are often camouflaged by a covering of fat making it difficult to identify them during surgery and may be confused with surrounding fat. The parathyroid gland usually weighs around 29.5 mg ± 17.8 (mean ± standard deviation), with a reported upper limit of 65 mg (Dufour & Wilkerson, 1983). However, the weight of the normal parathyroid glands removed at surgery in patients with primary hyperparathyroidism may be greater than that reported in autopsy studies (Yao et al., 2004).

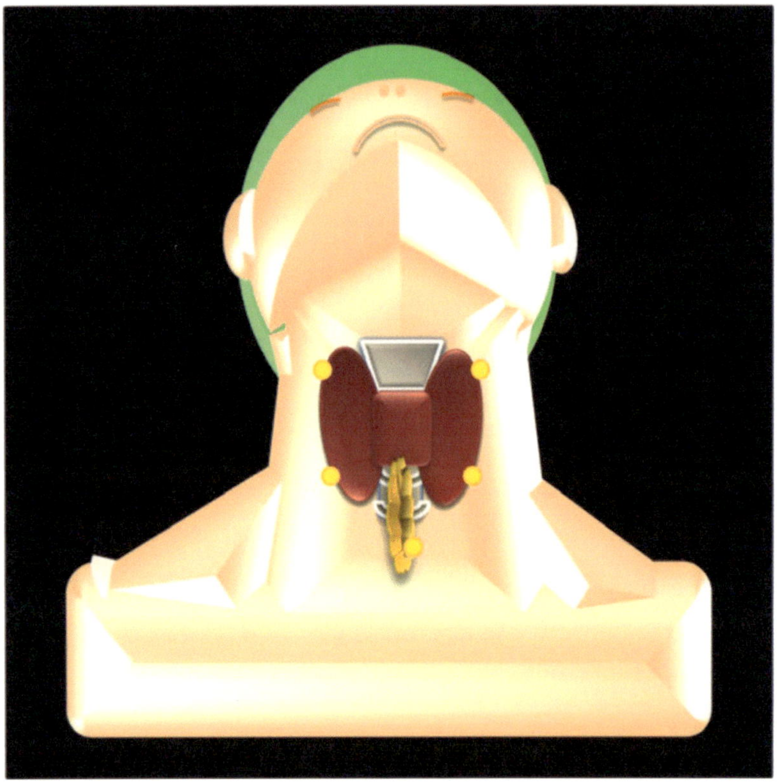

Fig. 1. The normal location of paired parathyroids and a supernumerary fifth gland within the thymus.

The inferior parathyroid gland derives its blood supply from the inferior thyroid artery. In about 10% of patients, the inferior thyroid artery may be absent, in which case the superior thyroid artery supplies the inferior parathyroids (Delattre et al, 1982). The superior parathyroid gland is also usually supplied by the inferior thyroid artery or from an anatomizing artery joining the superior and inferior parathyroid arteries. In about 20-45% of cases, the superior parathyroid glands receive their blood supply from a posterior branch of the superior thyroid artery (Bonjer & Bruining, 1997; Nobori et al., 1994). There often exists a good collateral arterial supply from the tracheal vessels and therefore adequate parathyroid function persists even if all four major thyroid arteries are ligated.

About 15-19 % of the glands can be found in ectopic locations and distant from the thyroid lobes, mostly posterior alongside the esophagus, in the upper anterior mediastinum encapsulated in the thymus, and within the carotid sheath or even rarely (0.5-4%) embedded within the thyroid itself. (Wang, 1981; Feliciano, 1992). The ectopic or aberrant locations of the parathyroid gland are related to discrepancies during embryological development and descent.

Key points-1

- In 80% of cases parathyroids are normal in position, symmetrical and paired.
- About 20% of the parathyroids are ectopic.
- 65mg is the upper normal weight limit for a single gland.
- Supernumerary glands may be commonly found within thymus (*"para-thymus"*).
- Collateral blood supply from tracheal vessels is protective to the parathyroids.
- Intra-thyroidal location of the parathyroid is rare.

2.2 Applied surgical embryology of the parathyroids

Although functionally independent, the development of thyroid, parathyroid and the thymus are closely related to one another. The parathyroid glands develop from the cranial portions of the third and fourth pharyngeal (branchial) pouches on either side of the embryo and are therefore designated as *parathyroid glands III* and *parathyroid glands IV* respectively. Since these pouches are bilateral they should normally yield four parathyroid glands.

The **parathyroid III (the future inferior parathyroids**) and the thymus arise from the third branchial pouch from its dorsal and ventral wings respectively [figure2]. The downward descent of the thymus pulls the parathyroid III along with it. But parathyroids usually halt at the dorsal surface and outside the fibrous capsule of the thyroid gland while the thymus descends further beyond. This embryonic descent therefore places the parathyroid IIIs inferior to the parathyroid IVs in the neck, thereby designating them as inferior and superior parathyroids respectively. Discrepancies in this course of normal descent can cause the parathyroid IIIs to be situated at levels higher up in the neck (sometimes referred to as *'undescended parathymus'*).

The **parathyroid IV glands (the future superior parathyroids**) and the ultimobranchial bodies are derived from the fourth pharyngeal pouch and migrate together. The superior parathyroid glands travel with the ultimobranchial bodies and consequently migrate a shorter distance than the inferior glands. They therefore remain in contact with the posterior part of the middle third of the thyroid lobes and are in a comparatively more constant position in the neck.

Key points-2

- The superior parathyroids are more constant in location.
- The inferior parathyroids are more prone to become ectopic.
- The superior parathyroid glands are typically located about 1 cm superior to the intersection of the inferior thyroid artery and the recurrent laryngeal nerve.[along the posterior border of the thyroid].

- The inferior glands are commonly found near the lower pole of the thyroid more often in an anterior plane.

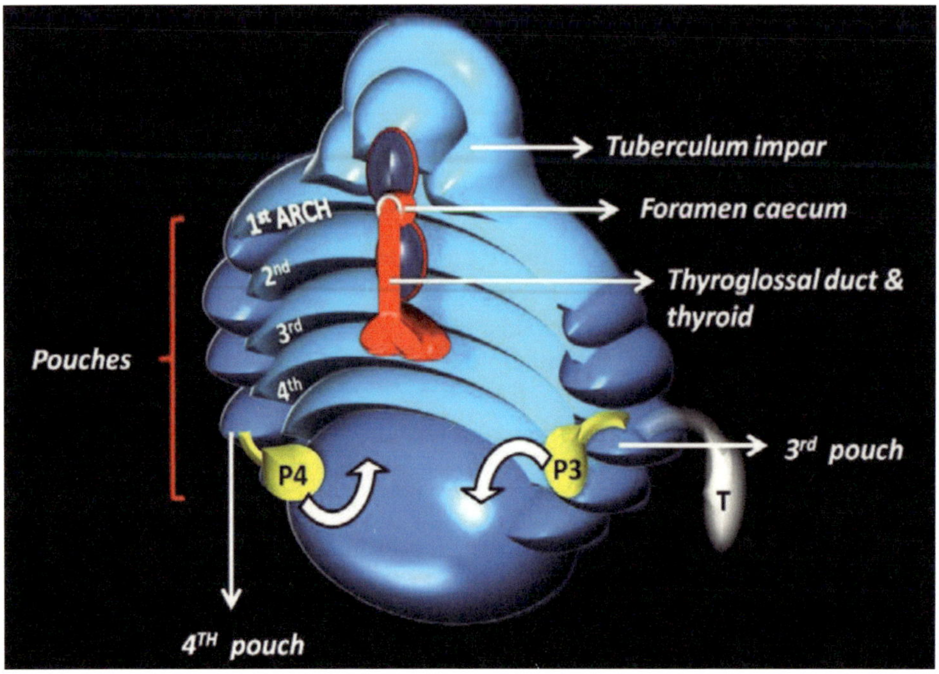

Fig. 2. The developing branchial complex demonstrating the parathyroid III (P3) and thymus (T) budding from the third branchial pouch on the dorsal and ventral aspects respectively. Pathways of parathyroids III (P3) and IV (P4) denoted by arrows.

3. Primary hyperparathyroidism

Primary hyperparathyroidism (PHPT) is a hypercalcaemic state caused by excessive unregulated production of parathyroid hormone, resulting in defective calcium homeostasis. The secretion of parathyroid hormone is regulated directly by the plasma concentration of ionized calcium. The exact cause of spontaneous hyperfuctioning of the parathyroids is unknown and it is often recognized due to peripheral or systemic effects of the excess hormone.

PHPT can be regarded as a relatively recent disease owing to the fact that the parathyroid glands were the last major organ to be recognized in humans. (Elaraj & Clark, 2008). Ivar Sandström, a Swedish medical student, in 1879 was the first to describe the parathyroid glands. (Eknoyan, 1995)

3.1 The spectrum of parathyroid disease

Parathyroid disease usually manifests in three forms namely **primary, secondary** and **tertiary** hyperparathyroidism. **Primary hyperparathyroidism (PHPT)** is a relatively common endocrine disorder and is the commonest reason for surgical exploration. The other two forms are consequences of other disease processes.

TYPE	CAUSE	TREATMENT
Primary HPT	Unregulated overproduction of parathyroid hormone resulting in abnormal calcium homeostasis, due to adenoma, hyperplasia or carcinoma, familial syndromes(MEN 1 or MEN 2a), familial isolated hyperparathyroidism (FIHPT) etc.	Surgery: open / minimal access Parathyroidectomy
Secondary HPT	Excessive production of parathyroid hormone secondary to a chronic abnormal stimulus such as chronic renal failure and vitamin D deficiency.	Primarily medical management
Tertiary HPT	Autonomous hypersecretion of parathyroid hormone causing hyperalcaemia often seen in chronic secondary hyperparathyroidism (prolonged compensatory stimulation) and often after renal transplantation.	Total parathyroidectomy with auto transplantation, subtotal parathyroidectomy

Table 1. The spectrum of hyperparathyroidism

3.2 Incidence

There is a wide variation in the incidence of PHPT geographically. This variation is most markedly seen in between the western world and developing countries. It is a common endocrine disease in countries where hyperalcaemia is detected at an early stage due to routine biochemical screening (Bilezikian et al, 2002). The exact incidence of PHPT is difficult to define since many patients remain asymptomatic and the reported incidence varies according to the population studied. In the United States, the incidence of primary hyperparathyroidism is 2 to 3 per 1000 women and approximately 1 per 1000 men. The incidence increases to 2% after the age of 55 years. It is more commonly seen in postmenopausal woman older than 50 years. With the advent of multichannel biochemical screening in the 1970s, the incidence of PHPT increased around the world especially in western countries and this brought to light the existence of the entity referred to as 'asymptomatic PHPT'.

3.3 Etiopathogenesis

The exact cause of primary hyperparathyroidism is not clear and may possibly due to an underlying primary pathology of the parathyroid gland itself.The pathogenesis of PHPT may be sporadic or familial. Normally the parathyroid glands are composed of chief cells, oxyphil cells, and transitional oxyphil cells mixed with adipose tissue. Chief cells secrete parathyroid hormone. Sporadic PHPT involves abnormal tissue in the parathyroid gland [figure 3].

The pathological lesions responsible for PHPT include **solitary adenomas** (>80%); **double adenomas** (2–3%) **multigland hyperplasia** (15%) and **carcinoma** (1-2%).**(Kaplan et al,1992)**

Inherited disorders include familial hyperparathyroidism, multiple endocrine neoplasia syndrome (MEN type 1 and 2A), and hyperparathyroidism-jaw tumor syndrome and these account for roughly about 10% of PHPT. Other suggested causes include over expression of PRAD1 oncogene and also low dose irradiation to the neck during childhood.

3.4 Double parathyroid adenomas -"fact or fiction"?

Double parathyroid adenomas account for only a small percentage of the lesions associated with PHPT. Controversy still exists as to whether double adenomas are a distinct entity or part of four gland hyperplasia presenting metasynchronously. There is no reliable method to accurately distinguish adenoma from hyperplasia. Some authors feel that the most reliable clinical criteria to document double adenomas, is the absence of recurrent hyperparathyroidism on follow up of at least 5 years following selective gland excision (Baloch & LiVolsi., 2001). Meanwhile some others have authoritatively documented the existence of double adenoma as a separate entity and are not simply missed cases of four-gland hyperplasia. (Abboud et al., 2005). Neonatal convulsions as the initial presentation of maternal PHPT due to double parathyroid adenomas has also been described (Zachariah & Thomas, 2010).

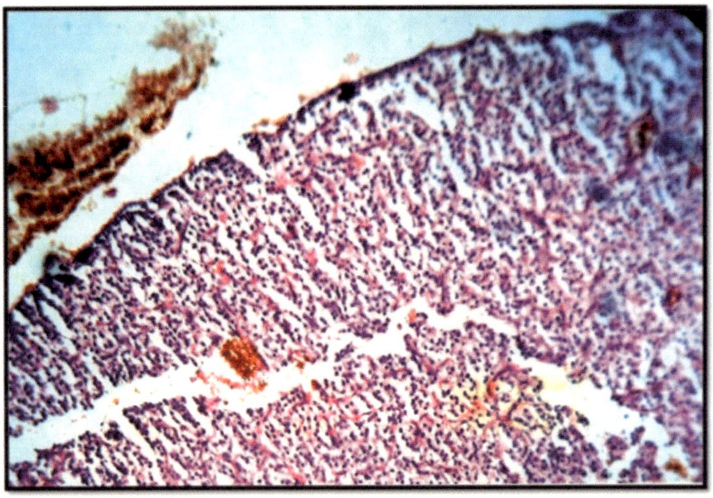

Fig. 3. Photomicrograph of a solitary parathyroid adenoma showing hypercellular parathyroid tissue, absence of fat cells and surrounding capsule (Haematoxylin & Eosin *40)

3.5 Clinical features

It is now well known or well phrased that *"The clinical presentation of PHPT has changed from a symptomatic to an asymptomatic disease"*. Patients with severe symptoms have become exceedingly rare. To make the discussion simpler, PHPT can be broadly classified into two types-namely symptomatic and asymptomatic PHPT, a view also supported by a National Institutes of Health consensus panel. (Bilezikian et al., 2002; Kearns & Thompson, 2002)

Clinical features are associated to the direct and indirect effects of excess parathyroid hormone on the skeleton, kidneys, and intestine may include bone resorption of calcium and phosphorus, enhanced intestinal absorption of calcium, renal tubular reabsorption of calcium, and hypercalciuria

3.5.1 Asymptomatic PHPT

Asymptomatic PHPT (APHPT) is the commonest form of the disease and therefore the most common clinical presentation of primary hyperparathyroidism is asymptomatic hyperalcaemia and this accounts for 75% to 80% of cases. However it should be understood that absence of any of the obvious classical clinical presentations is what is commonly referred to as asymptomatic disease. In such patients the symptoms are mild and nonspecific, often underestimated. But studies have shown that the so called asymptomatic patients will often have symptoms or metabolic complications when carefully evaluated with standardized health questionnaires. (Burney et al., 1999; Talpos et al., 2000). Patients may have weakness, fatigue, mild depression, anorexia, and often increased absence from work. These patients have mild and sometimes only intermittent hypercalcemia. In most of these cases, the mean serum calcium concentration is less than 1.0 mg/dL (0.25 mmol/L). Truly asymptomatic PHPT is therefore rare, occurring in only 2% to 5% of patients. (Chan et al, 1995; Clark et al, 1991) The importance of APHPT is that the surgical management of asymptomatic patients has been controversial and this very aspect has encouraged the formulation of treatment guidelines.

3.5.2 Symptomatic PHPT

This was the original form of the disease and is still at large in developing countries. The signs and symptoms of hyperparathyroidism largely reflect the effects of hypercalcemia and may involve multiple organ systems (Taniegra, 2004).

Classical symptoms of PHPT popularly summed up as "*bones, stones, abdominal groans and psychic moans*" are hardly ever encountered today. (Silverberg et al, 1999) This may be true in the western world. Conversely, in developing countries classic and severe forms of the disease are still the presenting features and asymptomatic PHPT is probably a rarity. Some of the classical radiological findings are shown in figure 4.

Bone related problems were the first to call attention to the disease and include manifestations of selective cortical bone loss. The high incidence of bone disease in patients with PHPT in developing countries has been attributed to associated vitamin D and dietary calcium deficiency (Harinarayan, 1995). The various classical clinical features are summed up in [Table 2]. Cardiovascular manifestations include hypertension, bradycardia, shortened QT interval, and left ventricular hypertrophy. It should be remembered that the symptoms may not be proportional to magnitude of hypercalcaemia.

In developing countries the scenario and spectrum of the disease are therefore different. In a systematic review of data of 858 patients with PHPT, from India, showed that majority of the patients (71.5%) were less than 40 yrs of age, (whereas patients from developed nations are diagnosed in the fifth and sixth decades) (Pradeep et al, 2011). Interestingly, 5 to 33% had a clinically palpable parathyroid gland. Also, the incidence of parathyroid carcinoma causing PHPT in the various series has been 2.6 to 6%, which is higher than in developing countries. Moreover in India, asymptomatic presentation is virtually unheard of. The symptomatic disease is identified much later after a series of management for fractures and renal stones. Another study also showed similar results, where in, 67% had bone disease, 48% had fractures, 21% had stone disease, 23% had psychiatric symptoms and 15% had peptic ulcer disease (Bhansali et al, 2005).

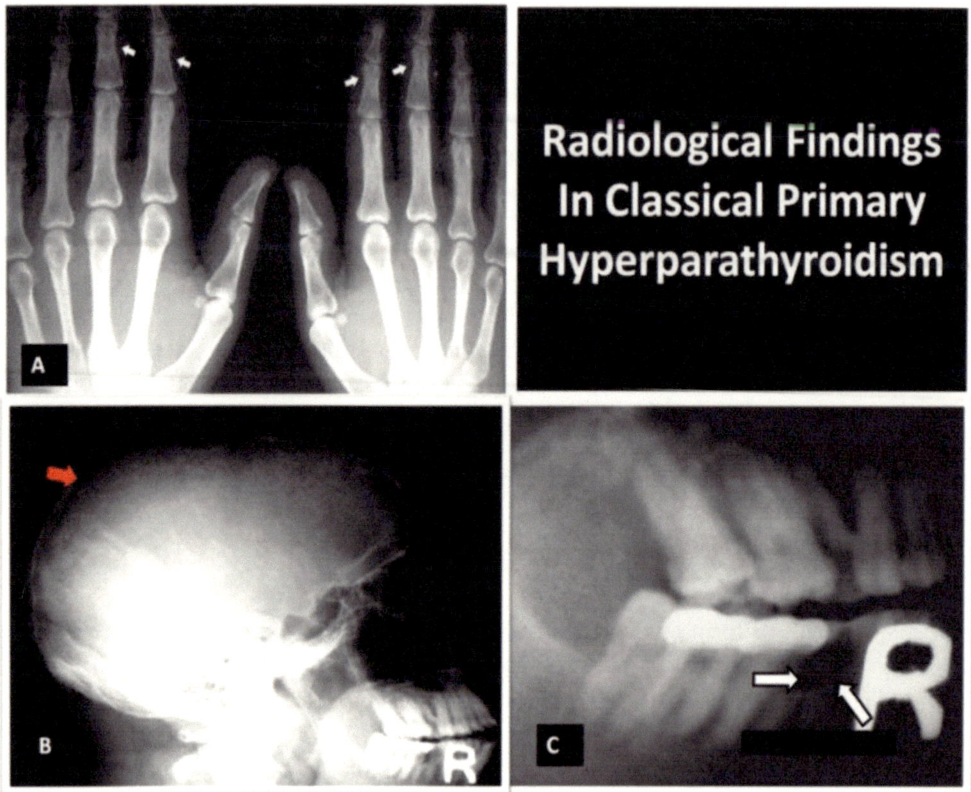

Fig. 4. SYMPTOMATIC PHPT: (A) Xray of the hands showing subperiosteal bone resorption over the middle phalanges (white arrows). (B) Showing *"salt and pepper"* appearance of the skull. (C) Showing a dental cystic lesion over the mandible.

SYMPTOMATOLOGY	ORGAN SYSTEM INVOLVED	FEATURES
Bones	Skeletal And Neuro-Muscular	Bone & Joint Pain; Osteoclastic Bone Resorption,Pseudo-gout; Chondrocalcinosis;Brown tumour, Bone cysts
Stones	Renal	Polyuria; Haematuria; Graveluria; Recurrent urinary tract infections Nephrolithiasis (35-50%); Nephrocalcinosis (rare: 3-5%) Hypercalciuria
Abdominal Groans	Gastro-Intestinal	Anorexia;Vomiting;Abdominal Cramps;Constipation;Acid Peptic Disease; Acute Pancreatitis Cholelithiasis (25-30%)
Psychic Moans	Psychological Manifestations	Depression; Poor Libido; Memory Loss,Lack of concentration

Table 2. Clincal features of classical disease

The association between pancreatitis and hyperparathyroidism was first reported in 1940 by Smith and Cooke. (Bess et al, 1980). The commonest manifestation of pancreatic disease with PHPT is the history of recurrent upper abdominal pain. A high concentration of serum calcium may responsible for the increased incidence of gall stone disease in PHPT and this is seen especially in developing countries

4. Making the diagnosis of primary hyperparathyroidism

4.1 Laboratory diagnosis

The diagnosis of PHPT is based on the documentation of elevated serum calcium in combination with elevated serum parathyroid hormone (PHT) levels. The initial finding of an elevated serum calcium (ionized fraction) level should always raise the suspicion of PHPT and in such cases hypercalceamia should be confirmed by a repeat test. In such cases, other causes of hypercalcaemia should be excluded (history of vitamin D intake, thiazide diuretics and family history of hypercalcemia). Elevated parathyroid hormone levels in the presence of persistent hypercalcemia confirms the diagnosis of primary hyperparathyroidism. Inorder to eliminate the variations that can occur with respect to time, blood volume, and dietary intake the PTH and serum calcium levels should be measured simultaneously.

The first generation parathyroid hormone assays is becoming obsolete. Second-generation parathyroid hormone assays (known as 'intact'), and third-generation parathyroid hormone assays (known as 'whole or bio-intact') are becoming more popular.

4.2 Additional investigations

The concentration of serum phosphate varies between 2.5 and 4.5 mg/100ml. About half the patients with PHPT have hypo-phosphataemia provided they do not have significant renal impairment. Also, 10-40% of patients have elevated levels of serum alkaline phospatase and almost all these patients have significant bone invovelment. Imaging studies have no role in the diagnosis of primary hyperparathyroidism and are mainly used for localization.

Recently a new clinical phenotype of PHPT has been identified known as **normocalcemic PHPT. Eucalcemic primary hyperparathyroidism** may represent the earliest manifestation of primary hyperparathyroidism. As for now more information is needed on this entity to consider its routine evaluation in PHPT (Peacock et al, 2005; Lowe et al, 2007).

5. The surgical management of PHPT

Surgery provides the only available cure for primary hyperparathyroidism. Although operative management is clearly indicated for all patients with symptomatic PHPT (classic symptoms or complications of PHPT), the role of surgery for asymptomatic PHPT is still controversial.

5.1 Decision making: "Current indications and guidelines"

There is no doubt patients with **symptomatic PHPT** should undergo surgery as there is enough evidence of symptomatic improvement and reversal of the effects of PHPT (such as improvement in bone density, reduction in fractures, reduced frequency of kidney stones, and improvements in some neurocognitive elements and sense of well being).

Controversy still exists as whether patients with **asymptomatic PHPT** should undergo surgery. Data increasingly appears to support parathyroidectomy in all patients with PHPT because it is associated with a quantifiable improvement in health related quality of life. (Sheldon et al, 2002).

However, among the so called 'asymptomatic patients' only about 2-5% are truly asymptomatic. Inorder to address this issue and set down guidelines, three conferences have been held on the management of asymptomatic PHPT during the past 18 years. The most recent conference (the third) was held in 2008 from which summary of guidelines are available for reference. Important aspects based on the current guidelines for surgical intervention and for medical surveillance, for patients with asymptomatic hyperparathyroidism are listed in table 3. (Bilezikian et al, 2009). As for now the surgical treatment should definitely be based on these guidelines.

FACTOR	CRITERIA
Asymptomatic	No Kidney Stones, Nephrocalcinosis, Fractures, Or Other Symptoms
Age	<50 years
Serum Calcium	>1 mg/dl Above Normal Upper Limit Of Normal
Creatinine Clearance	<60 ml/Min
Bone Mineral Density (BMD)	T-Score<-2.5 At Lumbar Spine, Hip, Or Forearm
24 hr Urine Calcium	Not Indicated (Hypercalciuria By Itself Is Not Considered An Indication For Surgery)
Asymptomatic PHPT who do not meet above criteria(1,2,3,4,5,6)	Medical surveillance (Can be safely managed without surgery) Monitor: serum calcium levels biannually Serum creatinine levels-annually BMD 1-2 years at three sites

Table 3. Current guidelines for surgical management of asymptomatic PHPT

5.2 Pre-operative localization: "Chasing the target"

Once we have confirmed the diagnosis of primary hyperparathyroidism from the laboratory and clinical information, the next and one of the most important step is to identify the source of the disease process.

In the past the only way of identifying an abnormal gland was at the time of bilateral neck exploration and the best tool available was an experienced surgeon!! This is aptly reflected in the words of Doppmann *"in my opinion, the only localizing study indicated in a patient with untreated hyperparathyroidism is to localize an experienced parathyroid surgeon."*(Doppmann, 1986).

The argument was that, in the hands of an experienced parathyroid surgeon, 95%to 97% of the cases could be resolved by a single neck exploration. Thus, in the past, the only indication for preoperative localization was re-exploration following an unsuccessful parathyroidectomy. The various modalities for preoperative location are listed in table.

IMAGING MODALITY	COMMENTS
Ultrasonography (USG)	Cheap & non invasive, no radiation, can localize upto 80% of adenomas. Not very useful for ectopic parathyroids USG guided FNAC can help confirm an adenoma preoperatively Reported accuracy 75%-80%
Computed Tomography Scan(CT)	Expensive. Useful for localizing ectopic glands Thin-section contrast-enhanced CT is reported to have a sensitivity ranging from 46% to 87%.
Magnetic Resonsce Imaging (T2-Weighted MRI)	Expensive. Useful for localizing ectopic glands Sensitivity of MRI is about 65% to 80%
Tc99m Sestamibi Scanning	The 'trend setter' and breakthrough investigation. "The preoperative localization investigation of choice in parathyroid disease" positive sestamibi does not improve surgical outcome Negative sestamibi scan is a predictor of those patients that are less likely to be cured.(Allendorf et al,2003) Combined with single photon-emission computed tomography (SPECT) can localize 90% of adenomas including ectopics.(Ho Shon et al,2001)
Combined USG + Tc99m Sestamibi Scanning	Ultrasound scan (USG) and Technetium (Tc ^{99m}) sestamibi scanning are combined, localization of a parathyroid adenoma is accurate in over 95% of cases (Miura et al,2002) Allows preoperative skin marking of the parathyroid position.

Table 4. Techniques of preoperative localization.

The interest in preoperative localization techniques is being given even more importance now, as more and more minimal access techniques are being developed for parathyroidectomy. Therefore it would be logical if the offending gland could be accurately localized as a part of preoperative planning. Preoperative localization would be advantageous for a single gland disease, but its utility in multi-gland disease is questionable. At present no single method of parathyroid localization matches to the unguided neck exploration by an experienced surgeon.

Key points-3

- Preoperative localization studies help plan the operative approach in patients who have biochemically confirmed diagnosis of primary hyperparathyroidism.
- Imaging studies are mainly used for localization and they have no role in the diagnosis.
- A single site positive imaging result does not rule out the possibility of multiglandular disease.
- Tc-99m sestamibi-SPECT scanning has been shown to be the best imaging modality to localize parathyroid adenomas.

5.3 Parathyroidectomy: "The dawn of a new concept"

Felix Mandl performed the first successful parathyroidectomy in Vienna in 1925. (Mandl, 1925). Thereafter and for a considerably long time the standard accepted procedure was wide exposure, for bilateral neck exploration and evaluation of all the four parathyroids.

The surgical treatment for PHPT has undergone a dramatic change in the last decade owing to the development of better localization techniques. The standard treatment advocated and practiced for years could be considered as a source control operation involving routine bilateral exploration of the neck with an attempt to identify and eliminate the offending gland or glands. These surgeries were elaborate, time consuming and the success rates depended on the experience of the surgeon. When performed by experienced surgeons, cure rates with parathyroidectomy are 95% to 98%, and complication rates are 1% to 2%. (Schell & Dudley, 2003; Clark, 1997) Of late, certain novel and more patient -friendly techniques such as minimally invasive surgery and targeted selective gland excision are being performed with reportedly excellent outcomes.

The present era of 'minimal access surgery' has made considerable progress in the field of parathyroid surgery too. The recent trend is to develop procedures that require significantly smaller incisions for performing the same procedure. The routinely performed parathyroid exploration which made use of the large Kocher cervicotomy can be now be conveniently referred to as the, 'conventional' or 'standard parathyroidectomy'. Any other surgical method or access entailing a smaller incision could therefore be referred to as minimal access parathyroidectomy **(MAP)** or minimally invasive parathyroidectomy **(MIP).**

The protocol of bilateral neck exploration was challenged initially in the 1980s, when a unilateral approach was advocated in an attempt to avoid the need for contralateral exploration and its associated risks (Wang, 1985; Tibblin, et al., 1982; Russell et al., 1990).

There was a dramatic change in concept following the introduction of Tc^{99m}-sestamibi parathyroid scanning especially with reports such as simultaneous sestamibi and ultrasound of the neck could localize an enlarged parathyroid gland with almost 95% accuracy. The rationale was that if the abnormal parathyroids could be localized accurately then they could be appropriately targeted and removed through very small incisions, thereby offering the proclaimed advantageous of minimally invasive surgery in a general perspective. This thought paved the way for developing minimal-access parathyroid surgeries.

Many studies have shown that minimally invasive parathyroidectomy offers advantages like reduced hospital costs, shorter hospital stays, a lower incidence of hypocalcemia, and equally high cure rates with lower complication rates (Udelsman R, 2002; Bergenfelz et al., 2002; Goldstein et al., 2000).

An average Kochers collar incision was usually about 8-10cm long. With time surgeons learned to perform the conventional bilateral exploration utilizing smaller incisions of about 4.1 cm (Brunaud et al, 2003). The point at which the procedure becomes a minimal-access operation probably is best defined by the length of the incision. It has been suggested that the procedure can be referred to as MAP when the inscion length is less than 2.5cm for a patient with BMI of less than 30.

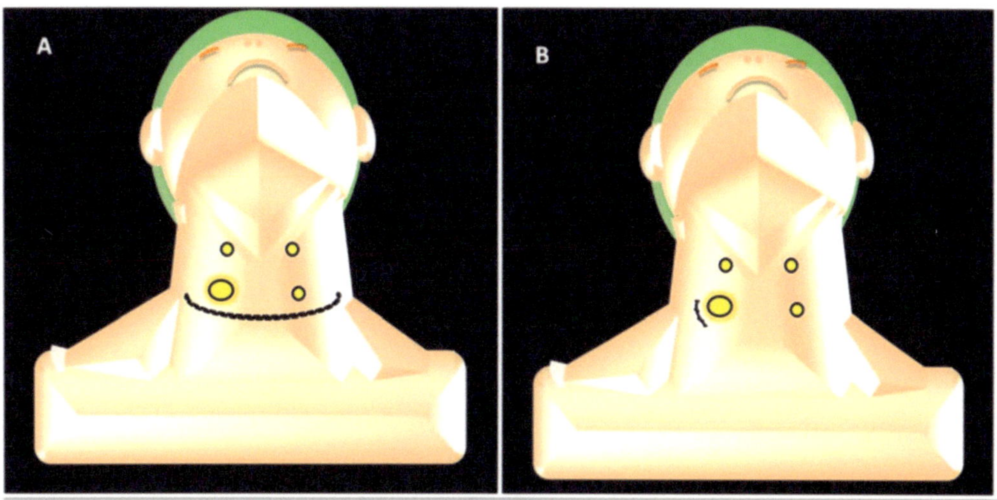

Fig. 5. Schematic representation comparing length of incisions of conventional (A) and minimally invasive parathyroidectomy (B).

5.4 Types of minimal access surgeries for parathyroid -"An overview of assortments"

5.4.1 Unilateral neck exploration (UNE)

The feasibility of unilateral neck exploration is based on the fact that that 85-90% of patients have single gland disease which could be preoperatively accurately localized by 99mTc sestamibi scanning and/or ultrasound. Therefore such patients require excision of only one gland to achieve a cure. The unilateral approach to the solitary parathyroid adenoma was advocated by Wang and later refined by Tibblin et al.

A meta-analysis of 99mTc sestamibi scanning has revealed a sensitivity and specificity of 90.7% and 98.8% respectively suggesting that the majority of patients may be suitable for unilateral exploration (Denham & Norman, 1998). A prospective randomized trial compared unilateral versus bilateral neck exploration in 91 patients. There was no statistically significant difference in the incidence of multiglandular disease, costs, or cure rate (95.1% vs. 97.5%) between unilateral versus bilateral exploration. However patients who underwent unilateral neck exploration had a lower incidence of biochemical and early severe symptomatic hypocalcaemia compared to patients who underwent bilateral exploration (Bergenfelz et al, 2002).

In another series of 184 patients who underwent scan-directed UNE, long term cure rates of 98.4% were reported (Sidhu et al, 2003)

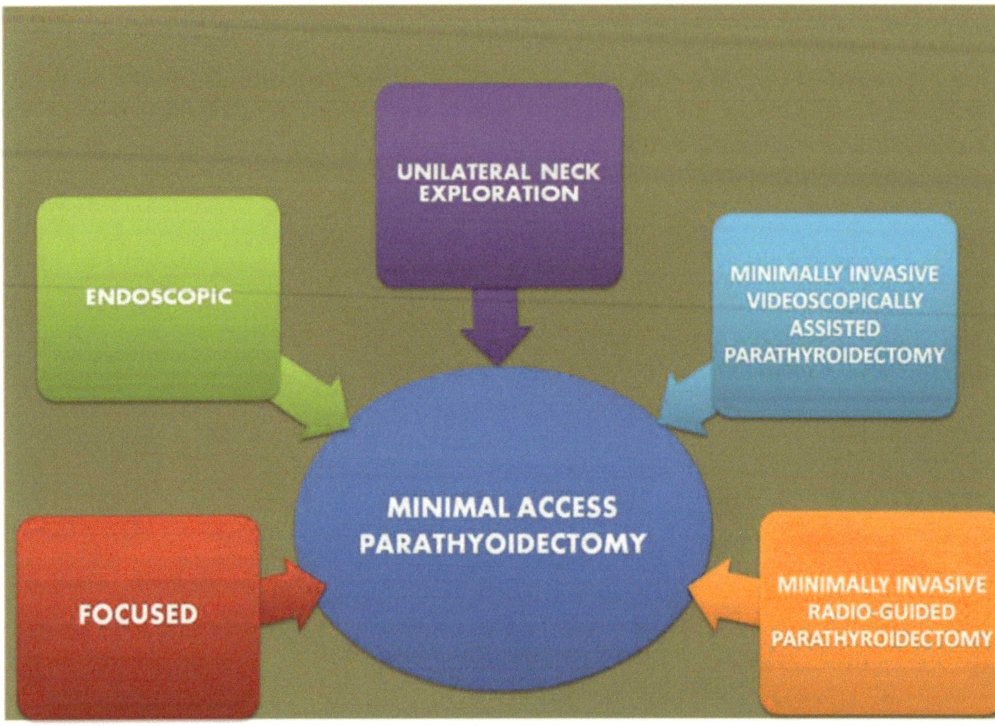

Fig. 6. Chart showing types of minimal access procedures for parathyroidectomy

5.4.2 Focused parathyoidectomy (FNE)

Also known as focused neck exploration(FNE). FNE can be performed as a day-case surgery and either under general anesthesia, cervical block, local anesthesia and sedation (Agarwal et al, 2002). Following 150 MIPs, 74 patients were discharged the same day and a further 70 were discharged the following day (within 23 h) (Mihai et al, 2007).

The technique usually makes use of a small (2cm) lateral incision to enter the space between the lateral border of the strap muscles and sternomastoid and thereby reach the lateral border of the thyroid gland and gain direct access to the parathyroid bearing areas. An FNE can be performed in as little as 12 minutes (Delbridge, 2003) and is achieved fully maintaining the principles, established with conventional parathyroid surgery.

Similar conclusions were drawn from a retrospective study comparing 255 focused lateral approaches to 401 bilateral neck explorations ,where there was no significant difference in surgical success (99% versus 97%) or complication rates (1.2% versus 3%). However a favorable reduction in the operating time from 2.4 hours to 1.3 hours for MIP was demonstrated.

As with FNE the obvious advantages are that these explorations are suitable for those patients who may otherwise be high risk candidates for general anesthesia.

5.4.3 Endoscopic parathyroidectomy / Minimally invasive endoscopic parathyroidectomy (MIEP)

Minimally invasive endoscopic parathyroidectomy **(MIEP)** is now regarded as a feasible surgical procedure. Early work on endoscopic approach to parathyroid disease was first described by Gagner. (Gagner, 1996)

The neck is obviously a small area, and therefore the major technical challenge of an endoscopic approach to parathyroidectomy was creation of enough working space to obtain adequate exposure and freedom of movement.

Enthusiasts have tried and tested various approaches including a three-port lateral approach along the anterior border of the sternomastoid muscle (Henry et al,1999) to a midline suprasternal port and two lateral ports on the same or opposite sides of the neck, in front or behind the sternomastoid muscle (Gauger et al, 1999). Irrespective of the port placement, the technique is essentially an endoscopic lateral approach. [Figure 7& 8] An axillary approach has also been described, inserting three trocars through the axilla. This completely avoids any scars in the neck or anterior chest.

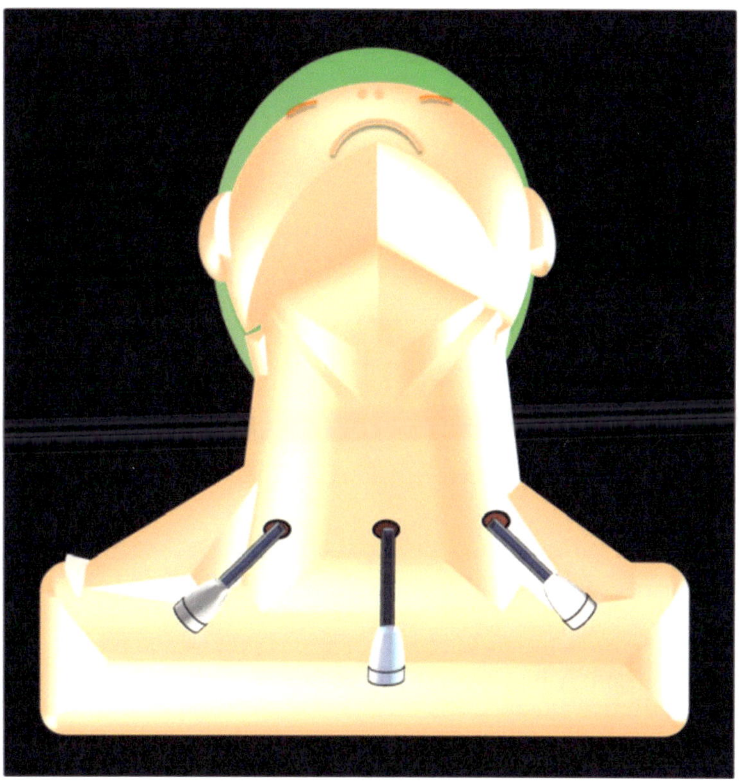

Fig. 7. Port positions in endoscopic parathyroidectomy using central access technique

5.4.4 Minimally invasive videoscopically assisted parathyroidectomy (MIVAP)

Miccoli P et al developed and described this gaseless procedure in 1998. The localized adenoma is approached via a 1.5 cm suprasternal incision, through which 5 mm endoscope is inserted, dissection is carried out with 2 mm spatulas and forceps. The rest of the operation follows the standard principles of open parathyroid surgery, with recurrent laryngeal nerve (RLN) identification and ligation of the parathyroid vascular pedicle MIVAP offers advantages over the endoscopic approach, with the preservation of tactile contact and a considerably smaller insicon.

5.4.5 Minimally invasive radio-guided parathyroidectomy (MIRP) – (*gamma probe assisted parathyroidectomy)*

A hand held gamma probe is used to determine the position of the incision and guide the dissection (20 mCi of Technetium 99msestamibi is injected intravenously, two to four hours prior to the surgery) the principle is similar that of sentinel lymph node biopsy.

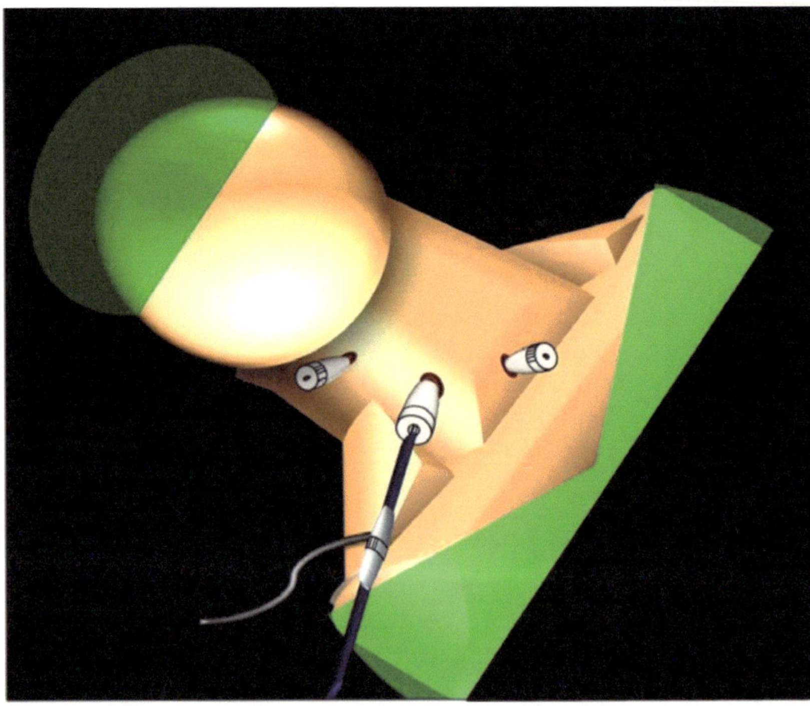

Fig. 8. Schematic representation of endoscopic parathyroidectomy: lateral access technique

With the continued improvements in parathyroid imaging techniques, minimally invasive parathyroidectomy is rapidly becoming the procedure of choice in patients with PHPT.

5.4.6 Intra-operative PTH (IOPTH) measurement

IOPTH measurements were first introduced in 1990, and represent an alternative to four-gland visualization. (Irvin GL., 1999) This is regarded as an important advancement in the development of unilateral surgery, replacing the need for visualisation of all glands, and has been referred to as biochemical "frozen section". During surgery, blood is drawn for PTH assays before (baseline) and after the excision of a hyperfunctioning gland. The removal of the diseased hyperfunctioning parathyroid tissue is predicted by a fall of PTH by more than

50% of its preoperative (baseline) value, within 10 to 15 minutes. Studies have reported that a 50% reduction from pre-excision PTH values within 5-10 minutes of adenoma excision can accurately predict post-operative normocalcaemia. (Inabnet et al, 1999). In other words, a decrease of more than 50% from the baseline value at 5–10 minutes after resection is suggestive of a single gland disease (solitary adenoma). However, if such a drop does not occur, then the possibility of multi gland disease is likely, and a conversion to bilateral neck exploration should be considered.

OUTCOMES	COMMENTS
Cure rates	Similar cure rates between MAP and conventional parathyroidectomy 95%-100%
Complications	Similar complication rates between minmal access parathyroidectomy and conventional parathyroidectomy(Starker et al 2011) Recurrent laryngeal nerve injury and transient hypoparathyroidism <1% Post operative haemorrhage (0.2%-0.5%)
Cosmesis	Definitive evidence of smaller scars Some opine that centrally placed scars appear better than lateral scars Concern of central scar more prone to keloid formation Axillary approach avoids unsightly scars in visible areas of the neck & torso
Hospital stay	Shorter hospital stay < 23 hrs Day case surgery especially if performed under local anaesthesia

Table 5. Overview of outcomes in minimal access parathyroidectomy

The disadvantages described include its cost,and interaction with anesthetic drug propofol (which should be stopped 5-10 minutes before blood sampling). The full potential of IOPTH needs further study. The role of intra-operative radioguided technique is controversial. Some are of the opinion that radioguided techniques rarely provide any additional information over the sestamibi scan itself and should not be routinely used during parathyroid operations.

All patients may not be candidates for directed or targeted minimal access approaches. Patients with mutigland disease, MEN-related hyperplasia, and renal disease may not be suitable candidates for MAP. Whether the long term outcomes of MAP will be comparable to the best results obtainable with a conventional bilateral exploration remains to be proven.

KEY POINTS-4

- Since majority of the patients have only a single-gland disease, bilateral neck exploration is not routinely necessary, in all patients.
- The term MAP/MIP should be reserved for parathyroidectomies performed through inscions less than 2.5 cm.

- Cure rates are equivalent to those of a bilateral neck exploration for single gland disease.
- Advantages include avoidance of general aneasthesa and overnight admission, good cosmesis.
- Minimal access approach may be best suited for single adenomatous disease.
- Surgical expertise is still an important factor.

6. Conventional parathyroidectomy: "Identification and dissection of the parathyroid glands"

The three important goals in parathyroid surgery are-

1. Recognizing the normal from abnormal parathyroids.
2. Identifying and protecting recurrent laryngeal nerves.
3. Searching for parathyroids in predictable locations.

The initial operative steps are similar to that for thyroidectomy. The corresponding thyroid lobe is elevated and the structures lying under this region are carefully inspected first. The normal parathyroids and the fat in this region may appear similar initially and moreover the parathyroids may be covered by a globule or layer of adipose tissue.

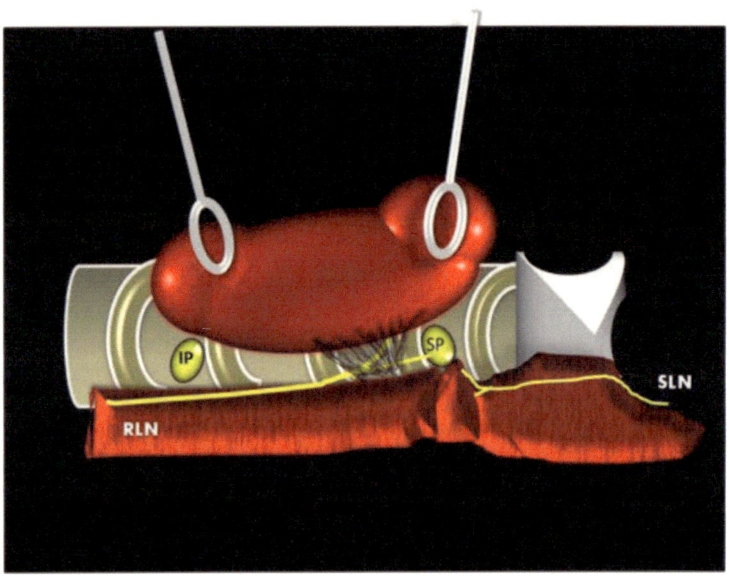

Fig. 9. Schematic representation of the expected anatomy during conventional parathyroidectomy. The thyroid lobe is mobilized .The recurrent laryngeal nerve(RLN) lies in the trachea-oesophageal groove. The commonest position of the superior parathyroid gland (SP) is posterior to the superior or middle third of the thyroid lobe and that of the inferior parathyroid gland(IP) is anterior, lateral, or posterior to the inferior third of the thyroid lobe with the nerve passing obliquely between them.

A small pledget can be used to tease way cobweb like fascia lying in close proximity to the posterolateral surface of the elevated thyroid lobe. This will most often bring into view the locations of the superior and inferior parathyroids. The presence of globular fat deposits might create some amount of confusion. The normal parathyroids are soft and can be present in different shapes and may be sometimes very much flattened like a disc by the overlying fascial layer. Once the fascia is teased away the glands will appear to be more globular. The gland will also have a network of fine capillaries on the surface [figure 10] and a biopsy might cause it to bleed (in contrast to fat). Lymph nodes and thyroid nodules may add to confusion too but these are often palpably firm.

The recurrent laryngeal nerve typically runs in the tracheo-esophageal groove with the superior parathyroids more anteriorly and inferior parathyroids more posterior in relation to this nerve. Capsular rupture of the abnormal gland should be avoided to prevent implantation of parathyroid cells in the operative site. Histological confirmation by frozen section examination is often valuable.

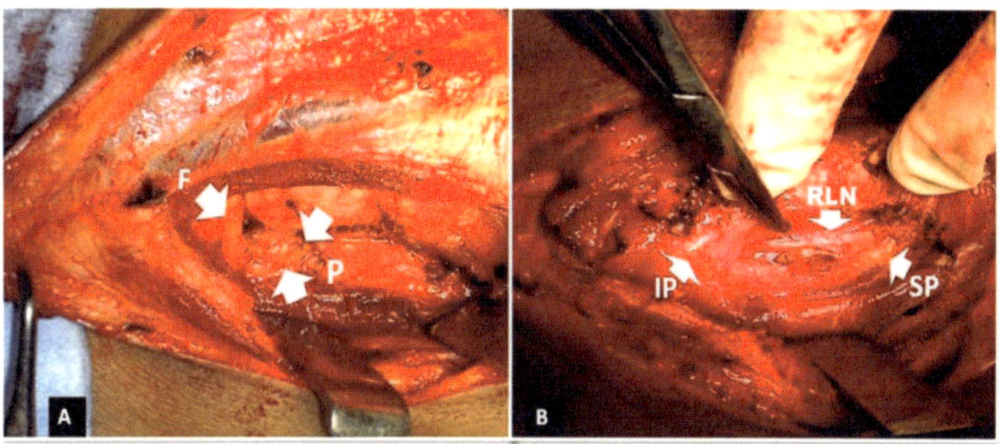

Fig. 10. (A) Operative photograph showing the parathyroid (P) which can be differentiated from fat (F) by the presence of fine blood vessels on the surface of the gland. (B) Operative photograph depicting normal relationships between recurrent laryngeal nerve (RLN), and superior(SP) and inferior parathyroid(IP) glands.

7. Ectopic parathyroids: "The hunt for the elusive parathyroids"

Sometimes, all the parathyroid glands cannot be identified readily. A systematic search is performed; based on the knowledge of the path of descent of superior and inferior parathyroid glands. The table gives a brief description of the places to look for in such cases.

The superior parathyroid glands are normaly located on the posterior aspect of the superior or middle third of the thyroid lobe in more than 90% of the cases. The location of an ectopic superior parathyroid gland may be above the upper pole of the thyroid lobe (<1%); posterior to the pharynx or esophagus, in either the neck or the superior mediastinum (1%-4%); or intrathyroidal (<3%) (Eslamy & Ziessman, 2008).

The ectopic inferior parathyroid glands may be found, inferior to the lower pole of the thyroid lobe, either in the thyrothymic ligament or associated with the cervical portion of the thymus (26%); on or adjacent to the posterior aspect of the middle third of the thyroid lobe (7%); in the anterior mediastinum (4%-5%); intrathyroidal (<3%); or along the carotid sheath (<1%-2%).

Gland	Where to look for
Superior parathyroids	adjacent to the superior thyroid vessels the carotid sheath or posterior to the esophagus or pharynx (retroesophageal) the capsule of the thyroid gland
Inferior parathyroids	thyrothymic ligament. the thymus anterior mediastinum carotid sheath capsule of the thyroid

Table 7. Locations of ectopic parathyroid s

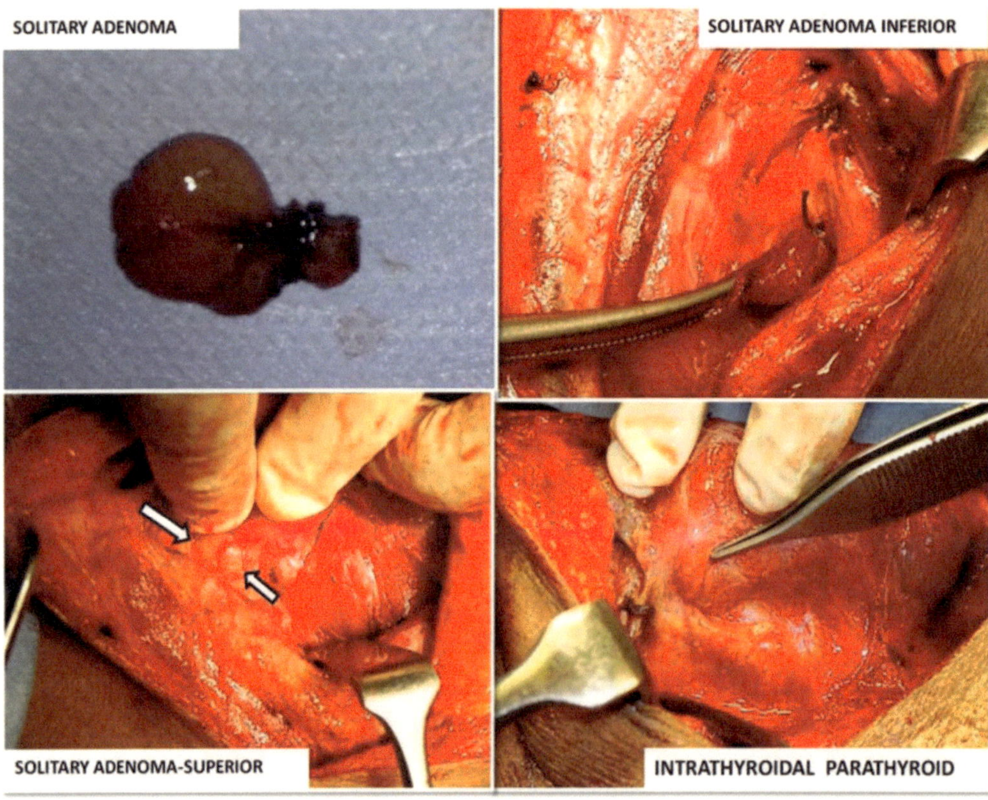

Fig. 11.

8. Conclusion - "The future"

As the patients are often asymptomatic, the diagnosis of primary hyperparathyroidism is based principally on laboratory findings of elevated serum calcium and serum parathyroid hormone levels. Asymptomatic disease is the commonest form of presentation in the developed nations. Symptomatic disease is very common in developing parts of the world.

Surgery is the only, definitive treatment for symptomatic disease. Since majority of cases of primary hyperparathyroidism, are due to a single parathyroid adenoma, selective gland excision is a better option. This should be facilitated with appropriate preoperative localization techniques such as with (Tc^{99m}) sestamibi scanning alone or combined with other modalities wherever possible. Intra-operative parathyroid hormonal monitoring may be a useful adjunct and can predict possibility of multigland disease and the need for converting the procedure to a bilateral neck exploration. The new surgical procedures are here to stay. Minimally access parathyroid surgery is feasible and should probably be increasingly offered to select group of patients. Conversion to bilateral neck exploration should not be regarded as a complication.

The final statement is that: "the success of both conventional and minimal access parathyroidectomy is dependent on the surgeon's hard earned experience and nothing can substitute that. "

9. References

Abboud, B., Sleilaty, G., Helou, E., Mansour, E., Tohme, C., Noun, R. & Sarkis, R. (2005), *Existence and Anatomic Distribution of Double Parathyroid Adenoma.* The Laryngoscope, 115: 1128–1131. doi: 10.1097/01.MLG.0000163745.57542.FE

Agarwal G, Barraclough BH, Reeve TS & Delbridge LW.(2002). *Minimally invasive parathyroidectomy using the "focused" lateral approach. II. Surgical technique.* Aust N Z J Surg;72:147–51

Akerström G, Malmaeus J & Bergström R.(1984). *Surgical anatomy of human parathyroid glands. Surgery.*;95(1):14-21

Allendorf J, Kim L, Chabot J, DiGiorgi M, Spanknebel K & Logerfo P. (2003).*The impact of sestamibi scanning on the outcome of parathyroid surgery.* J Clin Endocrinol Metab; 88:3015–8.

Baloch ZW & LiVolsi VA. (2001).*Double adenoma of the parathyroid gland; Does the entity exist?* Arch Pathol Lab Med 125:(2)178–179

Bergenfelz A, Lindblom P, Tibblin S, et al. (2002). *Unilateral versus bilateral neck exploration for primary hyperparathyroidism – a prospective randomized controlled.* Ann Surg.;236:543–551.

Bergenfelz A, Lindblom P, Tibblin S, Westerdahl J. (2002). *Unilateral versus bilateral neck exploration for primary hyperparathyroidism: a prospective randomized controlled trial. Ann Surg.* Nov;236(5):543–51.

Bess MA, Edis AJ, & von Heerden JA.(1980). *Hyperparathyroidism and pancreatitis. Chance or a causal association*? JAMA; 243: 246–7.

Bhansali, S. R. Masoodi, S. Reddy et al.(2005), "Primary hyperparathyroidism in north India: a description of 52 cases," Annals of Saudi Medicine, vol. 25, no. 1, 29–35,.

Bilezikian JP, Khan AA, & Potts JT Jr(2009). (Third International Workshop on the Management of Asymptomatic Primary Hyperparathyroidism). Guidelines for the management of asymptomatic primary hyperparathyroidism: summary statement from the Third International Workshop. *J Clin Endocrinol Metab.*;94:335-339.

Bilezikian JP, Potts JT, Jr, El-Hajj Fuleihan G, et al.(2002).*Summary statement from a workshop on asymptomatic primary hyperparathyroidism: a perspective for the 21st century.* J Bone Miner Res.;17(suppl 2):N2-N11

Bonjer HJ & Bruining HA. (1997) The technique of parathyroidectomy. In: Clark O, Duh Q, eds. Textbook of Endocrine Surgery. Philadelphia, Pa: WB Saunders;.

Brunaud L, Zarnegar R, Wada N, Ituarte P, Clark OH & Duh QY.(2003). *Incision length for standard thyroidectomy and parathyroidectomy. When is it minimally invasive?* Arch Surg;138:1140–3.

Burney RE, Jones KR & Christy B(1999). *Thompson NW. Health status improvement after surgical correction of primary hyperparathyroidism in patients with high and low preoperative calcium levels.* Surgery ;125(6):608-14.

Chan AK, Duh QY, Katz MH, Siperstein AE & Clark OH.(1995). *Clinical manifestations of primary hyperparathyroidism before and after parathyroidectomy. A case-control study.* Ann Surg.;222(3):402-12; discussion 412-4.

Clark O.(1997). *What's new in endocrine surgery.* J Am Coll Surg;184:126–36.

Clark OH, Wilkes W, Siperstein AE & Duh QY. (1991). *Diagnosis and management of asymptomatic hyperparathyroidism: safety, efficacy, and deficiencies in our knowledge.* J Bone Miner Res; 6 Suppl 2:S135-S42; discussion S151-2.

Delattre JF, Flament JB, Palot JP &Pluot M.(1982).*Variations in the parathyroid glands. Number, situation and arterial vascularization. Anatomical study and surgical application.* J Chir (Paris);119(11):633-41.

Delbridge LW. (2003). *Minimally invasive parathyroidectomy: the Australian experience.* Asian J Surg;26(2):76–81.

Denham DW & Norman J.(1998). *Cost-effectiveness of pre-operative sestamibi scan for primary hyperparathyroidism is dependent solely on surgeon's choice of operative procedure.* J Am Coll Surg; 186: 293-304.

Dufour DR & Wilkerson SY.(1983).*Factors related to parathyroid weight in normal persons.* Arch Pathol Lab Med; 107(4): 167–172

Eknoyan G.(1995).*A history of the parathyroid glands.* Am J Kidney Dis;26(5):801–7.

Elaraj DM & Clark OH (2008).*Current status and treatment of primary hyperparathyroidism.* Perm J. Winter; 12(1):32-7.

Eslamy HK, & Ziessman H. (2008). *Parathyroid scintigraphy in patients with primary hyperparathyroidism:* ^{99m}Tc sestamibi SPECT and SPECT/CT. Radiographics28:1461–1476.

Feliciano DV. *Parathyroid pathology in an intrathyroidal position.* Am J Surg; 164(5):496-500.

Gagner M.(1996). Endoscopic parathyroidectomy. Br J Surg;83:875.

Gauger PG, Reeve TS & Delbridge LW. (1999) *Endoscopically assisted, minimally invasive parathyroidectomy.* Br J Surg;86(12):1563–6.

Goldstein RE, Blevins L, Delbeke D, et al. (2000*). Effect of minimally invasive radioguided parathyroidectomy on efficacy, length of stay, and costs in the management of primary hyperparathyroidism.* Ann Surg.;231:732–742

Harinarayan CV, Gupta N & Kochupillal N.(1995).*Vitamin D status in primary hyperparathyroidism in India.* Clin Endocrinol (Oxf); 43: 35 1-8.

Henry JF, Defechereux T, Gramatica L & De Boissezon C. (1999). *Endoscopic parathyroidectomy via a lateral neck incision.* Ann Chir;53:302–6.

Ho Shon IA, Bernard EJ, Roach PJ & Delbridge LW.(2001). *The value of oblique pinhole images in pre-operative localiasation with 99Tc-MIBI for primary hyperparathyroidism.* Eur J Nucl Med;28:736–42.

Hooghe L, Kinnaert P & Van Geertruyden J.(1992). *Surgical anatomy of hyperparathyroidism.* Acta Chir Belg.; 92(1):1-9.

Inabnet WB, Fulla Y, Richard B, Bonnichon P, Icard P & Chapuis Y.(1999). *Unilateral neck exploration under local anaesthesia: the approach of choice for asymptomatic primary hyperparathyroidism. Surgery;* 126: 1004-1010

Irvin GL. (1999) *Presidential address: chasin' hormones.* Surgery;126(6):993–7.

Kaplan EL, Yashiro T & Salti G.(1992). *Primary hyperparathyroidism in the 1990s. Choice of surgical procedures for this disease.* Ann Surg. Apr;215(4):300-17.

Kearns AE & Thompson GB. (2002). *Medical and surgical management of hyperparathyroidism* [published correction appears in Mayo Clin Proc. 2002;77:298]. Mayo Clin Proc.;77:87-91.

Lee F. Starker, Annabelle L. Fonseca, Tobias Carling, & Robert Udelsman,((2011). *"Minimally Invasive Parathyroidectomy," International Journal of Endocrinology,* vol. 2011, doi:10.1155/2011/206502

Lowe H, McMahon DJ, Rubin MR, Bilezikian JP & Silverberg SJ.(2007). *Normocalcemic primary hyperparathyroidism: further characterization of a new clinical phenotype.* J Clin Endocrinol Metab.;92:3001-3005

Mandl F.(1925).*Therapeutischer Versuch bei Ostitis fibrosa generalisata mittels Exstinpationeines Epithelkorperchentumours. (Therapeutic attempt for osteitis fibrosa generalisata via the excision of parathyroid tumours).* Wien Klin Wochenschr 38:1343–4

Mihai, R., Palazzo, F.F., Gleeson, F.V. & Sadler, G.P. (2007). *Minimally invasive parathyroidectomy without intraoperative parathyroid hormone monitoring in patients with primary hyperparathyroidism.* British Journal of Surgery, 94, 42-47.

Miura D, Wada N, Arici C, Morita E, Duh QY & Clark OH. (2002). *Does intraoperative quick parathyroid hormone assay improve the results of parathyroidectomy?* World J Surg; 26(8):926–30.

Nobori M, Saiki S, Tanaka N, Harihara Y, Shindo S & Fujimoto Y.(1994).*Blood supply of the parathyroid gland from the superior thyroid artery.* Surgery; 115(4):417-23.

Peacock M,Bilezikian JP, Klassen PS, Guo MD, Turner SA & Shoback D.(2005). *Cinacalcet hydrochloride maintains long-term normocalcemia in patients with primary hyperparathyroidism.* J Clin Endocrinol Metab.;90:135-141

Pradeep P. V., Jayashree B., Mishra A, &. Mishra S. K.."*Systematic Review of Primary Hyperparathyroidism in India: The Past, Present, and the Future Trends,*" International Journal of Endocrinology, vol. 2011, Article ID 921814, 7 pages, 2011. doi:10.1155/2011/921814

Russell, C.F., Laird, J.D. & Ferguson, W.R. (1990). *Scan-directed unilateral cervical exploration for parathyroid adenoma: a legitimate approach?* World Journal of Surgery, 14, 406-409.

Schell SR & Dudley NE.(2003). *Clinical outcomes and fiscal consequences of bilateral neck exploration for primary idiopathic hyperparathyroidism without preoperative radionuclide imaging or minimally invasive techniques.* Surgery;133(1):32–9.

Sheldon DG, Lee FT, Neil NJ & Ryan JA.(2002) *Surgical treatment of hyperparathyroidism improves health related quality of life.* Arch Surg;137: 1022–8.

Sidhu S, Neill AK, Russell CFJ. (2003). *Long-term outcome of unilateral parathyroid exploration for primary hyperparathyroidism due to presumed solitary adenoma.* World J Surg; 27: 339-342

Sidhu, S., Neill, A.K. & Russell, C.F. (2003). *Long-term outcome of unilateral parathyroid exploration for primary hyperparathyroidism due to presumed solitary adenoma*. World Journal of Surgery, 27, 339-342.

Silverberg SJ, Shane E, Jacobs TP, Siris E & Bilezikian JP (1999). *A 10-year prospective study of primary hyperparathyroidism with or without parathyroid surgery*. N Engl J Med 341: 1249-1255.

Talpos GB, Bone HG 3rd, Kleerekoper M, et al.(2000). *Randomized trial of parathyroidectomy in mild asymptomatic primary hyperparathyroidism: patient description and effects on the SF-36 health survey*. Surgery; 128(6):1013-20;discussion 1020-1.

Taniegra ED. (2004).*Hyperparathyroidism*. Am Fam Physician.; 69:333-339.

Tibblin S, Bondeson AG & Ljungberg O. (1982). *Unilateral parathyroidectomy in hyperparathyroidismdue to parathyroid adenoma*. Ann Surg 195:245–52.

Udelsman R. (2002). *Six hundred fifty-six consecutive explorations for primary hyperparathyroidism*. Ann Surg.;235:665–670.

Wang C.(1981).*Hyperfunctioning intrathyroid parathyroid gland: a potential cause of failure in parathyroid surgery*. J R Soc Med.;74(1):49-52.

Yao K, Singer FR, Roth S, Sassoon A, C Ye, & Giuliano A E.. (2004). *Weight of Normal Parathyroid Glands in Patients with Parathyroid Adenomas*. The Journal of Clinical Endocrinology & Metabolism;vol. 89 no. 7:3208-3213

Zachariah S K & Thomas P. A. (2010) Primary hyperparathyroidism: A report of two unusual cases. *Indian Journal of Surgery* 72:2, 135-137

12

Treatment Modalities in Thyroid Dysfunction

R. King and R.A. Ajjan
Division of Cardiovascular and Diabetes Research, Leeds Institute of Genetics Health and Therapeutics, Faculty of Medicine and Health, University of Leeds, Leeds UK

1. Introduction

Thyroid dysfunction is a common condition mainly affecting women, with a male to female ratio of around 1:10. An organ-specific autoimmune response is the underlying cause in the majority and susceptibility to thyroid autoimmunity is believed to be influenced by an interaction between genetic predisposition and environmental factors, in addition to endogenous factors such as age and sex (Vanderpump 1995).

Autoimmune hyperthyroidism, or Graves' disease (GD), affects around 2% of the female population and is characterised by the presence of thyroid stimulating antibodies (TSAb), which mimic the action of thyroid stimulating hormone (TSH), resulting in uncontrolled thyroid hormone production. TSAb also contribute to extra-thyroidal manifestation of the disease, including thyroid eye disease (TED), although the exact mechanistic pathways are not entirely clear. At the other end of the spectrum, autoimmune hypothyroidism (AH) affects up to 5% of women and is characterised by the presence of thyroid peroxidase (TPO). These antibodies do not seem to have a direct functional role but are implicated in perpetuating the intrathyroidal inflammation and tissue destruction (Ajjan & Weetman 2008).

In this Chapter, we discuss the various therapies used in hyper- and hypothyroidism, and address management of special cases.

2. Aetiology of hyperthyroidism

GD is by far the commonest cause of hyperthyroidism accounting for around 80% of cases (Weetman 2000). It is frequently seen in multiple family members indicating a genetic predisposition, commonly seen in organ-specific autoimmune conditions.

The second commonest cause is a solitary toxic nodule or multinodular goitre accounting for 15-20% of cases (Orgiazzi & Mornex1990). Toxic multinodular goitres tend to occur insidiously in elderly patients with a longstanding nodular goitre. Toxic adenomas result from benign monoclonal proliferation producing a single autonomously functioning nodule, typically greater than 2.5cm in diameter. Goitres of any nature are more prevalent in iodine deficient areas and are more common in females (Reinwein et al 1988).

There are other rare causes for hyperthyroidism, which should be kept in mind when assessing the patient and these are summarised in Table 1.

Cause of hyperthyroidism	Frequency and aetiology	Diagnosis
Graves' disease	99%, thyroid stimulating antibodies	Clinical examination (Smooth goitre, extrathyroidal complications) Thyroid autoantibodies Thyroid uptake scan in difficult cases
Toxic nodule or toxic multinodular goitre	15%, activating mutations in TSH receptor and Gsα protein	Clinical examination Thyroid uptake scan
Thyroiditis	3%, autoimmune, viral or drug-related (amiodarone)	Clinical examination Thyroid uptake scan ESR
TSH-secreting tumour	<1%	Raised TSH and thyroid hormones Pituitary imaging
Exogenous thyroid hormone administration	Variable, excess ingestion of thyroid hormones	Clinical assessment
Hyperemesis gravidarum Choriocarcinoma	Rare, raised hCG	Clinical assessment Absence of thyroid autoimmunity Known pregnancy Imaging of the pelvis
Struma ovarii	Rare, ectopic ovarian thyroid tissue	Clinical assessment Thyroid/pelvic uptake scan Imaging of the pelvis
Thyroid hormone resistance	Rare, pituitary resistance to thyroid hormones	Clinical assessment Family history

Table 1. Hyperthyroidism: aetiology and diagnosis.

2.1 Diagnosis of hyperthyroidism

Main symptoms and signs of hyperthyroidism are summarised in Table 2. Careful history and examination will typically point towards a diagnosis of hyperthyroidism and its underlying cause. Biochemical confirmation is required and enables the clinician to monitor response to treatment. Levels of thyroid stimulating hormone (TSH) are suppressed (<0.03miu/l) together with elevated levels of circulating thyroid hormones, L-thyroxine (T4) and/or L-triidothyronine (T3). Measurement of TSH and free T4 (FT4) is usually sufficient to confirm a diagnosis of thyrotoxicosis, but FT3 levels should be measured when TSH levels are suppressed with normal FT4 levels as roughly 5% of all cases may only have elevated levels of T3 (Singer et al 1995).

The diagnosis of GD is usually based on clinical and biochemical thyrotoxicosis in the presence of a smooth goitre with or without extrathyroidal manifestation of the disease. In some cases, the cause of hyperthyroidism is unclear and additional biochemical and/or imaging tests may be needed.

The presence of thyroid autoantibodies supports the diagnosis of thyroid autoimmunity. Antibodies (Ab) against TPO are frequently checked in clinical practice, although these are only detected in 80% of individuals with GD (Ajjan & Weetman 2008). Antibodies against thyroid stimulating hormone receptor (TSHR) are detected in 95-99% of patients with GD (depending on the sensitivity of the test used) and therefore these are more informative than TPO-Ab in cases of uncertain aetiology (Ajjan&Weetman 2008; Matthews & Syed 2011).

Radioisotope uptake scans using 99mtechnetium or 131iodine, will show an increase in uptake and a diffusely enlarged thyroid in GD. Toxic MNG will show multiple nodules with increased uptake. A solitary nodule with increased uptake and suppressed function in the remaining, normal tissue is seen in a toxic adenoma (Cooper 2003). All forms of thyroiditis can be differentiated by low or absent uptake.

Symptoms	Frequency
Nervousness, irritability, heat intolerance, palpitation	>90%
Weight loss, increased appetite, fatigue, loose stool	>80%
Eye symptoms (TED)	>50%
Menstrual irregularities, insomnia, polyuria	>25%
Signs	**Frequency**
Hyperkinetic behaviour, fast speech, tachycardia, tremor, goitre, tachycardia or atrial fibrillation, moist skin	>90%
Thrill/bruit over the thyroid	>70%
Eye signs (in GD), thinning of hair, hyperreflexia	50%
Pretibial myxoedema and acropachy (in GD), onycholysis	5%

Table 2. Main symptoms and signs in Graves' disease. TED: thyroid eye disease, GD: Graves' disease.

2.2 Management of hyperthyroidism

There are three main treatment modalities for hyperthyroidism, which include medical therapy, radioactive iodine and surgery. In addition, supportive therapy is sometimes required to control symptoms. Treatment options for hyperthyroidism are summarised in Figure 1.

2.2.1 Medical

Control of hyperthyroidism. Anti thyroid drugs (ATD), known as thionamides, are commonly prescribed to control the excessive production of thyroid hormone and include carbimazole, its active metabolite methimazole and propylthiouracil (PTU). Use of these agents varies worldwide; methimazole and PTU are preferred in the USA, carbimazole is widely used first line in the United Kingdom and Methimazole is preferred in the rest of Europe and Asia (Weetman 2000). Methimazole or Carbimazole is often preferred to PTU as it has a longer half life and is therefore given once a day whereas PTU needs to be taken 2 or 3 times a day (Franklyn 1994). They should generally be instituted in patients with a confirmed diagnosis of hyperthyroidism, but may not be necessary if definitive treatment is planned early and hyperthyroidism is mild (Weetman 2000). Thionamides can be used in the short term to induce euthyroidism prior to more definitive treatment such as radio-iodine or surgery or in the medium term in case of GD with the aim of inducing remission. Long term treatment is reserved for patients in whom definitive treatment is relatively contraindicated, such as elderly, frail patients

T4 and T3 molecules are formed within the thyroid gland by the coupling of iodotyrosine residues, which in turn have been formed from the binding of iodine and tyrosine within thyroglobulin, an action catalysed by TPO (Cooper 2005). The thionamides act by inhibiting the formation and coupling of these iodotyrosine residues and thus reduce T4 and T3 concentrations. Propylthiouracil also has the action of inhibiting the peripheral conversion of T4 to T3.

Carbimazole is usually commenced at a dose of 20-40mg once a day, depending on the severity of thyrotoxicosis. Regular monitoring of TSH and T4 is required every 4-6 weeks and the initial dose can be titrated as the thyroid function normalises and the patient becomes euthyroid. A drop in the T4 to low-normal levels or below the normal range indicates that a reduction in dosage or addition of levothyroxine is needed. The former scenario constitutes the "titration regime", whereas the latter is known as "block and replace regime". In the titration regime, the smallest dose of anti-thyroid drug is used to maintain thyroid function within the normal range. The levels of T4 and T3 will begin to reduce within 2-4 weeks of treatment, however the TSH may remain suppressed for significantly longer and hence TSH alone should not be used to guide and monitor treatment (British Thyroid Association guidelines [BTA] 2006, Bahn 2011).

If block and replace is used, which is usually reserved to individuals with GD, the patient is maintained on a high dose of carbimazole or propylthiouracil for 4-6 weeks and when the T4 levels fall to the normal range, Levothyroxine is commenced (usually 75-150 μg daily, according to patient weight) whilst continuing with the same dose of thionamide. Regular monitoring of TSH and T4 are required initially with alterations in the dose of thyroxine guided by T4 levels. Once established on a maintenance dose and TSH and T4 levels have normalised, the doses are unlikely to vary and so less frequent testing is possible (e.g. 6 monthly). Block and replace regimes should not be used in pregnant women (detailed below).

If thionamides are used to treat Graves' disease they can usually be discontinued after a course of treatment, ranging from 6-18 months, with approximately 50% of patients remaining in remission thereafter (Hedley et al 1989, Maugendre et al 1999). In most centres, titration regime is administered for 18 months, whereas block and replace is usually given for 6 months only (Abraham et al 2005). There does not appear to be a difference in remission rates between titration and block and replace regimes (Abraham et al 2005, Reinwein at al 1993). Higher rates of relapse typically occur with severe biochemical thyrotoxicosis at diagnosis, a large goitre, extrathyroidal complications, high anti-TSHR titres and in men (Vitti et al 1997). Thyrotoxicosis caused by nodular goitres does not undergo remission and generally requires a more definitive treatment once the initial thyrotoxicosis has been controlled.

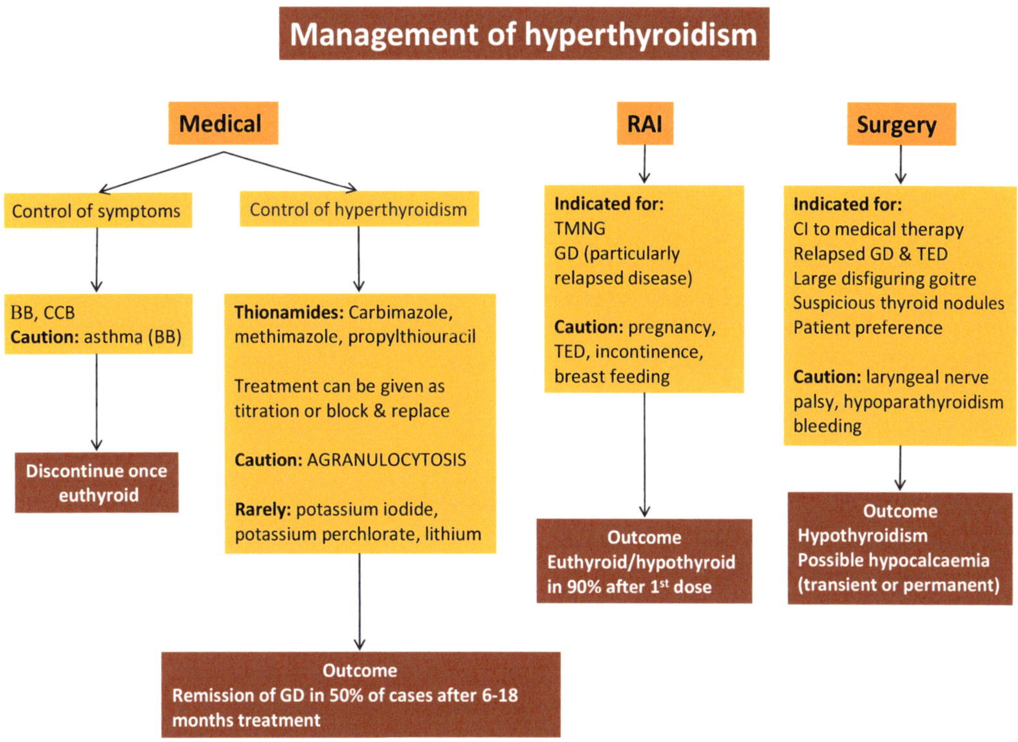

Fig. 1. Summary of the management of hyperthyroidism. BB: β-blockers, CCB: calcium channel blockers, GD: Graves' disease, TMNG: toxic nodular goitre, TED: thyroid eye disease, CI: contraindication.

Several side effects can be attributed to thionamide medication. Common adverse effects include nausea, gastrointestinal upset, headache, fever, rash, urticaria and arthralgia. Rarely, hair loss may occur as a result of carbimazole therapy, although this may also be a manifestation of thyrotoxicosis. More worrying but less frequent side effects include agranulocytosis, vasculitis, and hepatitis, with the latter being more of an issue with PTU (Cooper & Rivkees 2009). Agranulocytosis occurs in approximately 0.4-0.5% of cases. All patients are warned of this rare but serious side effect and asked to immediately report symptoms consistent with agranulocytosis such as severe sore throat, fever or mouth ulcers. Urgent full blood count is required in patients taking thionamide with such symptoms and treatment withheld until it is clear that white blood cells and neutrophil counts are normal. When such a complication develops, patients are admitted to hospital, given appropriate antibiotics and a haematology opinion is sought, particularly if they require granulocyte stimulating factor administration. Once a patient develops agranulocytosis to an antithyroid drug, it represents a contraindication to the use of other thionamides (Biswas 1991). However, in the presence of other adverse effects, swapping to another antithyroid medication is a possibility. For example, arthralgia induced by carbimazole does not necessarily occur with propylthiouracil treatment.

Supportive management. Some patients who present with significant thyrotoxic symptoms require supportive treatment whilst awaiting normalisation of thyroid hormone levels. Typically β-adrenergic blockers such as propranolol are used until thyroid function tests improve at which point they may be withdrawn (Franklyn 1994). Caution must be used in patients with a contra-indication such as heart failure and asthma. An alternative therapy would be a non-dihydropyridine calcium channel blockers such as diltiazem or verapamil

Other medical therapies. Treatments such as potassium iodide, potassium perchlorate and lithium are less conventional, but possible treatment options, particularly when agranulocytosis develops secondary to antithyroid drug treatment. When given in large enough quantities, potassium iodide blocks the synthesis and release of thyroid hormones from a thyrotoxic gland and results in an accumulation of iodide within the gland. A significant reduction in thyroid hormones can be seen as quickly as 2 days following administration, and is typically reserved for preparing thyrotoxic patients, who are unable to tolerate thionamide medication, for surgery. However, this treatment can only be given for a short period of time as the patient eventually "escapes" from the inhibitory effect of iodine (Philippou 1992).

Lithium acts by inhibiting the release of T4 & T3 and is generally used in similar circumstances to potassium iodide or in combination with a thionamide in patients who have needed recurrent doses of radioiodine as it is thought to help retention of I^{131} (Bal et al 2002, Bogazzi et all 1999). Potassium perchlorate is generally reserved for use in type 1 amiodarone induced thyrotoxicosis and requires similar monitoring to other anti-thyroid medication, with aplastic anaemia being the most serious side effect.

2.2.2 Radioactive Iodine (RAI)

Indications for RAI. This can be used as a primary treatment for hyperthyroidism or as a secondary option if anti-thyroid medication has failed to control hyperthyroidism. It is common practice for patients with GD to undergo a course of anti-thyroid medication initially. If this does not achieve long term euthyroidism, due to either the relapsing nature of the condition following withdrawal of ATD or treatment difficulties, then radioactive iodine is indicated as a definitive treatment due to long term morbidity and mortality associated with uncontrolled hyperthyroidism. Severe adverse events such as agranulocytosis and hepatic dysfunction caused by thionamides are also an indication for RAI (Royal College of Physicians [RCP] 2007). It is more commonly used in North America as a primary treatment in patients with GD (Solomon et al 1990), due to poor remission rates, and other factors including age, pre-existing medical conditions such as cardiovascular disease, availability of RAI and patient preference may influence this decision. RAI is recommended in patients with hyperthyroidism due to nodular goitres as antithyroid drugs do not result in long term cure of the disease.

RAI is successful in achieving long-term euthyroidism or hypothyroidism in approximately 90% of patients after a single dose of between 400-600MBq after 1 year (Regalbuto et al 2009). A minority will require a second dose and very rarely a third treatment with RAI.

Contraindications to RAI. Pregnancy and breastfeeding are absolute contraindications to RAI and pregnancy should be avoided for 6 months following treatment. Iodine is concentrated in milk and is able to cross the placenta, damaging the foetal thyroid. RAI should also be avoided in patients who are unable to comply with the safety regulations after administration. Current treatment with amiodarone (or within the preceding 12 months) is another contraindication as this reduces the uptake of RAI into the thyroid, greatly reducing its efficacy as is suspicion of thyroid malignancy. Caution is needed in patients incontinent of urine, which represents a relative contraindication and insertion of a urinary catheter or urinary pads with appropriate disposal facilities are ways to circumvent the problem (RCP 2007). Another relative contraindication is individuals with active eye disease. If RAI treatment is necessary in TED patients then concurrent oral glucocorticoids are effective in reducing development or progression of TED (Bartalena 2011). Some centres, including ours, advocate starting block and replace one week after RAI for 6 months after which antithyroid drugs can be withdrawn and levothyroxine continued. This helps in avoiding fluctuation in thyroid function, which can be associated with worsening of TED (Tallstedt et al 1994).

Precautions after RAI treatment. Most of the radioactivity is taken up by the thyroid, whilst some is excreted in urine and sweat. It is important that patients are able to comply with the necessary restrictions following RAI treatment to limit the radiation exposure of other members of the public. These include limiting close contact (less than 1m) with people, especially children under 3 years of age and pregnant women. The exact duration of the limitations will vary depending on the dose received, and can be up to 28 days (RCP 2007). Patients should be instructed to flush the toilet twice after passing urine and to wash their hands carefully. They should not share towels or face cloths and ensure that cutlery is thoroughly cleaned. Following RAI patients should be issued with a card outlining the details of their treatment and should carry this for 4 weeks or up to 6 months if they are travelling by plane as some airport security devices are able to detect levels of radioactivity this long after RAI (RCP 2007).

Follow up and monitoring. Careful follow up after RAI is essential to detect alterations in thyroid status. Patients treated with ATD and who are biochemically euthyroid prior to RAI are unlikely to require subsequent ATD unless the risk of recurrent hyperthyroidism is deemed unacceptable such as in the elderly or those with cardiovascular co-morbidity (RCP 2007). Patients should be warned that there is a risk of an increase in hyperthyroid symptoms in the first 1-2 weeks after treatment which often respond to β-blockers. Thyroid function tests (TFT's) should be performed around 6 weeks after RAI. Hypothyroidism within the first 6 months of RAI may be transient and thyroid replacement medication should only be commenced if there is a continual rise in TSH levels and falling freeT4 levels Aizawa et al 1997). If patients require re-commencement of ATD following RAI this should be gradually withdrawn over 3 to 5 months. If a patient remains euthyroid 6 weeks post RAI then further thyroid function tests should be performed at 12 weeks, 6, 9 and 12 months. In those who remain hyperthyroid 6 months post RAI, a second dose should be considered (RCP 2007). Annual TFT's are subsequently required to monitor for late onset hypo-, or hyperthyroidism (BTA 2006).

2.2.3 Surgery

Patient selection. Thyroid surgery, in various guises, has been performed since the 1860's as a treatment of goitres (Sawyers 1972). In the modern age there are a number of indications for thyroidectomy; relapse of GD following a course of ATD is one and patients who are unable to undergo RAI, i.e., pregnant women, those with small children who are unable to comply with restrictions, and those with severe ophthalmopathy can be offered surgery as are those who decline RAI. Similarly, patients who are hyperthyroid due to nodular goitre may be offered surgery as a definitive treatment due to the same reasons. Other indications include thyroid malignancy or uncertainty regarding thyroid malignancy and to alleviate compressive or respiratory symptoms due to large goitres (BTA 2006). Another indication for surgery is a cold nodule in a patient with GD, due to the relatively high risk of malignancy in such nodules (Abraham-Nordling et al 2005).

Preparation of patient for surgery. Euthyroid patients undergoing thyroid surgery require no special preparation prior to surgery. If they have had previous thyroid or parathyroid surgery, cervical disc operations or have a hoarse voice then direct or indirect laryngoscopy is recommended to identify previous recurrent laryngeal nerve palsy (Moorthy et al 2011). Thyrotoxic patients should be rendered euthyroid with ATD prior to surgery. Lugol's Iodine was used to be given pre-operatively, which along with reducing thyroid hormone secretion is also thought to reduce thyroid blood flow. However, this is now less common and provided the patient is euthyroid, such a treatment is not usually required (Feek et al 1980).

Post-operative complication. With careful pre-operative preparation and meticulous surgical technique, mortality from thyroid surgery should be <1% and similar to that of general anaesthesia alone (Weetman 2000). Complications do occur to varying degree and include thyroid storm, wound haemorrhage, hypoparathyroidism and recurrent laryngeal nerve injury. The incidence of thyroid storm as a result of thyroid surgery is now very low due to improved pre-operative treatment with ATD and post-operative management. Wound haemorrhage although rare, (occurring <1%) can be very serious and life threatening especially if there has been arterial bleeding causing tracheal compression. Any sign of wound haemorrhage causing respiratory compromise requires urgent intervention Schwartz et al 1998). The occurrence of hypoparathyroidism post-operatively can be either permanent or temporary and is rarely due to mistaken removal of all four parathyroid glands, but rather interruption to their blood supply (Pattou et al 1998). In the hands of experienced surgeons performing a total thyroidectomy, the risk is thought to be between 0-3% (Schüssler-Fiorenza et al 2006). New techniques such as auto transplantation of parathyroid glands during surgery are effective at reducing these rates further (Testini et al 2007). Injury to the recurrent laryngeal nerve is also thought to be around 1-2% and is also higher when surgery is performed for thyroid malignancy. Some return of function to the vocal cords can be expected within the first few months and possibly up to 12 months. Beyond this time it is likely that injury will be permanent.

2.3 Special cases of hyperthyroidism

2.3.1 Amiodarone induced thyrotoxicosis

Treatment of amiodarone induced thyrotoxicosis (AIT) can be challenging, due in most part to the degree of overlap between type1 and type 2 AIT. The first step in the treatment of either case is to discontinue amiodarone if it is safe to do so, for which a cardiology opinion is usually sought. The attending physician attempt to distinguish whether the patient has type 1 or type 2 AIT (summarised in Table 2). Type 1 AIT is due to increased production of thyroid hormones, and so treatment with a thionamide should result in lowering of thyroid hormone levels. Occasionally potassium perchlorate can be added or substituted if there is no response. If successful the dose of thionamide is tapered and the thyroid function tests are monitored. If there is little to no response from first line treatment for type 1 AIT, this may raise the possibility that type 2 AIT is the predominant aetiology. Type 2 AIT is more of an inflammatory response to the drug itself leading to an increase in release of thyroid hormone rather than excessive production. Main treatment involves glucocorticoids, usually prednisolone at a dose of 0.5-1.0 mg/kg/day which is tapered over several months according to response. If hyperthyroidism persists despite these measures, in both type 1 and 2 AIT, then referral for thyroidectomy should be considered as RAI is unlikely to be of benefit due to reduced uptake secondary to amiodarone therapy. In clinical practice, it may be difficult to differentiate between type 1 and type 2 AIT, and sometimes both may occur together. Therefore, a pragmatic approach is frequently adopted by treating for both types of AIT simultaneously using antithyroid drugs and steroids.

2.3.2 Thyroid storm

Although thyroid storm is becoming increasingly less common due to improved diagnosis and treatment of hyperthyroidism, it remains a potentially life threatening emergency that requires urgent attention in an intensive care setting. Early supportive measures are important including fluid resuscitation, correcting electrolyte imbalances, supplemental oxygen, active cooling, and sedation if delirium is difficult to manage. Other treatments are based on clinical findings, such as broad spectrum intravenous antibiotics if infection is suspected and treating dysrhythmia or heart failure. More focused therapy includes ATD and typically PTU is preferred as it helps to lower T3 levels quicker that carbimazole due to its added effect of preventing peripheral conversion of T4 to T3 (Cooper & Rivkees 2009). PTU is given 6 hourly initially and usually oral administration is sufficient. Nasogastric tube may be required in individuals too ill to swallow and the drug can be administered intravenously if there are concerns over drug absorption. Unless contraindicated, propranolol is used to settle tachycardia and anxiety. Once ATD have been instituted, potassium iodide can be added, usually 1 hour after ATD and continued at a dose of 100 mg every 12 hours. The use of glucocorticoids is generally accepted, especially if there is a suspicion of concomitant adrenal insufficiency and may have the additional benefit of lowering T3 levels by preventing peripheral conversion of T4 to T3 (Bahn 2011). In extreme circumstances if there has not been a satisfactory response to treatment, procedures such as dialysis and plasma exchange can reduce levels of thyroid hormone, but in practice are very rarely required (Alfadhi & Gianoukakis 2011).

	Type 1 AIT	Type 2 AIT
FH of thyroid autoimmunity	Possible	Usually absent
Goitre	Yes	No
Thyroid antibodies	Yes	No
Vascularity of thyroid gland assessed by ultrasound	Increased	Decreased
Raised inflammatory markers (IL-6, CRP)	No	Yes

Table 2. Differentiation of type1 and type 2 amiodarone-induced thyrotoxicosis (AIT). FH: family history, IL: interleukin, CRP: C-reactive protein.

2.3.3 Pregnancy

Patients who are receiving treatment with ATD should receive pre-conceptual advice with a view to optimal preparation prior to pregnancy. This includes ensuring they are euthyroid prior to conception and altering medication to PTU which is felt to be superior to carbimazole during pregnancy, especially in the first trimester due to reduced incident of aplasia cutis (Bowman et al 2011). Current evidence suggests that following organogenesis, carbimazole or methimazole should be re-introduced due to a possible increased risk of hepatitis with PTU (Lazarus 2011). Those on a block and replace regime should also be swapped to PTU alone as thionamides will cross the placenta but levothyroxine will not, thus increasing the risk of foetal goitre and hypothyroidism (Weetman 2000). Pregnant patients taking ATD should have frequent TFT's throughout pregnancy (monthly) and the dose reduced to the lowest possible to maintain euthyroidism with T4 at the upper limit of the reference range (Lazarus 2011). Doses of ATD are reduced in the latter stages of pregnancy, and not infrequently stopped altogether as the condition undergoes remission. If hyperthyroidism is secondary to GD (or patient has had previous definitive treatment such as surgery or RAI) then TSH receptor antibodies should be measured as high titres can indicate intrauterine or neonatal thyrotoxicosis (Laurberg et al 1998). TSHR antibodies should not be checked in euthyroid patients previously treated with antithyroid drugs only.

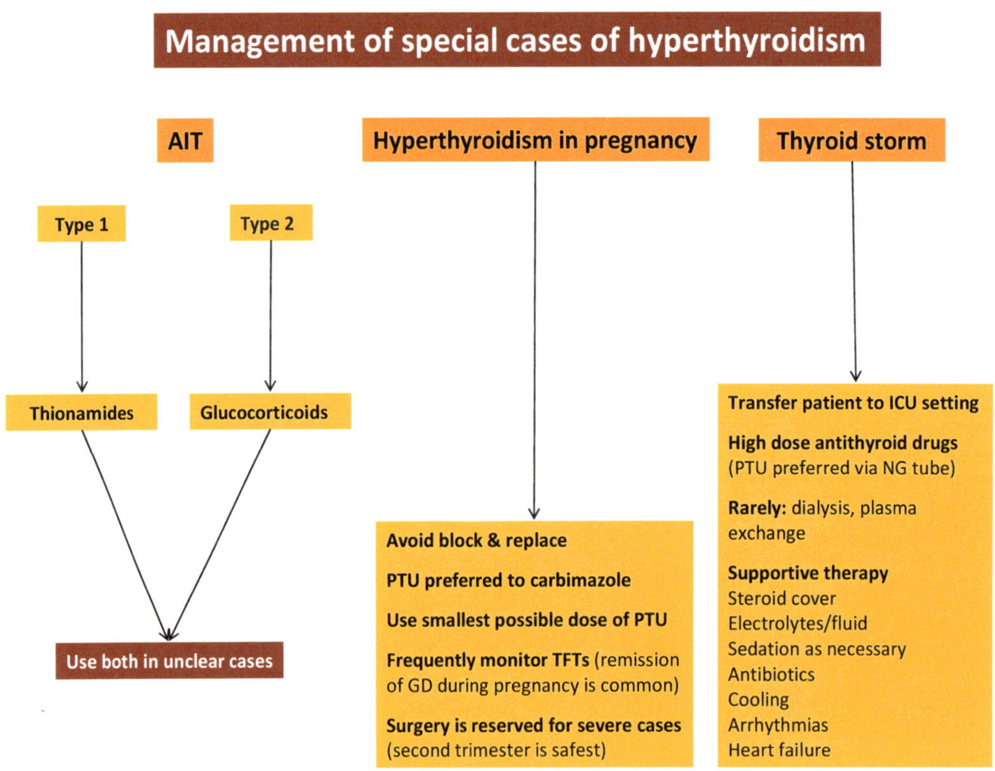

Fig. 2. Management of special cases of hyperthyroidism. AIT: amiodarone induced thyrotoxicosis, GD: Graves' disease, PTU: propylthiouracil, NG: nasogastric, TFT's: thyroid function tests. ICU: intensive care unit.

All euthyroid patients who have previously received treatment for hyperthyroidism should have TFT's checked in each trimester and importantly after delivery as there is an increased risk or recurrence post-partum. If surgery is required, due to allergy or adverse effect of ATD, it is safest to be performed in the second trimester.

2.3.4 Subclinical hyperthyroidism

Subclinical hyperthyroidism is defined as a low TSH level, which is below the reference range (<0.1-0.4 mU/l), in the presence of a normal T4 and T3 concentration. It has become an increasingly problematic clinical entity following the introduction of new and more sensitive serum TSH assays. Patients usually exhibit non-specific symptoms or have no symptoms at all. There remains much debate regarding the correct management of such patients, with a lack of firm evidence to support treatment at present. The ultimate goal of treating these patients early (with the same treatment options as discussed above) is to prevent progression to overt hyperthyroidism, to reduce the risk of developing atrial fibrillation (AF) and ostoeporotic fractures and reduce mortality (Vanderpump 2011). A serum TSH level of between 0.1 and 0.4mU/l carries a very low risk of progression to overt hyperthyroidism, and so treatment need only be considered for those with a persistently suppressed TSH, especially in the presence of cardiovascular disease (Bahn 2011). Given the lack of supporting evidence advocating treatment, a pragmatic approach may be required, balancing the morbidity of hyperthyroid treatment against the risks of developing conditions such as AF, ostoeporotic fractures and overt hyperthyroidism (Vanderpump 2011).

3. Aetiology of hypothyroidism

The causes of hypothyroidism can be differentiated into primary thyroid failure or secondary central hypothyroidism caused by pituitary or hypothalamus failure. In clinical practice most cases are primary in nature, due to chronic autoimmune thyroiditis, which can be goitrous (Hashimotos thyroiditis) or non-goitrous (atrophic thyroiditis). Iatrogenic hypothyroidism is usually caused secondary to treatment of hyperthyroidism. Transient hypothyroidism may be seen following a post-partum thyroiditis or viral induced sub-acute thyroiditis as the thyroid begins recovery after a destructive phase in which stored thyroid hormone is released (Franklyn 1994). Causes of primary hypothyroidism are summarised in Table 3.

3.1 Diagnosis of hypothyroidism

Symptoms of hypothyroidism are numerous and are often also found in patients who are euthyroid, whilst some hypothyroid patients will complain of no symptoms at all. Clinical signs are also very variable, but if present give a strong suspicion of the disease. However the absence of signs cannot be relied upon to exclude a diagnosis. Thyroid function testing is vital to make a diagnosis and include the measurement of TSH and T4 levels. The presence of TSH >10mU/l and free T4 levels below the normal reference range indicate overt hypothyroidism and requires treatment with thyroid replacement hormone. Subclinical hypothyroidism is classified by TSH level above the normal reference range with normal T4. The majority of patients (>95%) with hypothyroidism due to thyroid autoimmunity have detectable TPO antibodies, which aid the diagnosis and help to differentiate from other causes of low thyroid hormone levels. The main clinical symptoms and signs of hypothyroidism are summarised in Table 4.

3.2 Management of hypothyroidism

Treatment of individuals with hypothyroidism is relatively easy and consists of replacement with thyroid hormones. In frank hypothyroidism the decision to start treatment is straightforward but in subclinical disease, criteria to start treatment are more complex (detailed below). Management of hypothyroidism is summarised in Figure 3.

Cause of hypothyroidism	Aetiology	Permanent?
Primary Myxoedema	Autoimmune	Yes
Hashimotos thyroiditis	Autoimmune	Yes
Silent Thyroiditis	Autoimmune	No
Postpartum thyroiditis	Autoimmune	No (30% may develop permanent hypothyroidism)
Subacute thyroiditis	Viral	No
Post-surgery	Iatrogenic	Yes
Following RAI	Iatrogenic	Yes
Drug induced	Iatrogenic	Reversible if drug discontinued
Iodine deficiency or excess		Reversible

Table 3. Causes of primary hypothyroidism.

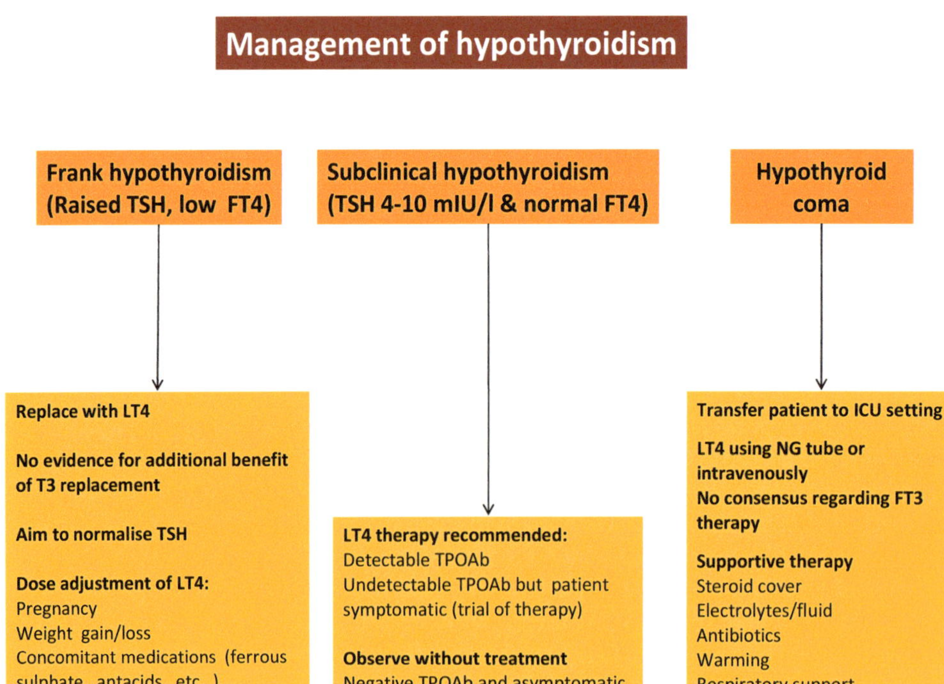

Fig. 3. Management of hypothyroidism. LT4: levothyroxine, TSH: thyroid stimulating hormone, TPOAb: thyroid peroxidise antibodies, ICU: intensive care unit.

3.2.1 Levothyroxine replacement

In non-elderly individuals with no history of cardiovascular disease, levothyroxine can be commenced at a dose of 50-100mcg daily, otherwise low doses are started initially (25 mcg evey day or every other day). It is estimated that most individuals require roughly 1.4-1.6 mcg/kg and so frequently doses will need to be titrated further, which can be done in increments of 25-50 mcg. Free T4 and TSH should be measured 8-12 weeks after commencing levothyroxine and after a change in dose. Until patients are on a stable dose of thyroxine, TSH and T4 should be checked together, after which annual check of TSH is sufficient. Controversy remains as to what value of TSH should be the target in hypothyroid patients treated with levothyroxine (Wartofsky & Dickey 2005). There does appear to be a lack of evidence supporting improved patient well being from maintaining TSH at the lower end of the reference range (BTA 2006), however many physicians continue to advocate this along with a lowering of the upper limit of the reference range for TSH to 2.5mu/L, given that >95% of euthyroid individuals have a TSH between 0.4mU/l to 2.5 mU/L (Gursoy et al 2006). A pragmatic approach which our centre follows is to aim for a TSH in the lower reference range by adjustment of levothyroxine dose if a patient remains symptomatic. The suppression of TSH is certainly not recommended due to fears of osteoporosis and atrial fibrillation (BTA 2006).

Assuming that a patient's weight remains stable, with no alterations to their medication or change in co-morbidities, the dose of levothyroxine should in theory remain stable. There are several factors that require alterations in doses such as pregnancy, malabsorption and medication.

Any state that produces intestinal malabsorption, such as coeliac disease, may lead to reduced uptake of thyroxine and hence a need to increase thyroxine dose. It is important to be weary of individuals who suddenly need an increase in thyroxine and who complain of gastrointestinal symptoms. Many medications can interfere with the absorption of thyroxine, such as ferrous sulphate, calcium carbonate, proton pump inhibitors, orlistat and cholestyramine (BTA 2006). Patients prescribed these medications should be advised to take them at least 2-4 hours apart from their thyroxine. In rare circumstances, TSH levels remain raised despite replacement therapy, usually due to compliance issues that the patient typically denies. Provided malabsorption is ruled out, a large dose of supervised levothyroxine replacement (1 mg/week) can be attempted, which fixes the problem in the majority (Grebe et al 1997).

Symptoms	Frequency
Weakness, lethargy, slow speech and dry/coarse skin	>90%
Cold intolerance, facial oedema, coarse hair	>80%
Weight gain, constipation, hair loss, memory problems	>60%
Anorexia, impaired hearing, dyspnoea, menorrhagia	>30%
Emotional instability, chest pain, dysphagia	10%
Signs	**Frequency**
Dry/coarse skin, facial oedema, thick tongue	>80%
Bradycardia, skin pallor, slow relaxing reflexes	>65%
Pericardial effusion	30%
Ascites, pleural effusion, carpal tunnel syndrome	<10%

Table 4. Main symptoms and signs in autoimmune hypothyroidism

3.2.2 T3 replacement therapy

The use of tri-iodothyronine, either alone or in addition to levothyroxine remains controversial (Escobar-Morreale et al 2005). LT-3 has a much shorter half life than T4 and so repeated doses are needed throughout the day, and this can also impair measurement of free T3. Measurement of free T4 when T3 is used alone is of no benefit, and similarly to T4 treatment, the aim is for TSH within the normal range. There is currently no consistent evidence that combination therapy of T4 and T3 is superior to T4 treatment alone, and therefore this therapy is not generally advocated (BTA 2006).

3.3 Special cases of hypothyroidism

3.3.1 Myxoedema coma

Myxoedema coma is a very rare complication of untreated hypothyroidism but is associated with significant mortality. Patients with severe long standing hypothyroidism suddenly become unable to maintain homeostasis, usually due to a precipitating event such as infection, heart failure, stroke, gastrointestinal bleeding or medications (mainly sedatives and analgesics). Prompt treatment with intravenous levothyroxine is required, initially with a loading dose, followed by smaller maintenance doses which can be given orally if the patient is able. No consensus exists as to whether T3 treatment should commence at the same time, or indeed if T3 alone is all that is required (Kwaku & Burman 2007). Caution is needed in the elderly, or those with cardiovascular disease due to increased risk of myocardial infarction and tachyarrhythmia. Concurrent use of intravenous glucocorticoids are usually required during initiation of thyroxine treatment due to the potential for evoking an adrenal crisis in the first few days as the hypothalamic-pituitary-adrenal axis is usually impaired in severe hypothyroidism. Other supportive measures include blankets to warm the patients slowly, cautious use of intravenous fluid to treat hypotension and a low threshold for broad spectrum antibiotics if infection is thought to be implicated. Consideration should be given early to intubation and mechanical ventilation if deemed appropriate, especially in a comatose patient.

3.3.2 Pregnancy

During pregnancy, it is common for thyroxine requirements to increase by roughly 50%, and it is essential therefore that all pregnant ladies on thyroxine are reviewed regularly during pregnancy so that dose alteration can be made. It is recommended that TSH is maintained at the lower end of the reference range during pregnancy, with the free T4 at the upper range of normal (Lazarus 2011). It is particularly important during the first trimester, before the foetal thyroid is formed, that normal maternal levels of T4 are maintained as they play a vital role in foetal neurological development (Williams 2008). TSH and T4 should be checked pre-conceptually, at antenatal booking, within each trimester and 4-6 weeks post-partum, at which point the dose of thyroxine can usually be reduced to pre-pregnancy levels (Lazarus 2011).

3.3.3 Subclinical hypothyroidism

This relatively common clinical scenario can cause management confusion. It is recommended that replacement therapy is started in those with TSH between 4 and 10 mIU/L and positive TPO antibodies as these individuals usually progress to overt hypothyroidism. In those with similar TSH levels, symptoms of hypothyroidism but negative TPOAb, a 6 months trial of replacement therapy is advocated with reassessment as to whether this therapy is needed. In asymptomatic individuals with negative TPOAb, simple observation with repeat TFT's is probably all that is required (BTA 2006).

4. Conclusion

Thyroid dysfunction can represent a wide spectrum of disease and the consequences of under treatment are evident with the two extremes of thyroid storm and myxoedema coma. Treatment options of both hypo- and hyperthyroidism are generally well established but are not perfect and there remain several unanswered questions regarding both forms of management, such as the optimal range of TSH with thyroxine replacement, the duration of ATD for GD, and whether to treat subclinical disease. Ongoing research into such areas is likely to provide further insight into the conditions and new therapies. Even with an expansion of the evidence base, clinical experience is likely to remain an invaluable asset in many instances. Regardless of treatment, lifelong follow up is required to maintain euthyroidism.

5. References

Abraham-Nordling M, Törring O, Hamberger B. (2005). Graves' disease: a long-term quality-of-life follow up of patients randomized to treatment with antithyroid drugs, radioiodine, or surgery. *Thyroid.* 15, 1279-1286.

Abraham P, Avenell A, Park CM, Watson WA, Bevan JS. (2005). A systematic review of drug therapy for Graves' hyperthyroidism. *Europ J Endocrinol* 153, 489-498

Aizawa Y, Yoshida K, Kaise N et al (1997). The development of transient hypothyroidism after iodine–131 in hyperthyroid patients with Graves' disease: prevalence, mechanism and prognosis. *Clin Endocrinol.* 461–5

Ajjan RA, Weetman AP.(2008).Techniques to quantify TSH receptor antibodies. *Nat Clin Pract Endocrinol Metab.*4, 461-8

Alfadhli E, Gianoukakis AG. (2011) Management of severe thyrotoxicosis when the gastrointestinal tract is compromised *Thyroid.* 21,215-20

Association for Clinical Biochemistry and British Thyroid Association (2006) UK Guidelines for the Use of Thyroid Function Tests. Available from: http://www.british-thyroid-association.org/info-for-patients/Docs/TFT_guideline_final_version_July_2006.pdf

Bahn RS, Burch HB, Cooper DS, Garber JR, Greenlee MC, Klein I, Laurberg P, McDougall IR, Montori VM, Rivkees SA, Ross DS, Sosa JA, Stan MN. (2011) Hyperthyroidism and other causes of thyrotoxicosis: management guidelines of the American Thyroid Association and American Association of Clinical Endocrinologists. *Thyroid.* 21, 593-646

Bal CS, Kumar A, Pandey RM (2002). A randomized controlled trial to evaluate the adjuvant effect of lithium on radioiodine treatment of hyperthyroidism. *Thyroid.* 12, 399–405

Bartalena L. (2011). The dilemma of how to manage Graves' disease in patients with associated orbitopathy. *J Clinb Endocinol Metab.* 96, 592-599.

Biswas N, Ahn Y-H, Goldman JM, Schwartz JM. (1991) Case report: Aplastic anemia associated with antithyroid drugs. *Am J Med Sci.* 301, 190-194.

Bogazzi F, Bartalena L, Brogioni S et a (1999). Comparison of radioiodine with radioiodine plus lithium in the treatment of Graves' hyperthyroidism *J Clin Endocrinol Metab.* 84, 499–503

Bowan P, Osborne NJ, Sturley R, Vaidya B. (2011) Carbimazole embryopathy: implications for the choice of antithyroid drugs ion pregnancy. *Q J Med.* [Epub ahead of print]

Cooper DS. (2003). Hyperthyroidism. *Lancet.* 362, 459-468

Cooper DS. (2005). Antithyroid drugs. *N Engl J Med.* 352, 905-917

Cooper DS, Rivkees SA. (2009). Putting propylthiouracil in perspective. *J Clin Endocrinol Metab.* 94, 1881-2.

Costagliola S, Morgenthaler NG, Hoermann R, et al (1999). Second generation assay for thyrotropin receptor antibodies has superior diagnostic sensitivity for Graves' disease. *J Clin Endocrinol Metab.* 84, 90-97

Escobar-Morreale HF, Botella-Carretero JI, Gómez-Bueno M, Galán JM, Barrios V, Sancho J. (2005). Thyroid hormone replacement therapy in primary hypothyroidism: a randomized trial comparing L-thyroxine plus liothyronine with L-thyroxine alone. *Ann Intern Med.* 15, 412-24

Feek CM, Sawers JSA, Irvine WJ, Beckett GJ, Ratcliffe WA, Toft AD. (1980). Combination of potassium iodide and propranolol in preparation of patients with Graves' disease for thyroid surgery. *N Engl J Med* .302, 883-885

Franklyn JA (1994). The management of hyperthyroidism. *N Engl J Med.* 330, 1731-173

Grebe SK, Cooke RR, Ford HC, et al.(1997) Treatment of hypothyroidism with once weekly thyroxine. *J Clin Endocrinol Meta.* 82,870–5

Gurosy A, Ozduman Cin M, Kamel N, Gullu S. (2006) Which thyroid-stimulating hormone level should be sought in hypothyroid patients under L-thyroxine replacement therapy?. *Int J Clin Pract.*60, 655-9

Hedley AJ, Young RE, Jones SJ, Alexander WD, Bewsher PD (1989). Antithyroid drugs in the treatment of hyperthyroidism of Graves' disease: long-term follow-up of 434 patients. *Clin Endocrinol.* 31, 209-218

Kwaku MP, Burman KD. (2007) Myxedema coma. *J Intensive Care Med.* 22, 224-31

Laurberg P, Nygaard B, Glinoer D, Grussendorf M, Orgiazzi, J (1998). Guidelines for TSH-receptor antibody measurements in pregnancy; results of an evidence-based symposium organized by the European Thyroid Association. *Eur J Endocrinol.* 139: 584-590

Lazarus JH. (2011). Thyroid function in pregnancy. *British Medical Bulletin.* 97, 137-148.

Matthews DC, Syed AA (2011) The role of TSH receptor antibodies in the management of Graves' disease..*Eur J Intern Med.* 22, 213-6

Maugendre D, Gatel A, Campion L, et al (1999). Antithyroid drugs and Graves' disease -- prospective randomised assessment of long-term treatment. *Clin Endocrinol.* 50, 127-132

Moorthy R, Balfour A, Jeannon JP, Simo R. (2011) Recurrent laryngeal nerve palsy in benign thyroid disease: can surgery make a difference?.*Eur Arch Otorhinolaryngol.* 21

Orgiazzi J, Mornex R: Hyperthyroidism. In: Greer M ed. *The thyroid gland.* New York: Raven Press 442, 1990.

Pattou F, Combemale F, Fabre S, et al. (1998) Hypocalcemia following thyroid surgery: Incidence and prediction of outcome. *World J Surg* . 22, 718–724.

Philippou G, Koutras DA, Piperingos G, Souvatzoglou A, Moulopoulos SD (1992). The effect of iodide on serum thyroid hormone levels in normal persons, in hyperthyroid patients, and in hypothyroid patients on thyroxine replacement. *Clin Endocrinol.* 36, 573-578

Royal College of Physicians. (2007). Radioiodine in the management of benign thyroid disease. Clinical guidelines Report of a Working Party. *Royal College of Physicians, London*

Regalbuto C, Marturano I, Condorelli A, Latina A, Pezzino V (2009) Radiometabolic treatment of hyperthyroidism with a calculated dose of 131-iodine: results of one-year follow-up. *J Endocrinol Invest.* 32, 134–138

Reinwein D, Benker G, Konig MP, et al. (1984). The different types of hyperthyroidism in Europe. Results of a prospective survey of 924 patients. *J Endocrinol Invest.* 11,193-200.

Reinwein D, Benker G, Lazarus JH, Alexander WD (1993). A prospective randomized trial of antithyroid drug dose in Graves' disease therapy. *J Clin Endocrinol Metab.* 76, 1516-

Sawyers JL, Martin CE, Byrd BF Jr, Rosenfeld L.(1972). Thyroidectomy for hyperthyroidism. *Ann Surg.* 175, 939-947

Schüssler-Fiorenza CM, Bruns CM,Chen H. (2006). The Surgical Management of Graves' Disease. *Journal of Surgical Research.* 133, 207-214

Schwartz AE, Clark O, Ituarte P, LoGerfo P. (1998). Therapeutic controversy. Thyroid surgery: The choice. *J Clin Endocrinol Metab* 83, 1097 1105.

Singer PA, Cooper DS, Levy EG, et al. (1995). Treatment guidelines for patients with hyperthyroidism and hypothyroidism. *JAMA.* 273, 808-812

Solomon B, Glinoer D, Lagasse R, Wartofsky L. (1990). Current trends in the management of Graves' disease. *J Clin Endocrinol Metab.* 70, 1518-1524

Tallstedt L, Lundell G, Blomgren H et al. (1994). Does early administration of thyroxine reduce the development of Graves' ophthalmopathy after radioiodine treatment? *Eur J Endocrinol,* 130, 494–7.

Testini M, Gurrado A, Lissidini G, Nacchiero M. (2007). Hypoparathyroidism after total thyroidectomy. *Minerva Chin.* 62, 409-15

Vanderpump MPJ, Tunbridge WMG, French JM. (1995). The incidence of thyroid disorders in the community; a twenty-year follow up of the Whickham survey. *Clin Endocrinol.* 43, 55-68

Vanderpump MP (2011). Should we treat mild subclinical/mild hyperthyroidism? No .*Eur J Intern Med.* 22, 330-3

Vitti P, Rago T, Chiovato L, et al (1997). Clinical features of patients with Graves' disease undergoing remission after antithyroid drug treatment. *Thyroid*. 7, 369-75

Weetman AP (2000). Graves' disease. *N Engl J Med*. 343, 1236-1248

Wartofsky L, Dickey RA (2005). The evidence for a narrower thyrotropin reference range is compelling. *J Clin Endocrinol Metab*. 90, 5483–8.

Williams GR. (2008) Neurodevelopmental and neurophysiological actions of thyroid hormone. *J Neuroendocrinol*. 20, 784-194.

13

New Technologies in Thyroid Surgery

Bahri Çakabay and Ali Çaparlar
Ankara University, Faculty of Medicine Department of Surgery
Turkey

1. Introduction

One of the earliest references to a successful surgical attempt for the treatment of goitre can be found in the medical writings of the Moorish physician Ali Ibn Abbas. In 952 A.D., he recorded his experience with the removal of a large goitre under opium sedation using simple ligatures and hot cautery irons as the patient sat with a bag around his neck to catch the blood. The first accounts of thyroid surgery for the treatment of goiters were given by Roger Frugardi in 1170. In response to failure of medical treatment, two setons were inserted at right angles into the goiter and tightened twice daily until the goiter separated. The open wound was treated with caustic powder and left to heal. The first successful typical partial thyroidectomy was performed by the French Surgeon, Pierre Joseph Desault, in 1791 during the French Revolution. Dupuytren followed in 1808 with the first total thyroidectomy, but the patient died 36 hours after the operation.

Despite these limited descriptions of early successes, the surgical approach to goitre remained shrouded in misunderstanding and superstition. Thyroid surgery in the 19th century carried a mortality of around 40% even in the most skilled surgical hands, mainly due to haemorrhage and infection. The French Academy of Medicine actually banned thyroid surgery in 1850 and German authorities called for restrictions on such 'foolhardy performances'. Leading surgeons avoided thyroid surgery if at all possible, and would only intervene in cases of respiratory obstruction. Samuel Gross wrote in 1848: "Can the thyroid gland when in the state of enlargement be removed…? If a surgeon should be so foolhardy as to undertake it. .every step he takes will be environed with difficulty, every stroke of his knife will be followed by a torrent of blood and lucky it would be for him if his victim lives long enough to enable him to finish his horrid butchery. No honest and sensible surgeon would ever engage in it."

Early surgical approaches for treatment of thyroid disorders were associated with high rates of mortality and morbidity due to hemorrhage, asphyxia, air embolism, and infection. Surgical approach to thyroid disease was seen as the last resort. It was not until the late 1800s after the advent of ether as anesthesia, antiseptic technique, and effective artery forceps that allowed Theodor Kocher to perfect the technique for thyroidectomy. Kocher used the technique of precise ligation of the arterial blood supply to perform an unhurried, meticulous dissection of the thyroid gland, decreasing the morbidity and mortality associated with thyroid surgery to less than 1% (Giddings,1998).

Advancements could only take place in the field of thyroid surgery with the introduction of improved anaesthesia, antiseptic techniques, and improved ways of controlling haemorrhage during surgery. The first thyroidectomy under ether anaesthesia took place in St Petersburg in 1849; the second half of the 19th century saw the introduction of Lister's antiseptic techniques through Europe, and the development of haemostatic forceps by such figures as Spencer Wells in London led to much better haemostasis than could be achieved by crude ligatures and cautery.

The most notable thyroid surgeons were Emil Theodor Kocher (1841–1917) and C.A. Theodor Billroth (1829–1894), who performed thousands of operations with increasingly successful results. However, as more patients survived thyroid operations, new problems and issues became apparent. After total thyroidectomy, patients became myxedematous with cretinous features. Myxedema effectively treated in 1891 by George Murray and Edward Fox. In 1909, Kocher was awarded the Nobel Prize for medicine in recognition "for his works on the physiology, pathology, and surgery of the thyroid gland."

The thyroid gland is removed traditionally through a small curvilinear incision approximately 3 cm above the sternal notch. While these original incisions allow for optimal exposure and successful removal of the diseased organ, they tend to subject the patients to lengthy hospital stays,significant postoperative pain, and in some cases, cosmetically undesirable results.

By the end of the twentieth century, laparoscopy was already accepted worldwide for a large number of operations in general surgery. By minimizing the size of the skin incisions while still permitting superior visualization of the operative field, laparoscopy was proven for certain operations to lessen postoperative pain, improve cosmesis, and shorten postoperative hospital stays.

As minimally invasive surgery became more popular,surgeons realized some true limitations. Sensory information is limited due to lack of tactile feedback and restriction to a two-dimensional (2D) image. In addition, compared to the human hand in an open case,laparoscopic instruments have restricted degrees of freedom mainly due to the lack of a wrist-like joint in the instrument tip and the lack of maneuverability due to a fixed axis point at the trocar (Hansen et al., 1997).

The advent of robot-assisted laparoscopic surgery seems to deal with many of the recognized limitations of hand-held laparoscopic surgery. In general, robots reduce the natural tremor of the human hand, reestablish comfortable ergonomics, reducing stress and surgeon fatigue, and,in certain cases, reestablish the three-dimensional (3D) view of the surgical field. In addition, surgical robots have the potential to be more precise and permit greater accuracy when it comes to suturing tasks and careful perivascular dissections. (Jacob et al., 2005)

2. Surgical instrumants for improved hemostasis

Thyroid surgery involves meticulous devascularization of the thyroid gland, which has one of the richest blood supplies of all organs, with numerous blood vessels and plexuses enteringits parenchyma. Therefore, hemostasis is of paramount importance when dividing the various vessels before excising the gland(Çakabay et al., 2009).

Although nearly a century has passed since Halstead and Kocher first described thyroidectomy, it has changed little until recently, and is a procedure that is performed extensively. Two of the most commonly used techniques for hemostasis are suture ligation and electrocoagulation. The disadvantage of suture ligation and electrocoagulation techniques is the prolonged operating time. Recently, a number of innovative methods of hemostasis in thyroid surgery have been tested, with promising results. New techniques developed over the past decade include hemostatic clipping, laser, LigaSure diathermy (ValleyLab, CO, USA) (or the LigaSure vessel sealing system), and ultrasonic instrumentation. Clips work for large vessels and are subject to dislodgment; whereas staples are wasted and costly for multiple single-vessel applications. Lasers are hindered by the risk of injury to many vital structures (such as the recurrent nerves) in the operative field, and bipolar electrocautery does not give the surgeon the freedom of applicability at different angles (Kennedy et al., 1998).

There have been significant advances in vessel sealing systems for the occlusion of blood vessels during general and gynecological surgical procedures. Two such devices are now commonly used in thyroid surgery: a bipolar energy sealing system and ultrasonic coagulation (Rahbari et al., 2011).Thyroid surgery is the most common endocrine surgical operation. Like all surgical procedures, the basic tenant of good exposure and hemostasis apply to thyroid surgery.

2.1 LigaSure

LigaSure (ValleyLab, CO, USA) is a bipolar diathermy system that seals vessels with reduced thermal spread. The device has been used successfully in abdominal surgery and has been introduced as a new method for hemostasis during thyroidectomy. The LigaSure diathermy system enables simultaneous selective sealing and division of a vessel without dispersion of the electric power, and with less heat production. The device is used in abdominal surgery and has proved suitable for use in thyroid surgery(Çakabay et al., 2009).

Any new surgical technology or operating technique should yield similar or improved patient outcomes and similar or lower rates of complications, compared with conventional methods. LigaSure, allowing vessel sealing and division with no dispersion of the electric power and with little or no heat production, has been widely used in diverse fields of surgery for its efficiency and safety. However, in thyroid surgery,where a considerable amount of minute vessels must be divided and hence microsurgical techniques required, LigaSure is also preferred for its further efficiency by shortening the duration of the operation.

Various specialties have reported shorter operating times with LigaSure (Lee et al., 2003,Levy et al., 2003,Jayne et al., 2002). However, in the literature, the postoperative outcome of thyroidectomy with LigaSure is controversial. Some studies (Petrakis et al., 2004) reported fewer complications and shorter operating times in the LigaSure , while others (Kiriakopoulos et al., 2004) did not observe a reduction in operating time for patients who underwent total or near-total thyroidectomy with LigaSure. According to two studies (Kirdak et al., 2005,Shen et al., 2005) the operating time was reduced substantially and the reduction in operating time in the LigaSure group was most probably a reflection of changes in operating technique (Shen et al., 2005).They reported that this change in technique facilitates dissection of the thyroid lobes and helps to reduce operating time and results ina decreased requirement for lateral skin etraction;the reduction in incision length in the

LigaSure group is probably a result of this decreased need for lateral retraction.The reduced operating time may result in decreased postoperative pain. The cause of postoperative pain is hyperextension of the neck (Defechereux et al., 2003); therefore, the pain can be reduced if the operating time is minimized. We found (Çakabay et al., 2009) that the use of the LigaSure significantly reduced the operating time for both total and one side total+other side subtotal thyroidectomy. The reduction in operating time was greatest in the total+subtotal thyroidectomy group. This is probably the result of faster but equally safe dissection of the thyroid gland compared with the conventional clamp-and-tie technique. In our experience, thyroid surgery using LigaSure does not require a significant learning period.

The major complications of thyroidectomy are laryngeal nerve injury and hypocalcemia. The reported permanent RLN palsy rate is 0%-14%. The use of LigaSure did not increase the RLN palsy risk(Çakabay2 et al., 009). Iatrogenic injury to the parathyroid glands resulting in hypocalcemia can occur from direct damage through inappropriate manipulation of surgery.

The cost of the LigaSure device is an important issue. According to some studies (Kirdak et al., 2005) the use of LigaSure is more expensive than the other conventional techniques. They reported that a cost-benefit analysis of this instrument may be helpful when choosing one of these techniques over the other. However, as the LigaSure device is produced to be disposable, the costeffectivenessof LigaSure can be increased by using one device for several patients. The reuse of LigaSure hand pieces decreases its cost of purchase (Dilek et al., 2005). In our exprience,we found that the additional cost of using LigaSure was $95 per operation, and our observations indicate that the same device will provide safe hemostasis for no more than 10 patients .

2.2 Harmonic scalpel

New techniques, such as hemostatic clipping, monopolar/bipolar diathermy, and laser and ultrasonic instrumentation, have been developed over the past decade. Of these, the harmonic scalpel is the most frequently used. The harmonic scalpel uses high-frequency mechanical energy to cut and coagulate tissues at the same time ,and it is widely used in otorhinolaryngological, cardiac, gastrointestinal, vascular, hemorrhoid, laparoscopic, obstetric, and gynecological surgery. The main advantages of ultrasonic coagulating /dissecting systems compared with a standard electrosurgical device are represented by minimal lateral thermal tissue damage (the harmonic scalpel causes lateral thermal injury 1-3 mm wide, approximately half that caused by bipolar systems),less smoke formation, no neuromuscular stimulation, and no electrical energy to or through the patient (Roye et al., 2000). Since its introduction, the harmonic scalpel has also gained popularity in thyroid and neck surgery. The proposed advantages of the harmonic scalpel include less lateral thermal tissue damage with no electrical energy transferred to the patient, as in electrocautery. In addition, the harmonic scalpel has some advantages over conventional techniques, particularly in terms of operative time, intraoperative bleeding, and hospitalization time.

The harmonic scalpel is a new surgical device for thyroid surgery and, to the best of our knowledge, studies in the English-language literature have been undertaken to compare harmonic scalpel versus conventional techniques. The characteristics of these studies summarized in Table1. The majority of these studies compared operative time, hospitalization time, drain use, incision size, postoperative pain, cosmetic results, cost analysis, and RLNP and other postoperative complications. The main advantage of using the harmonic scalpel in thyroid surgery is the reduction in operative time. Studies showed that the use of a harmonic scalpel significantly decreased the operative time (Yildirim et al., 2008, Voutilainen et al., 2000).

Some studies shown that no difference (Siperstein et al., 2002) was observed between the two techniques (harmonic scalpel and conventional techniques) regarding the amount of blood loss,others (Miccoli et al., 2006,Kilic et al., 2007, Yildirim et al., 2008) have shown that drainage volume is significantly lower in patients treatment with a harmonic scalpel compared to those treated with conventional techniques.

Despite the safety demonstrated by harmonic scalpel in several studies, specific training and experience in the use of the device are necessary because the active blade in inexperienced hands can easily injure surrounding vital structures. Approximately 10 h of experience are required (Voutilainen et al., 2000).The majority of transient and permanent complications occurred in the period of early training. Hypocalcemia and nerve palsy rates will decrease in time as our experience with the harmonic scalpel technique increases.

	References	**Year**	**Type of study**	**Number of patients (HS/CSL)**	**Summary of studies**
1	Voutilainen et al.,	2000	Prospective	19/17	Hospitalization time, postoperative drainage, and intraoperative bleeding were similar between groups. Operative time was shorter in the HS group than in the CSL group.
2	Shemen	2002	Retrospective	105/20	The incision length was shorter and the operating time was reduced in the HS compared to CSL group. Bleeding was negligible and complications were few.
3	Siperstein et al.,	2002	Retrospective	86/85	Operative time was shorter in the HS group than in the CSL group. Thyroid size tended to be larger in the HS group than in the CSL group. The two groups were similar regarding blood loss.
4	Ortega et al.,	2004	Prospective	100/100	The operative time was shorter in the HS group than in the CSL group. Hospitalization was similar between groups, but the global cost per patient was significantly less in the HS group. Postoperative complications were similar between groups.

	References	Year	Type of study	Number of patients (HS/CSL)	Summary of studies
5	Cordon et al.,	2005	Prospective	30/30	Operative time and number of ligatures were significantly reduced in the HS group compared to the CSL group. Drainage and postoperative pain were similar between groups. No episode of persistent RLNP or hypoparathyroidism occurred in either group.
6	Miccoli et al.,	2006	Prospective	50/50	Postoperative pain, operative time, drainage volume, and transient hypocalcemia decreased significantly in the HS group compared to the CSL group.
7	Karvounaris et al.,	2006	Prospective	150/150	No significant difference was observed in terms of postoperative blood loss, temporary hypoparathyroidism, or RLNP, although use of the HS significantly decreased operative time.
8	Koutsoumanis et al.,	2007	Prospective	107/88	Use of the HS decreased operative time, but increased the cost of surgery.
9	Kilic et al.,	2007	Prospective	40/40	Use of the HS in thyroid surgery resulted in decreased operative time, number of ligatures, total drain time, average incision length, and number of blood-soaked gauzes; it also produced better cosmetic results, but did not increase postoperative complications.
10	Hallgrimsson et al.,	2008	Prospective	27/24	Operative time was significantly shorter in the HS group than in the CSL group.
11	Lombardi et al.,	2008	Prospective	100/100	Operative time and total operating room occupation time were significantly shorter in the HS group than in the CSL group. The cost of the disposable materials was significantly higher in the HS group.
12	Leonard et al.,	2008	Prospective	21/31	The two groups were similar regarding operative time and incision size. This was the first reported series in which HS usage did not reduce operative time.

	References	Year	Type of study	Number of patients (HS/CSL)	Summary of studies
13	Yildirim et al.,	2008	Prospective	50/54	Use of the HS in thyroid surgery decreased operative time, mean blood loss, drain usage, number of ligatures, and amount of bleeding, and did not increase postoperative complications.
14	Manouras et al.,	2008	Prospective	144/90	The operative time was shorter in the HS group than in the CSL group. The rate of postoperative complications and hospitalization time were similar between groups.
15	Sebaq et al.,	2009	Prospective	50/50	The two groups were similar regarding hospitalization time and operative cost. Operative time decreased significantly in the HS group compared to the CSL group.

Table 1. A summary of studies on the use of harmonic scalpel(HS) versus conventional suture ligation(CSL)

3. Endoscopic techniques

Neck surgey is one of the newest and most interesting applications of minimally invasive surgery.Several approaches have ben proposed in the application of endoscopic thyroidectomy. The primary aim of all these different approaches has been to improve the cosmetic results of conventional surgery. Endoscopic thyroidectomy has been divided into two types, videoassisted and total endoscopic. Others classified it as with CO2 insufflation or gasless.

Minimally invasive video-assisted thyroidectomy (MIVAT) is characterized by a single access of 1.5 cm in the middle area of the neck, approximately 1-2 cm above the sternal notch; the midline is incised, and a blunt dissection is carried out with tiny spatulas to separate the strap muscles from the underlying thyroid lobe. From this point on the procedure is performed endoscopically on a gasless basis with an external retraction. An laparoscope of 5 mm, 30 degrees, is used. After the insertion of laparoscope through the skin incision, the lobe was completely dissected from the strap muscles with 2-mm-diameter laparoscopic instruments and other instruments regularly used. The optical magnification allows an excellent vision of both the external branch of the superior laryngeal nerve and the recurrent nerve, which are prepared together with the upper parathyroid gland. The vessels are ligated between clips or with the harmonic scalpel until the lobe, completely freed, can be extracted by gently pulling it out through the skin incision.The isthmus is then dissected from the trachea and divided. After checking the recurrent laryngeal nerve once again, the lobe is finally removed (Miccoli et al., 2001). In this technique, no subplatysmal flaps are raised and no muscules are divided, resulting in reduced tissue edema when compared with conventional surgery.I nitial experiences published on MIVAT underlined the advantages of the procedure in terms of a better cosmetic result and less postoperative pain when compared with conventional surgery.

Endoscopic lateral cervical approach used for hemithyroidectomy, two 2-5 mm trocars an done 10-mm trocar are inserted along the anterior border of the sternocleidomastoid muscle on the ipsilateral side and using endoscopic instruments specially designed fort his procedure. An additional advantage of this technique over endoscopically assisted midline technique was that no additional assistants were requred to hold retractors(Palazzo et al., 2006).

Total endoscopic thyroidectomy is a more sophisticated variation of minimally invasive thyroid. Using special instrument and technique, part or all of the thyroid gland can be removed through small puncture site, avoiding any incision on the neck whatsoever . Various approaches have been devised and improved further to fulfill this goal, mainly including the cervical approach, anterior chest approach, axillary and breast approach. However, none of these approaches is exclusively advantageous and universally accepted. (Irawati, 2010). The cervical approach and anterior chest approach are minimally invasive, but not cosmetically excellent. The axillary and breast approaches have maximized cosmesis, but meanwhile cause much invasiveness. Furthermore, the axillary approaches is not suitable for bilateral manipulation and even more technically challenging with abnormal anatomic vision. Therefore, an axillary-bilateral-breast approach (ABBA) has been developed, which is actually a combination of the procedure. Bilateral-axillary-breast approach (BABA) was introduced later and was claimed be easily applied for thyroid cancer as well. Whereas applicability of the endoscopic-assisted approach is limited by the size of the gland, the investigators noted that this constraint does not exist for BABA, as even large glands are easily retrieved through the axillary port (Becker et al., 2008). This technique now is even improved by using Da Vinci robotic system (Eun Lee et al., 2009). The endowrist function of the instrument is beneficial in doing complex tasks in difficult areas with limited access.

Disadvatages of endoscopic thyroidectomy include the requirement for additional equipment, namely high-resolution endoscopes and monitors for video-assisted techniques and insufflation units for purely endoscopic approaches. In addition,there is a distinct learning curve, which is more pronounced with purely endoscopic approaches.While video-assisted techniques clearly result in limited surgical dissection, purely endoscopic approaches, by virtue of their remote approaches, result in an equivalent amount of dissection. Because of this, most description include the routine use of drains, which may increase the lenght of hospitalization (Becker 2008).The increased chest-wall dissection can result in hypoesthesia in this area, and cases of pneumothorax have been described (Choe et al., 2007).Operative time for endoscopic approaches may be up to %30 longer than they are for traditional approaches (Terris et al.,2007).

4. Robotic surgery

Robots have been in the operating room for approximately 15 years now, but their use in assisting laparoscopic endocrine surgery is very new. With the refinement of the technology, easier set up, better image quality, and smaller robotic systems, there has been an interest in using the robot for more general surgical laparoscopic procedures as well as for thyroid surgery. Thyroid surgery procedures are excellent targets for robotic instrumentation when compared with the conventional endoscopic techniques, since it requires to work in a small space, significantly limiting the type of equipment that can be used. In spite of its deficiencies and unanswered questions especially about cost efectiveness, robotic technology seems to overcome the limitations of conventional laparoscopic technology in thyroid surgery.

The Da Vinci Surgical System consists of a "surgeon console" and a "surgical arm cart.". The surgical arm cart holds the robotic instruments and the endoscopic camera. The endoscope for the Da Vinci system is a specially designed 12 mm dual-camera endoscope that is capable of sending a 3D image to a specialized viewing screen in the console called the InSite Vision System. By looking into this 3D-image system, which eliminates all extraperipheral images other than those on the screen, the surgeon immerses himself in the operative field. The camera and instruments are both controlled by maneuvering the joysticks on the console. To alternate the digital handle's control back and forth between control of the camera and control of the instruments, the surgeon taps a foot pedal at the base of the console. At the current time there are 18 different robotic instruments in the Da Vinci system, which are appropriately called "endowrist instruments."

Once immersed in the Da Vinci's virtual field, the surgeon inserts his fingers into the handles, sits in an ergonomically correct position, and then maneuvers the endowrist instruments with up to 7 degrees freedom: yaw (side-to-side), pitch (up/down), insertion (in andout), grip, and three additional degrees of freedom provided by the second joint in the instrument tip. In effect, maneuvering the Da Vinci instruments is like miniaturizing your hands and wrists and placing them into cavities they normally could never fit into, thus permitting the performance of delicate, precise dissection and suturing in the smallest cavity—all through small skin incisions (Jacob BP& Gagner M,2004).

Once the system was on the market, Intuitive continued perfecting it, and the second generation—the da Vinci S—was released in 2006 (Figure 1). The latest version, the da Vinci Si became available in April 2009 with improved full HD camera system, advanced ergonomic features, and most importantly, the possibility to use two consoles for assisted surgery.

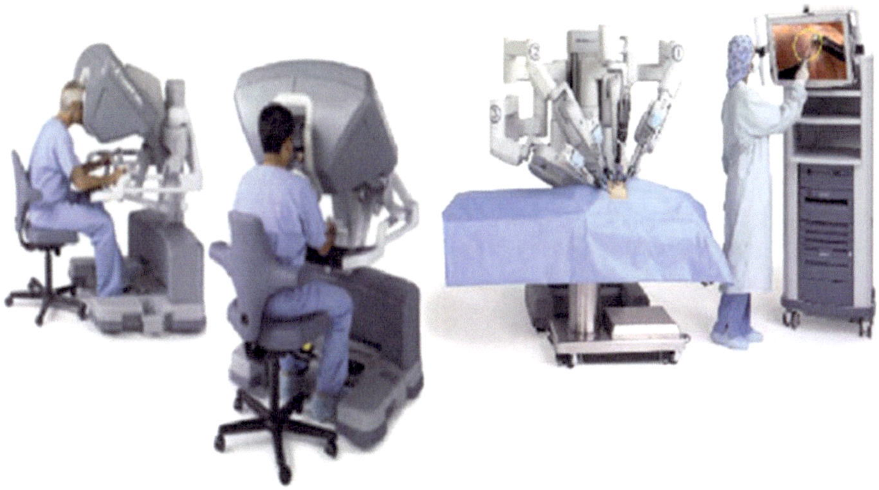

Fig. 1. Master controllers and the patient side manipulators of the new Da Vinci Si surgical system. (Photo: Intuitive Surgical Inc.)

The Zeus Robotic Surgical System also has two components: the surgeon console and the robotic instrument arms connected by a computer interface that can filter tremor and adjust the movement and rotational scale of the instruments. Unlike the Da Vinci system, the Zeus robotic arms are not on a cart, but instead can be attached directly to the operating room table. A second difference between the Zeus and the Da Vinci is that the Zeus uses a oiceactivated camera control system called the AESOP Robotic Endoscope Positioner. Instead of requiring a special 12 mm endoscope as with the Da Vinci, the Zeus allows the use of routine 5 or 10 mm endoscopes with the AESOP arm. With this system the surgeon can continuously maneuver the camera's position with simple voice commands like "camera in, camera out." The third difference between the two robotic surgery systems is that currently the Zeus system uses robotic laparoscopic instruments that mimic the hand-held laparoscopic instruments, thus lacking the additional degrees of freedom that you would get with an "endorist" instrument tip designed to mimic the human hand. Like standard laparoscopic instruments, these current Zeus instruments have only 5 degrees of freedom.

As the robotic technology is advancing rapidly, the Zeus is already in its third phase of design and is now available with instruments called "Microwrist technology." These new instruments, like the Da Vinci, have tips that offer a second joint mimicking the movements of the human wrist. Because this technology has just become available, there are no studies or published results demonstrating their efficiency, but the ability to perform wrist-like articulations inside the abdomen through small skin incisions is obviously promising.

The Zeus robot proved to be a solid platform to test and experiment different telesurgical scenarios. Between 1994 and 2003 the French Institut de Recherche contre les Cancers de l'Appareil Digestif (IRCAD) (Strasbourg, France) and Computer Motion Inc. Worked together in several experiments to learn about the feasibility of long distance telesurgery and effects of latency, signal quality degradation (Fig. 2).

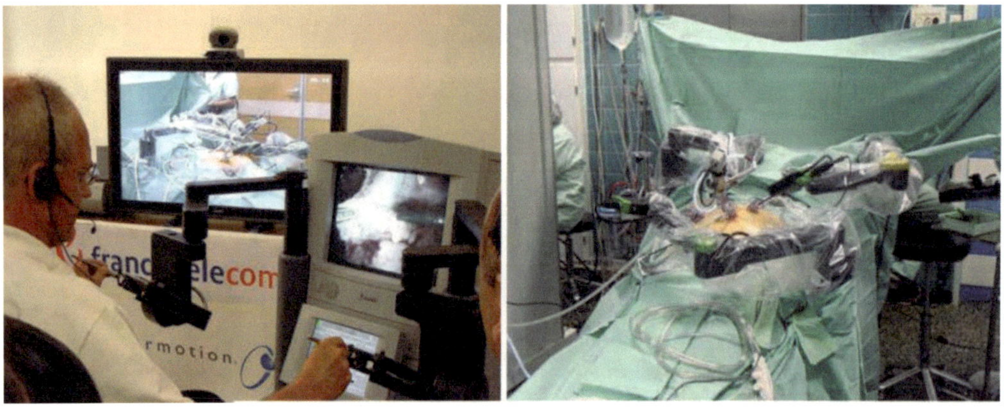

Fig. 2. The Zeus robot during the first intercontinental surgery, the colecystectomy was performed on the patient in Strasbourg from New York. (Photo: IRCAD)

Each robotic system has been used for a large number of different surgical procedures. The Da Vinci surgical robot system provides a three dimensional field of view and a more accurate sense of perspective (Ballantyne et al., 2007, Hartmann et al., 2008,Jacobsen et al., 2004).Moreover, because this system can magnify target structures, it more easily enables the preservation of the parathyroid and recurrent laryngeal nerves. The robot arm can be driven in multi-angular motions with seven degrees freedom. This enables safe and complete central compartment node dissection in the deep and narrow operation space (Jacob et al., 2003). The hand-tremor filtration, the fine motion scaling, the negative motion reversal of the robot system (providing minute and precise manipulations of tissue), and the ergonomically designed console means that surgeons experience less fatigue (Gutt et al., 2004, Savitt et al., 2005, Link et al., 2006).

Despite these various advantages of the Da Vinci surgical robot system, it may prove cost inhibitive when factors such as general cost, fees of disposables, and maintenance are taken into consideration. Additionally, the large room space it requires may be another factor thatlimits its widespread use in thyroid surgery (Link et al., 2006).

The early surgical outcomes of robot-assisted endoscopic thyroidectomies were compared with the data for conventional open thyroidectomies. As described earlier, this transaxillary approach is a more time-consuming procedure than conventional open thyroidectomy. However,with accumulation of experience, the actual operation time is decreasing. The patients in the robotic group were highly selected for several reasons such as the expected risk group and the expensive operation fee, and the difference in operation method was expected. However, there was little difference in the retrieved lymph node numbers, postoperative hospital stays, and pain between the two groups. Moreover, the postoperative complications in the robotic group were somewhat fewer than in the conventional open thyroidectomy group.

Although robot-assisted endoscopic thyroid surgery showed cosmetic and various technical advantages for surgeons, the major concerns when a new treatment technique for malignant tumors is considered should be the safety and radicalness of the operation to prevent local recurrence and distant metastasis. The relative oncologic safety of endoscopic versus robot-assisted endoscopic thyroid surgery has not yet been established due to the newness of this technology. To prevent cancer cell dissemination and to minimize the possibility of local recurrence during endoscopic thyroidectomy, the safety of the operational methods and the degree of surgical skill are important. If the safety and radicalness of robotic thyroid surgery as a treatment for papillary thyroid microcarcinoma can be established by the performance of complete thyroidectomies with secure lymphadenectomies, then the application boundaries and development area of this technique can be gradually extended (Kang et al., 2009).

5. References

Ballantyne GH.(2007). Telerobotic gastrointestinal surgery: phase2 safety and efficacy. *Surg Endosc.*2007,21:1054–1062

Choe JH, Kim SW, Chung KW,at al.(2007). Endoscopic thyroidectomy using a new bilateral axillo-breast approach.*World J Surg.* 2007 Mar;31(3):601-6

Cordón C, Fajardo R, Ramírez J, Herrera MF. (2005). A randomized, prospective, paralel group study comparing the Harmonic Scalpel to electrocautery in thyroidectomy.*Surgery.* 2005 Mar;137(3):337-41.

Cakabay B, Sevinç MM, Gömceli I,et al. (2009).LigaSure versus clamp-and-tie in thyroidectomy: a single-center experience. Adv Ther. 2009 Nov;26(11):1035-41. Epub 2009 Dec 18

Defechereux T, Rinken F, Maweja S, et al.(2003). Evaluation of the ultrasonic dissector in thyroid surgery. A prospective randomisedstudy. *Acta Chir Belg*. 2003;103;274-227.

Dilek ON, Yilmaz S, Degirmenci B, et al. (2005).The use of a vessel sealing system in thyroid surgery. *Acta Chir Belg*.2005;105:369-372.

Eun Lee K, Rao J, Kyu Youn Y, et al.(2009). Endoscpic Thyroidectomy with the da-Vinci Robot System Unsing the BABA Technique- Our Initial Experience. *Surg Laparosc, Endosc & Percutan Tech* 2009; 19 (3): e71-5

Giddings AE.(1998). The history of thyroidectomy. *J R Soc Med*.1998;91 Suppl 33:3–6.

Gutt CN, Oniu T, Mehrabi A, Kashfi A, Schemmer P, Bu¨chler MW.(2004). Robot-ssisted abdominal surgery. *Br J Surg* .2004,91:1390–1397

Hallgrimsson P, Lovén L, Westerdahl J, Bergenfelz A.(2008). Use of the harmonic scalpel versus conventional haemostatic techniques in patients with Grave disease undergoing total thyroidectomy: a prospective randomised controlled trial. *Langenbecks Arch Surg*. 2008 Sep;393(5):675-80. Epub 2008 Aug 2.

Hansen P, Bax T, Swanstrom L.(1997). Laparoscopic adrenalectomy: history, indications, and current techniques for a minimally invasive approach to adrenal pathology. *Endoscopy* 1997; 29:309–314.

Hartmann J, Jacobi CA, Menenakos C, Ismail M, Braumann C.(2008).Surgical treatment of gastroesophageal reflux disease and upside-down stomach using the Da Vinci robotic system: a prospective study. *J Gastrointest Surg* 2008 .12:504–509

Irawati N.(2010).Endoscopic right lobectomy axillary-breast approach: a report of two cases. *Int J Otolaryngol*. 2010;2010:958764. Epub 2010 Dec 28.

Jacobsen G, Elli F, Horgan S.(2004). Robotic surgery update. *Surg Endosc* 18:1186–1191

Jacob BP, Gagner M.(2003). Robotics and general surgery. *Surg Clin North* Am 83:1405–1419

Jacob BP&Gagner M. (2004). Robotic Endocrine Surgery,In:*Endocrine Surgery*, Arthur E. Schwartz,Demetrius Persemlidis, Michel Gagner ,pp.(11-16), Library of Congress Cataloging-in-Publication Data, ISBN: 0-8247-4297-4,Canada

Jayne DG, Botterill I, Ambrose NS, et al. (2002).Randomized clinical trial of Ligasure versus conventional diathermy for day-case haemorrhoidectomy. *Br J Surg*.2002;89:428-432.

Kang SW, Jeong JJ, Yun JS, et al.(2009). Robot-assisted endoscopic surgery for thyroid cancer: experience with the first 100 patients. *Surg Endosc*. 2009 Nov;23(11):2399-406. Epub 2009 Mar 5.

Karvounaris DC, Antonopoulos V, Psarras K, Sakadamis A .(2006).Efficacy and safety of ultrasonically activated shears in thyroid surgery.*Head Neck*.2006;28;1028-1031

Kennedy JS, Stranahan PL, Taylor KD, Chandler JG. (1998).High-burst-strength, feedbackcontrolled bipolar vessel sealing. *Surg Endosc*. 1998;12:876-878.

Kilic M, Keskek M, Ertan T, et al. (2007). A prospective randomized trial comparing the harmonic scalpel with conventional knot tying in thyroidectomy.*Adv Ther*. 2007 May-Jun;24(3):632-8.

Kirdak T, Korun N, Ozguc H.(2005). Use of LigaSure inthyroidectomy procedures: results of a prospectivecomparative study. *World J Surg*. 2005;29:771-774.

Kiriakopoulos A, Dimitrios T, Dimitrios L. (2004). Use ofa diathermy system in thyroid surgery. *Arch Surg*.2004;139:997-1000.

Koutsomanis K,Koutras AS,Drimousis PG,et al.(2007). The use of aharmonic scalpel in thyroid surgery:report of a 3-year experience.*Am J Surg*.2007;193

Lee WJ, Chen TC, Lai IR, et al.(2003). Randomized clinical trial of LigaSure versus conventional surgery for extended gastric cancer resection.*Br J Surg*. 2003;90:1493-1496.

Levy B, Emery L.(2003). Randomized trial of suture versus electrosurgical bipolar vessel sealing in vaginal hysterectomy. *Obstet Gynecol*. 2003;102:147-151.

Leonard DS, Timon C.(2008).Prospective trial of the ultrasonic dissector in thyroid surgery. *Head Neck*. 2008 Jul;30(7):904-8.

Link RE, Bhayani SB, Kavoussi LR.(2006). A prospective comparison of robotic and laparoscopic pyeloplasty. *Ann Surg* 2006,243:486–491

Lombardi CP, Raffaelli M, Cicchetti A,et al.(2008). The use of "harmonic scalpel" versus "knot tying" for conventional "open" thyroidectomy: results of a prospective randomized study. *Langenbecks Arch Surg*. 2008 Sep;393(5):627-31. Epub 2008 Jul 15.

Manouras A, Markogiannakis H, Koutras AS, et al. (2008).Thyroid surgery: comparison between the electrothermal bipolar vessel sealing system, harmonic scalpel, and classic suture ligation.*Am J Surg*. 2008 Jan;195(1):48-52

Miccoli P, Berti P, Raffaelli M, et al.(2001). Comparison between minimally invasive video-assisted thyroidectomy and conventional thyroidectomy: a prospective randomized study. *Surgery*. 2001 Dec;130(6):1039-43

Miccoli P, Berti P, Dionigi GL, et al. (2006). Randomized Controlled Trial of Harmonic Scalpel Use During Thyroidectomy *Arch Otolaryngol Head Neck Surg*. 2006;132:1069-1073

Ortega J, Sala C, Flor B, Lledo S. (2004). Efficacy and cost-effectiveness of the UltraCision harmonic scalpel in thyroid surgery: an analysis of 200 cases in a randomized trial. *J Laparoendosc Adv Surg Tech A*. 2004 Feb;14(1):9-12

Palazzo FF, Sebag F, Henry JF. (2006).Endocrine surgical technique: endoscopic thyroidectomy via the lateral approach.Surg Endosc. 2006 Feb;20(2):339-42. Epub 2005 Dec 9.

Petrakis IE, Kogerakis NE, Lasithiotakis KG,et al. (2004). LigaSure versus clamp-and-tie thyroidectomy for benign nodulardisease. *Head Neck*. 2004;26:903-909.

Rahbari R, Mathur A, Kitano M et al.(2011). Prospective Randomized Trial of Ligasure Versus Harmonic Hemostasis Technique in Thyroidectomy. *Ann Surg Oncol* (2011) 18:1023–1027

Roye GD, Monchik JM, Amaral JF. (2000). Endoscopic adrenalectomy using ultrasonic cutting and coagulating. *Surg Technol Int*. 2000;IX:129-138.

Savitt MA, Gao G, Furnary AP, Swanson J, Gately HL, Handy JR. (2005) Application of robotic-assisted techniques to the surgical evaluation and treatment of the anterior mediastinum. *Ann Thorac Surg* 2005, 79:450–455

Sebag F, Fortanier C, Ippolito G, et al.(2009). Harmonic scalpel in multinodular goiter surgery: impact on surgery and cost analysis. *J Laparoendosc Adv Surg Tech A*. 2009 Apr;19(2):171-4.

Shemen L.(2002). Thyroidectomy using the harmonic scalpel: analysis of 105 consecutive cases. *Otolaryngol Head Neck Surg*.2002;127:234-238

Shen WT, Baumbusch MA, Kebebew E, Duh QY. (2005).Use of the electrothermal vessel sealing systemversus standard vessel ligation in thyroidectomy. *Asian J Surg*. 2005;28:86-89.

Siperstein AE, Berber E, Morkoyun E. (2002). The Use of the Harmonic Scalpel vs Conventional Knot Tying for Vessel Ligation in Thyroid Surgery *Arch Surg*. 2002;137:137-142.

Terris DJ, Chin E. (2006). Clinical implementation of endoscopic thyroidectomy in selected patients. *Laryngoscope*. 2006 Oct;116(10):1745-8

Voutilainen PE, Haglund CH. (2000). Ultrasonically activated shears in thyroidectomies: a randomized trial. *Ann Surg*. 2000;231:322-328.

Yildirim O, Umit T, Ebru M, et al. (2008). Ultrasonic harmonic scalpel in total thyroidectomies. *Adv Ther*. 2008 Mar;25(3):260-5.

14

Management of Primary Hyperparathyroidism

Jessica Rose and Marlon A. Guerrero
Department of Surgery, University of Arizona, Tucson, Arizona USA

1. Introduction

Primary hyperparathyroidism (PHPT) is caused by overproduction of parathyroid hormone (PTH) by at least 1 autonomously functioning parathyroid gland. Such overproduction results in increased blood calcium levels because of increased renal absorption, increased vitamin D synthesis (and calcium absorption in the gastrointestinal tract), and increased bone resorption. (Felger, Johnson) PHPT is caused by a single parathyroid adenoma 80% to 85% of the time. (Pyrah) Less frequently, it is caused by multiple adenomas or multigland hyperplasia (MGH). Intraoperatively, MGH may be difficult to differentiate from an adenoma, because hyperplasia may occasionally be asymmetric. (Kaplan) PHPT is generally a benign disease, but parathyroid carcinoma accounts for 0.5% of cases. The majority of PHPT cases are sporadic, but PHPT may also be associated with familial syndromes, including familial PHPT and multiple endocrine neoplasia type I and IIA. (Johnson)

2. Embryology

Most normal parathyroid glands (parathyroids for short) weigh between 35 and 50 mg, are under 5 mm in diameter, and are yellowish-brown. (Pyrah, Johnson) The upper parathyroids develop embryologically from the fourth branchial pouches. They descend with the thyroid into the neck and tend to have a fairly consistent location in the posterior portion of the middle third of the thyroid, just above the intersection of the inferior thyroid artery and recurrent laryngeal nerve. (Pyrah) Ectopic superior parathyroids may be found in the tracheoesophageal groove; in the retropharyngeal or retroesophageal space; posterior mediastinum; in the carotid sheath; or within the thyroid itself (intrathyroidal). (Johnson) Inferior parathyroids derive from the third branchial pouch, descend with the thymus, and are typically found on the posterior portion of the lower pole of the thyroid. However, *ectopic* inferior parathyroids may be submandibular, intrathymic, or intrathyroidal, or may be found in the thyrothymic ligament or anterior mediastinum. (Pyrah) Supernumerary parathyroids are found in 13% of cases; fewer than 4 of them are found in about 3% of cases. (Johnson)

3. Diagnosis

PHPT commonly affects individuals between the ages of 30 and 60 years—and women by a 3-to-1 ratio. (Kaplan) In outpatients, it is the most frequent cause of hypercalcemia. It is typically identified as hypercalcemia on routine laboratory evaluation in a seemingly asymptomatic individual. Symptoms may include weakness, easy fatigability, muscle aches, weight loss, irritability, depression, constipation, epigastric pain, nausea, vomiting, polyuria, renal colic, arthralgias, bony aches, pruritus, and paresthesias. Less common are the supposedly classic symptoms known by this rhyming mnemonic: stones, bones, groans, and psychic overtones (for renal calculi, osteoporosis, abdominal pain, and neuropsychiatric symptoms). If left untreated, patients with PHPT are at risk for hypertension, peptic ulcers, pancreatitis, nephrolithiasis, gout, and pathologic fractures. Patients typically present in one of three groups: those with osteitis fibrosa, those with nephrolithiasis, and those who are asymptomatic and whose disease is incidentally found. Those with osteitis fibrosa tend to have more symptoms and higher concentrations of PTH. (Mallette)

Most cases of PHPT are diagnosed incidentally, when hypercalcemia is identified on routine blood work. Hypercalcemia with an elevated PTH level confirms the diagnosis of PHPT. Some patients have a PTH level within the normal range, but the level is inappropriately high relative to the serum calcium level. (Mallette) In patients with symptoms suggestive of PHPT, the serum calcium level (corrected for albumin) should be checked and compared with the specific laboratory reference range. (Chan, Kaplan, Glendenning) The ionized calcium level may also be obtained, because that level is not affected by binding globulins, transfusions, venous stasis, or gadolinium. (Glendenning)

If the serum or ionized calcium level is elevated, other causes must be considered, such as milk-alkali syndrome, malignancy, sarcoidosis, hyperthyroidism, hypervitaminosis D, and many primary bone disorders. (Keating) In addition, the PTH level (via second- or third-generation assays) should be measured. (Chan AK, Bilezikian) In young patients and in patients of any age who have family members with hypercalcemia, the urinary calcium level should also be obtained, in order to evaluate for familial hypocalciuric hypercalcemia (FHH). (Kaplan) A Ca/Cr ratio of less than 0.01 is diagnostic of FHH; a ratio of more than 0.02 confirms PHPT. (Glendenning) Other laboratory abnormalities associated with PHPT include hypophosphatemia, hyperchloremic acidosis, hypomagnesemia, elevated alkaline phosphatase levels, and increased urinary calcium excretion. Moreover, 25-hydroxy vitamin D levels should be checked, in order to identify coexisting vitamin D deficiency. (Mallette)

Classic symptoms	Associated symptoms	Associated conditions
Renal calculi Osteoporosis Abdominal pain Neuropsychiatric symptoms	Weakness Easy fatigability Muscle aches Weight loss Irritability Depression Constipation Epigastric pain Nausea Vomiting Polyuria Renal colic Arthralgias Bony aches Pruritus Paresthesias	Hypertension Peptic ulcers Pancreatitis Nephrolithiasis Gout Pathologic fractures Osteitis fibrosa

Table 1. Symptoms of PHPT

4. Surgical indications

An operation can be helpful in patients with PHPT in order to restore their calcium balance and euparathyroid state. Postoperatively, most symptoms resolve, especially osteitis fibrosa. (Kaplan)

Preoperatively, all patients should begin, or continue, treatment for any concomitant diseases, such as angina, hypertension, and diabetes. They should be adequately hydrated, especially if they have significant hypercalcemia. In addition, their calcium level and renal function should be evaluated. It is also a good idea to assess bone mineral density, which gives an idea of the chronicity of a given patient's PHPT and the potential need for antiresorptive therapy postoperatively. (Davies)

4.1 Symptomatic PHPT

In patients with confirmed PHPT who can tolerate surgery, symptoms are one of the main indications. (Kaplan, Bilezikian) Those with renal involvement benefit from a parathyroidectomy, in order to reduce the risk of nephrolithiasis and to help improve renal function. Those with pancreatitis should be offered a parathyroidectomy; without one, the risk of disease recurrence and of significant complications is significant. Those with osteitis fibrosa and osteoporosis also benefit from a parathyroidectomy, which improves cortical and trabecular bone symptoms, though not always bone mineral density. A parathyroidectomy also decreases the risk of a pathologic fracture and lessens muscle weakness and fatigue. In addition, it helps avoid a hypercalcemic crisis. (Davies)

Reviewing the records of their own patients and other studies, Kaplan et al. found that 100% of patients with osteitis and pancreatitis saw improvement after a parathyroidectomy. And about 90% of patients with nephrolithiasis saw improvement, although renal function improved only variably (in 0% to 43% of patients). Other symptoms of PHPT also improved only variably, specifically peptic ulcers, hypertension, neuropsychiatric symptoms, and constipation. (Kaplan)

Renal involvement
Pancreatitis
Osteitis fibrosa
Osteoporosis
Bone Fracture
Muscle weakness
Fatigue
Hypercalcemic crisis

Table 2. Indications for surgery: *symptomatic* PHPT

4.2 Asymptomatic PHPT

In most asymptomatic patients, if they are not treated surgically, PHPT will eventually progress; in many of them, bone mineral density (BMD) will decrease. Such patients are also potentially at risk for cardiovascular and neurocognitive problems, and they have lower quality of life scores and more psychological symptoms. (Bilezikian)

Asymptomatic PHPT should be treated surgically if the patient meets the criteria set by the Task Force on Primary Hyperparathyroidism of the American Association of Clinical Endocrinologists and the American Association of Endocrine Surgeons (AACE/AAES). The criteria are as follows: patient age under 50 years, serum calcium level more than 1 mg/dL above the upper limit of normal, creatinine clearance less than 30% below age-matched norms, decreased BMD (T or Z score under -2.5), and difficulty with medical follow-up. (Felger, Bilezikian, Kukora)

In the past, hypercalciuria (excretion of more than 400 mg/day of calcium) was an indication for surgery--even in the absence of renal stones; it is no longer an indication, according to a summary statement from the Third International Workshop on Asymptomatic PHPT. (Bilezikian)

Most asymptomatic patients have improved symptoms postoperatively. (Felger) The reason is probably that many patients with hyperparathyroidism suffer preoperatively from weakness, easy fatigability, depression, neurocognitive dysfunction, and increased sleep requirements; still, it is impossible to predict which patients will benefit from surgery. (Bilezikian) Surgeons adhering to the National Institutes of Health (NIH) surgical indications criteria have noticed a cure rate of 95% to 98%, with a risk of complications of only 1% to 2%. (Sosa, Kukora) Some groups feel that the criteria for a parathyroidectomy are too limited, and that more patients would benefit from it. (Sywak)

Patient age < 50 years
Serum calcium level > 1 mg/dL above the upper limit of normal
Creatinine clearance < 30% below age-matched norms
Decreased BMD (T or Z score under -2.5)
Difficulty with medical follow-up

Table 3. Indications for surgery: *asymptomatic* PHPT

5. Preoperative imaging

The choice of preoperative imaging for patients with PHPT is often controversial. Without imaging, in the hands of an experienced surgeon, a patient undergoing a bilateral neck exploration for PHPT typically has a cure rate of 95% to 98%. (Shaha) But given the ability to perform minimally invasive surgery, preoperative imaging is gaining importance. (Shaha, Johnson) Such imaging can lead to the discovery of ectopic parathyroids and other pathology (such as other cervical masses). (Lumachi)

Imaging is most valuable for patients who require a reoperation for persistent or recurrent PHPT. Other populations who particularly benefit from preoperative localization via imaging include asymptomatic patients who previously underwent related neck surgery (such as a thyroidectomy or neck dissection); patients with difficult anatomic issues (such as those who are obese with a short neck); and patients at high operative risk. (Shaha)

Currently, sestamibi and ultrasound studies are the most common preoperative imaging modalities, but other imaging modalities are being more readily utilized.

5.1 Sestamibi scans

A sestamibi scan is a scintigraphic study; sestamibi was first noted to be taken up by the parathyroids when the study was used to evaluate cardiac perfusion. Since then, it has been thought to be a valuable tool for preoperative evaluation of the parathyroids. It uses technetium-99m hexakis-methoxyisobutyl isonitrile as the radionucleotide. The technetium is taken up by both the thyroid and parathyroids, so iodine (I^{123}) is used for thyroid subtraction. Initially, the study was performed with thallium technetium; however, sestamibi has a higher affinity for abnormal parathyroids. A sestamibi scan result is deemed positive if it pinpoints a "hot focus" on the initial and/or the delayed image of the parathyroids (but not on the thyroid scan). (Shaha)

One group noted that the accuracy of the sestamibi scan is 80% and the positive predictive value is 89%. (Shaha) Its sensitivity for identifying solitary adenomas ranges from 68% to 95%. (Johnson) However, it is able to identify only 30% of patients with double adenomas. As a single modality, it has a higher sensitivity than other imaging modalities for identifying solitary adenomas. However, false-positives may be due to thyroid nodules, lymph nodes, and brown adipose. (Mihai)

Using the sestamibi scan to preoperatively locate abnormal parathyroids is thought to improve the cure rate of PHPT, decrease operative time, and allow the possibility of a minimally invasive parathyroidectomy; however, such speculation is not always supported in the literature. Patients with negative sestamibi scan results are more likely to have lower operative cure rates (92%) than those whose scans showed a distinct adenoma (99%). (Allendorf) The scan result is more likely to be positive for adenomas in the face of higher calcium and PTH levels, higher oxyphil concentration, and vitamin D deficiency. Patients who are taking a calcium channel blocker are more likely to have a negative sestamibi scan result. Radiotracer retention is necessary in order for the sestamibi scan result to be positive; therefore, patients with high levels of P-glycoprotein (a multidrug resistance protein) are likely to have a negative result. (Mihai)

Pros	Cons
Highest sensitivity as single modality Positive results suggestive of higher cure Visualization of one focus allows facilitates minimally invasive parathyroidectomy	False-positives due to thyroid nodules, lymph nodes, and brown adipose False-negatives in patients on calcium channel blockers, high P-glycoprotein, and drug resistance genes

Table 4. Pros and Cons of Sestamibi Scans

5.2 Ultrasound (US) scans

An US study performed with a high-frequency transducer is used to comprehensively evaluate the neck from the hyoid bone to the thoracic inlet. The thyroid is imaged as well, looking for nodules or intrathyroidal parathyroids. Doppler is added to image the vascular structures and to visualize vessels supplying adenomas. In obese patients, graded compression can be used to assist in visualization. (Johnson)

US has a sensitivity for finding solitary adenomas of 72% to 89%. On US, adenomas appear homogenous and hypoechoic. They are most frequently seen if they are at least 10 mm.

Sometimes the blood supply of the adenoma can be visualized with Doppler: frequently a rim of vascularity at the periphery of the gland is seen. Normal parathyroids are small (about 5 mm) and are rarely seen on ultrasound. It can be difficult to diagnose hyperplasia with US, since the parathyroids are not markedly enlarged. Retrotracheal and mediastinal ectopic parathyroids are not well visualized on US. (Johnson)

Another difficulty is differentiating cervical lymph nodes from parathyroids; the two can be mistaken for each other. Nodes typically have a fatty hilum and are supplied by small hilar vessels. Thyroid nodules, especially those posteriorly located, can also be difficult to differentiate from parathyroids. Thyroid nodules do not typically display a vascular pattern. Intrathyroid parathyroids are also difficult to discern from thyroid nodules. (Johnson) Diagnostic fine-needle aspiration of thyroid nodules helps differentiate parathyroids from other cervical nodules. (Dimashkieh)

Individually, sestamibi and US studies have limited accuracy, but the use of both imaging modalities increases the ability to successfully identify a single adenoma: the reported combined sensitivity is 95%. (Lumachi, 2000) When the results of both the sestamibi and US studies are concordant, the accuracy for identifying a single adenoma can be as high as 98%. (Haciyanli)

Pros	Cons
Anatomic study Identifies concomitant thyroid disease Intraoperative use	Difficulty visualizing normal glands Mistaking of thyroid nodules and lymph nodes for adenomas Difficulty in identifying multigland disease

Table 5. Pros and Cons of US Scans

5.3 Computed tomography (CT)

CT of the neck and mediastinum is very good for recognizing enlarged glands, with sensitivity from 76% to 83%. Despite its accuracy, CT is infrequently used because of the associated radiation exposure and the need to give intravenous (IV) contrast. However, it can help predict four-gland hyperplasia (necessitating bilateral neck exploration) more frequently than other imaging modalities. It has also been shown to pick up some parathyroid adenomas previously missed on ultrasound scans. (Lumachi, 2004)

CT is efficacious when combined with sestamibi scans: their combined sensitivity nears 100%. (Lumachi, 2004)

SPECT/CT is an emerging technology that allows better definition of scintigraphic images; its sensitivity for defining parathyroid lesions preoperatively is close to 88%. (Neumann) (SPECT stands for single-photon- emission CT.) It is most beneficial when patients have had a prior operation and when anatomic details matched with functional information from sestamibi scans are required. It is also very useful for identifying ectopic parathyroids. (Krauz)

A new method, called 4D-CT, uses CT anatomic images combined with functional images. Its purported sensitivity is 88%, higher than the individual sensitivities of sestamibi and US scans. 4D-CT is very beneficial for identifying multigland disease. (Mihai)

5.4 Positron emission tomography (PET)

A newer form of PET called [18F]-2-fluorodeoxyglucose (FDG)-PET can be helpful with parathyroid imaging. FDG-PET uses a methionine-labeled radiotracer that has good specificity for hyperfunctioning parathyroid tissue. It is helpful in patients who have had a negative result on localization imaging studies or who need a reoperation. Its sensitivity is 86%, but increases to 92% when coupled with CT. (Mihai)

5.5 Magnetic resonance imaging (MRI)

MRI can be used in a similar manner to CT to diagnose the cause of PHPT. (Johnson) It has not been used frequently or studied extensively in patients with PHPT, but its sensitivity ranges from 71% to 100%. MRI may be especially useful if paired with a sestamibi scan or with a methoxyisobutylisonitrile (MIBI) scan for enhanced accuracy, though no protocols have yet been developed for such combinations. (Mihai)

Image Modality	Sensitivity
Sestamibi	68-95%
US	72-89%
CT	76-83%
PET	86%
MRI	70-100%
Combined Sestamibi and US	95%
Combined CT and Sestamibi	100%
Combined PET and CT	92%

Table 6. Sensitivities of Imaging Modalities

6. Adjuncts in parathyroid surgery

As minimally invasive procedures become more popular, the need becomes greater to provide minimally invasive parathyroidectomies. With a minimally invasive parathyroidectomy, as previously mentioned, preoperative imaging is necessary in order to determine which gland needs to be removed. Additionally, intraoperative adjuncts (described below) are frequently used in order to decrease operative time and increase operative success.

6.1 Intraoperative PTH monitoring

Intraoperative PTH (IOPTH) monitoring was developed to help guide the extent of surgical exploration and parathyroid resection. The most common reason for a failed initial operation is missed multigland disease. (Irvin, 1994) IOPTH monitoring is based on the assumption that removing the hyperfunctioning gland will cause the PTH level to fall appropriately. (Vignali) The half-life of PTH ranges from 3 to 4 minutes and can be measured easily with a quick immunoradiometric assay or with a two-site antibody immunochemiluminometric assay. (Irvin, 1994)

The Miami group was the first to describe IOPTH monitoring in conjunction with a minimally invasive parathyroidectomy. The PTH is measured twice before the parathyroid is resected (preincision and preexcision). The higher value of the two is used. Once the parathyroid is removed, the PTH is measured again at 5 and 10 minutes. PTH levels are drawn either from a peripheral vein or from an internal jugular vein. Additional intervals are also measured if deemed necessary by the operating surgeon. (Boggs) A successful resection is defined as a ≥ 50% drop in PTH from baseline at 10 minutes after parathyroid removal. (Boggs, Vignali, Irvin, 1994) A fall in PTH < 50% indicates inadequate resection and necessitates further exploration. (Boggs) The success of minimally invasive parathyroidectomies and IOPTH monitoring is now reported as 98%, a rate equivalent to the standard bilateral neck exploration. (Vignali) However, IOPTH also results in a false-positive rate of 3% to 24% (the rate is lower with adenomas and higher with multigland disease), leading to failed operations. (Yang)

IOPTH monitoring is an important adjunct to surgery, especially with negative or discordant results of preoperative imaging studies. (Gawande) It can guide the operation and minimize unnecessary bilateral neck dissections. It is also beneficial in reoperative parathyroidectomies, when it is necessary to find the source of disease. Higher success rates (from 76% to 94%) have been noted for reoperative parathyroidectomies that incorporate IOPTH monitoring. (Irvin, 1999)

6.2 Gamma probes

Minimally invasive radio-guided surgery is now performed for patients with PHPT. The technique involves preoperative IV injection of 37MBq of MIBI). (Rubello) Then the 11-mm gamma probe is used to scan the patient's neck, near the site of the presumed adenoma, in order to obtain a preoperative background gamma count. After the surgical field is exposed, the radioactivity of the parathyroid adenoma, thyroid, and surrounding area are all re-measured. An adenoma is defined as an ex-vivo parathyroid with at least 20% of the background radioactivity. The empty parathyroid bed is also checked for radioactivity, and any remaining tissue should only have up to 3% of the radioactivity of the adenoma. (Rubello, Howe) Some clinicians opt to perform *intraoperative* PTH measurements as well, to enhance their accuracy. (Rubello)

One of the benefits of using the gamma probe is that it assists in localizing ectopic adenomas and those located deep in the neck. It allows re-checking not only of the operative field for radioactivity after removal of the presumed source but also of the removed tissue, in order to be certain that the hyperactive adenoma has been removed. (Rubello) Technically, the gamma probe is also helpful with a very small incision, which makes visualization of glands much more difficult than in a traditional bilateral neck exploration. It is also helpful for reoperations, because scar tissue makes finding the adenoma of interest much more difficult. (Jaskowiak) Some clinicians find that the gamma probe is also more cost-effective in that it decreases the number of frozen sections. (Jaskowiak) However, most agree that it is possible to miss multigland disease with this technique. (Rubello) About 2% to 3% of patients require conversion to a bilateral neck exploration, most frequently because intraoperative PTH levels failed to decrease. (Rubello, Jaskowiak)

6.3 Intraoperative assessment

6.3.1 Frozen section analysis

Intraoperative frozen sections for PHPT are helpful in many situations. Parathyroids can be difficult to grossly differentiate from other tissues, such as fat, thymus, thyroid, and lymph nodes. Despite advances in preoperative imaging studies, their accuracy remains limited; sampling parathyroids intraoperatively, before excision, may be necessary to look for hypercellularity. (Osamura) Frozen section analysis allows for rapid confirmation of the tissue, and especially for differentiation between parathyroid and non-parathyroid tissue. Like any other test, frozen sections have limitations. During the freezing process, the tissue can be damaged and distorted, leading to a delay in diagnosis (while awaiting final pathology results) or to an error in diagnosis. In small glands, the sample may not be large enough for an adequate diagnosis (although this is not an issue with enlarged, abnormal glands). It can be very difficult to differentiate thyroid nodules from intrathyroidal parathyroids. (Westra) With the advent of minimally invasive parathyroidectomies, frozen sections are no longer used to assess non-affected glands. (Osamura)

At some institutions, instead of frozen section analysis, scrape cytology is performed to assess the parathyroids intraoperatively. Scrape cytology requires few instruments and little equipment, which makes it a more economical test. One study reported its sensitivity to be 86%. Its main drawback is that, in very small glands, obtaining an adequate sample may be more difficult. Occasionally, the sample is misinterpreted as thyroid tissue. Still, if frozen sections are not available, scrape cytology can be very helpful. (Rohaizak)

6.3.2 Needle aspiration and PTH analysis

An alternative to frozen section analysis for intraoperative identification of parathyroids is needle aspiration with rapid PTH analysis. This method is more cost-effective than frozen section analysis because it allows for intraoperative identification without the need for pathologic evaluation. It uses the same technique as IOPTH monitoring, but requires much less tissue for diagnosis. Some groups advocate this method for intraoperative confirmation of PHPT, while others use it to confirm that the removed tissue is parathyroid tissue. Some have raised the concern that this method can damage normal parathyroids, yet no evidence of this effect exists. Needle aspiration for PTH can also be used preoperatively by percutaneously aspirating a presumed parathyroid under imaging guidance, in order to confirm that a visualized neck nodule is a parathyroid. (Chan RK)

The technique for needle aspiration involves a 25-gauge needle on a 3-cc syringe filled with 1.0 mL normal saline solution. The PTH level is determined by the dual-antibody immunoassay for intact PTH. The PTH value of the thyroid is used as a control. Aspiration of parathyroids have reportedly produced a value greater than 1600 pg/mL; the average PTH of the thyroid is 87 pg/mL. (Chan RK) Some clinicians, while advocating similar methods of obtaining tissue, have shown that more needle passes (20 instead of 10) and a larger biopsy size (1.0-mm^3) increase accuracy. The method can be performed in vivo or ex vivo. Its sensitivity for identifying parathyroid tissue is 99%, using 1,000 pg/mL as the cutoff. (Conrad)

When this method is performed preoperatively, either a CT or ultrasound scan is obtained to identify cervical masses in patients with PHPT or in patients who have recurrent PHPT after an initial operation. Any level of PTH is considered a positive result, because no other tissue should contain PTH. Percutaneous aspiration can be performed safely with minimal associated complications. Although this method allows for accurate identification of parathyroid tissue, the false-negative rate is 13% (likely depending on the needle aspiration technique). (Sacks)

7. Operative techniques

7.1 Minimally invasive parathyroidectomy (MIP)

With technical advances in imaging and surgical adjuncts, PHPT is now commonly treated with a minimally invasive parathyroidectomy. Most clinicians agree that candidates for a minimally invasive parathyroidectomy need to have two concordant preoperative imaging studies (typically, sestamibi and ultrasound scans). The operation is usually performed with one of the aforementioned surgical adjuncts, which allow for a more focused operation, a smaller and more cosmetic incision, less operative risk, and outpatient surgery or the use of local anesthesia. Most patients have single-gland disease, so a minimally invasive approach seems preferable. (Lorenz)

7.1.1 Focused parathyroidectomy

A focused parathyroidectomy entails a targeted exploration, directed by the results of preoperative imaging, at the site of the suspected adenoma. All patients undergoing a focused parathyroidectomy were thought to possibly have single-gland disease, per preoperative imaging. The operation can be performed with IOPTH monitoring or the gamma probe. A 2-cm transverse incision is made over the site of the suspected adenoma, at the medial border of the ipsilateral sternocleidomastoid muscle. The sternocleidomastoid muscle and carotid artery are retracted laterally, and the thyroid is retracted anteromedially. If the adenoma is identified, it is circumferentially dissected. If the adenoma is not identified, the ipsilateral neck should be explored; conversion to a traditional bilateral exploration may be necessary. Although focused parathyroidectomy allows for a smaller cosmetic incision, the downside is that conversion to a bilateral neck exploration may require a second incision. (Lorenz)

7.1.2 Unilateral neck exploration

In a unilateral neck exploration, the incision is half the length of the traditional Kocher incision. The skin and subcutaneous layers are divided down through the platysma, and the subplatysmal flaps are raised. The median raphe of the strap muscles is divided; the ipsilateral strap muscles are retracted laterally; and the thyroid lobe is rotated anteromedially. Once the adenoma is identified, it is circumferentially dissected and resected. Both parathyroids on the ipsilateral side should be visualized: one normal and one abnormal gland should be visualized. However, if both those glands appear normal, or if an abnormal adenoma is not localized, the contralateral side must be explored. (Lorenz)

A unilateral exploration may be performed under local anesthesia. Frequently, this operation is coupled with intraoperative adjuncts to help guide the extent of resection. (Lorenz) Most groups report similar rates of disease recurrence after unilateral and bilateral neck explorations. The Michigan group reported no incidence of recurrent disease after unilateral neck explorations and a follow-up of 4 years. (Lucas)

7.1.3 Endoscopic parathyroidectomy

This type of neck exploration uses multiple small incisions to insert endoscopic instruments and a camera.(Lorenz) It has several advantages. First, it is a minimally invasive method that can treat multigland disease. Second, it magnifies all of the anatomy, making a nerve injury less likely. Third, it allows exploration of the mediastinum, if needed, for ectopic glands. (Gagner) Its downsides are that the surgeon is unable to use tactile sensation and that the patient is prone to hypercarbia and subcutaneous emphysema. (Naitoh)

An endoscopic parathyroidectomy can be performed in several different ways. Gagner et al. devised a method with CO_2 insufflation. They use a 2-cm suprasternal incision for a 5-mm trocar, and then place 2 to 3 needle trocars and one more 5-mm trocar on the medial aspect of the ipsilateral sternocleidomastoid muscle. The camera goes in the 5-mm trocars; the rest are working trocars. The area is insufflated to 15 mm Hg. Endoscopic scissors and dissectors are used to dissect out the borders of the thyroid and trachea. Clips are used to ligate vessels. The specimen is retrieved through an incision of 2 to 3 cm at the maxillary angle. Single adenomas as well as multigland disease can be effectively treated with this method.

Yeung et al. place an 11-mm trocar above the suprasternal notch. The platysma is incised, and CO_2 is insufflated to 6 to 8 mm Hg. Then a 5-mm trocar is placed near the lower edge of the sternocleidomastoid muscle, 2 cm above the incision on the opposite side of the lesion. A second 5-mm trocar is placed 2 to 3 cm lateral to the midline incision. One additional trocar, if needed, is occasionally placed. Endoscopic scissors are used to create a plane between the sternocleidomastoid and the strap muscles. The carotid sheath and thyroid lobe are exposed, and the fascia of the thyroid is incised, to mobilize the thyroid anteromedially after dividing the middle thyroid vein. Any abnormal parathyroids are identified and resected, then removed through the 11-mm port.

An endoscopic video-assisted parathyroidectomy is also possible. Miccoli et al. described a procedure using only CO_2 during the initial dissection, in order to avoid hypercarbia and subcutaneous emphysema. They make a 1.5-cm incision 1 cm above the sternal notch and incise the linea alba to insert a 12-mm trocar toward the side of the adenoma. The area is insufflated to 12 mm Hg, in order to dissect the strap muscles away. Then the CO_2 is turned off, and the space is maintained with retraction. A 5-mm camera is inserted in the same incision, as are skin retractors (one lifting the thyroid up and the other retracting laterally). The thyrotracheal groove is exposed, and the 2-mm instruments are inserted through a small lateral incision. The parathyroid of interest is identified and resected.

7.1.4 DaVinci-assisted parathyroidectomy

Robot-assisted parathyroidectomy was first used to assist with removing mediastinal parathyroids. (Harvey) The daVinci system has now been used for robotic transaxillary parathyroid surgery. A daVinci-assisted parathyroidectomy and an open operation have equivalent cure and complication rates. However, the advantages of a daVinci-assisted parathyroidectomy include cosmesis (it avoids neck scars), reduced operating times, shorter hospital stays, and decreased analgesia requirement. The robotic endoscope has magnification, enabling better visualization than traditional endoscopic procedures. Though robotic instrumentation allows more flexible motion than traditional endoscopic instruments, it is still more restricted than open surgery. Other limitations include difficulties with depth perception, less tactile feedback, and dependence on multiple assistants. (Tolley)

For a daVinci-assisted parathyroidectomy, the patient is positioned supine, with the neck extended and the shoulder bolstere. The initial incision is made below the ipsilateral clavicle to expose the sternoclavicular junction, long enough for a 12-mm trocar. Dissection continues cranially until exposure of the internal jugular vein, carotid artery, and omohyoid and sternohyoid muscles. A retractor is used to retract the strap muscles. At this point, the posterolateral border of the thyroid is exposed. The other three trocars are then inserted at the anterior axillary line. The camera is placed through the infraclavicular trocar. The daVinci instruments are placed through the axillary incisions (5-mm trocars). Then, the inferior thyroid pole, recurrent laryngeal nerve (RLN), and vascular pedicle of the parathyroid gland are exposed. A nerve stimulator may be used to continually identify the RLN. A harmonic scalpel is used to dissect the pathologic parathyroid free. Hemostasis is obtained, the trocars are removed, and the wounds are closed. (Tolley)

7.2 Conventional bilateral neck exploration

7.2.1 Surgical approach

A traditional bilateral neck exploration is performed through a transverse cervical incision (Kocher), about 2 cm above the sternal notch and just below the cricoid cartilage. The dissection is carried through the subcutaneous tissue and platysma down to the strap muscles, which are opened in the midline and retracted laterally. A self-retaining retractor is placed to assist with exposure. The strap muscles are separated from the thyroid. The right lobe of the thyroid is dissected bluntly and retracted medially, enabling the surgeon to look for the course of the recurrent laryngeal nerve. The middle thyroid vein is identified and ligated. The thyroid gland is rotated anteromedially, and the recurrent laryngeal nerve is identified near the middle thyroid artery. The superior parathyroid is found by slowly dissecting the loose tissue attaching the superior pole of the thyroid. The inferior gland is found in the same manner near the inferior thyroid artery. The procedure is repeated on the left side. All four glands are accessible through this incision and all four glands are viewed. (Johnson)

Once all four glands are identified, the extent of resection must be decided. If a single adenoma is found, it is removed. Two glands are removed if a double adenoma is visually confirmed. If all four glands are enlarged, indicating multigland hyperplasia, then a 3.5-gland resection is performed. All four glands can be biopsied to accurately distinguish single-gland from multigland disease. (Lorenz)

If the parathyroids are not found in their usual location, it is necessary to explore the common locations of ectopic glands. Ectopic *superior* glands may be found in the tracheoesophageal groove; in the retropharyngeal or retroesophageal space; posterior mediastinum; in the carotid sheath; or within the thyroid itself (intrathyroidal). (Johnson) Ectopic *inferior* parathyroids are typically on the posterior portion of the lower pole of the thyroid, but may be submandibular, intrathymic, or intrathyroidal, or may be found in the thyrothymic ligament or anterior mediastinum. (Pyrah) At this point, if the adenoma is still not localized, an ipsilateral thyroidectomy is performed. The success rate of a bilateral neck exploration is 95% when performed by an experienced endocrine surgeon. (Low)

7.2.2 Indications

A bilateral neck exploration should be performed when the results of preoperative localizing imaging studies are equivocal or discordant. (Lumachi, 2000) It is also recommended for patients with familial PHPT; patients with multiple endocrine neoplasia syndrome type I and IIA; and patients who may have a carcinoma. In addition, it should be performed when a thyroid resection is planned concomitantly. Obese patients may be more likely to require a bilateral neck exploration, because their body habitus may preclude a minimally invasive procedure. (Grant)

7.2.3 Indications for conversion from a minimally invasive parathyroidectomy

A minimally invasive parathyroidectomy is becoming more common in patients with single-gland disease. However, in some patients, it may be necessary to convert from a minimally invasive parathyroidectomy to a bilateral neck exploration. The most common reason for conversion is failure to appropriately identify a single abnormal gland. Conversion is also recommended when surgical adjuncts fail to indicate success (for example, the operation is unsuccessful when IOPTH monitoring shows a drop of < 50% in the PTH). Note that, if a unilateral neck exploration finds two normal or two abnormal glands, it, too, should be converted to a bilateral neck exploration. (Moalem)

For Initial Surgery
Equivocal or discordant preoperative imaging results
Familial PHPT
Multiple endocrine neoplasia syndrome type I and IIA
Carcinoma
Concomitant thyroid resection
Obesity
For Conversion from Minimally Invasive Surgery
Failure to identify a single abnormal gland
Multiple abnormal glands
Failure of adjuncts to indicate success

Table 7. Indications for Bilateral Neck Exploration

8. Complications

All operations on the parathyroids have potential complications, regardless of the surgical approach. Of most concern to patients is the risk of RLN injury leading to vocal cord paralysis on the side of the injury. The risk of RLN injury is about 1% in the hands of experienced surgeons. Rarely, both RLNs may be injured, resulting in airway obstruction, stridor, and the need for a tracheostomy. The superior laryngeal nerve can also be injured, which leaves patients hoarse and unable to change the pitch of their voice. (Fewins)

Another common risk is postoperative hypocalcemia, which occurs temporarily in 5% of patients (because of bone hunger or inadequate PTH secretion from the remaining parathyroids as a result of prolonged suppression). In 1% of patients, hypocalcemia is permanent, as a consequence of inadvertent injury to the remaining parathyroid(s). (Inabnet) Hypocalcemia typically involves perioral numbness or digit tingling and paresthesias, but can progress to tetany or stridor. Treatment requires calcium, and often vitamin D, supplementation. (Fewins)

Other, more rare complications include cervical hematomas, injury to the carotid artery, dysphagia, deep vein thrombosis, wound infection, and pneumothorax. (Low, Fewins) Hematomas are usually secondary to inadequate hemostasis. (Fewins) Symptoms can include pain, dysphagia, and respiratory distress. Such patients need to emergently undergo reexploration; however, the hematoma needs to be evacuated at the bedside if the patient is in respiratory distress. (Fewins) Complications specific to endoscopic parathyroidectomies include hypercarbia and extended subcutaneous emphysema. (Lorenz)

If the patient has significant comorbidities before surgery, the risks of anesthesia can also cause complications, including aspiration pneumonia, respiratory failure, cardiac events, and even death. (Low) It is important to note that, in the hands of experienced endocrine surgeons at high-volume parathyroidectomy centers, postoperative complication rates decrease. (Stavrakis)

Common Hypocalcemia Injury to the recurrent or superior laryngeal nerve
Rare Cervical hematomas Injury to the carotid artery Dysphagia Deep vein thrombosis Wound infection Pneumothorax

Table 8. Surgical Complications

9. Summary

PHPT is a common disease that is effectively treated by surgery. The many surgical options range from a minimally invasive parathyroidectomy to a bilateral neck exploration. Regardless of the surgical approach, the likelihood of success is highest with an experienced endocrine surgeon at a high-volume center. To reduce the chance of operative failure, knowledge of the anatomy and embryology of the parathyroids is paramount.

10. Acknowledgement

We would like to acknowledge and thank Mary Knatterud for her assistance in editing this chapter.

11. References

Allendorf J, Kim L, Chabot J, DiGiorgi M, Spanknebel K, Logerfo P. The impact of Sestamibi scanning on the outcome of parathyroid surgery. J Clin Endocrinol Metab, 2003; 88: 3015-3018.

Bergenfelz A, Kannigiesser V, Zielke A, Neis C, Rothmund M. Conventional bilateral cervical exploration versus open minimally invasive parathyroidectomy under local anesthesia for primary hyperparathyroidism. BJS, 2005; 92: 190-197.

Bilezikian JP, Khan AA, Potts JT. Guidelines for the management of asymptomatic primary hyperparathyroidism: Summary statement from the third international workshop. J Clin Endocrinol Metab, 2009; 94: 335-339.

Boggs JE, Irvin GL, Molinari AS, Deriso GT. Intraoperative parathyroid hormone monitoring as an adjunct to parathyroidectomy. Surgery, 1996; 120: 954-958..

Chan AK, Duh QY, Katz, MH, Siperstein AE, Clark OH. Clinical manifestations of primary hyperparathyroidism before and after parathyroidectomy: A case-control study. Ann. Surg., 1995; 222: 402-414.

Chan RK, Ibrahim SI, Pil P, Tanasijevic M. Validation of a method to replace frozen section during parathyroid exploration by using the rapid parathyroid hormone assay on parathyroid aspirates. Arch Surg. 2005; 140: 371-373.

Conrad DN, Olson JE, Hartwig HM, Mack E, Chen H. A prospective evaluation of novel methods to intraoperatively distinguish parathyroid tissue using a parathyroid hormone assay. Journal of Surgical Research, 2006; 133: 38-41.

Davies M, Fraser WD, Hosking DJ. Management of primary hyperparathyroidism. Clinical Endocrinology, 2002; 57: 145-155.

Dimashkieh H, Krishnamurthy S. Ultrasound guided fine needle aspiration biopsy of parathyroid glands and lesions. Cytojournal. 2006; 3: 6.

Felger EA, Kandil E. Primary hyperparathyroidism. Otolaryngol Clin N Am 43 (2010) 417-432.

Fewins J, Simpson CB, Miller FR. Complications of thyroid and parathyroid surgery. Otolaryngol Clin N Am., 2003; 36: 189-206.

Gagner M. Endoscopic subtotal parathyroidectomy in patients with primary hyperparathyroidism. Br J Surg., 1996; 83: 875.

Gawande AA, Monchik JM, Abbruzzese TA, Iannuccilli JD, Ibrahim SI, Moore FD. Reassessment of parathyroid hormone monitoring during parathyroidectomy for primary hyperparathyroidism after 2 preoperative studies. Arch Surg. 2006; 141: 381-384.

Glendenning P. Diagnosis of primary hyperparathyroidism: controversies, practical issues and the need for Australian guidelines. Intern Med J 2003; 33: 598–603.

Grant CS, Thompson G, Farley D, van Heerden J. Primary hyperparathyroidism surgical management since the introduction of minimally invasive parathyroidectomy. Arch Surg. 2005; 140: 472-479.

Haber RS, Kim CK, and Inabnet WB. Ultrasonography for preoperative localization of enlarged parathyroid glands in primary hyperparathyroidism: comparison with 99m technetium sestamibi scintigraphy. Clinical Endocrinology, 2002; 57: 241-249.

Haciyanli M, Lal G, Morita E, Duh QY, Kebebew E, Clark OH. Accuracy of preoperative localization studies and intraoperative parathyroid hormone assay in patients with primary hyperparathyroidism and double adenoma. J Am Coll Surg. 2003; 197: 739-46.

Inabnet WB, Fulla Y, Richard B, Bonnichon P, Icard P, Chapuis Y. Unilateral neck exploration under local anesthesia: the approach of choice for asymptomatic primary hyperparathyroidism. Surgery, 1999; 126: 1004-10.

Irvin GL, Deriso GT. A new, practical intraoperative parathyroid hormone assay. Am J Surg., 1994; 168: 466-468.

Irvin GL. Molinari AS, Figuroa C, Carniero DM. Improved success rate in reoperative parathyroidectomy with intraoperative PTH assay. Ann Surg. 1999; 229: 874-879.

Jaskowiak NT, Sugg SL, Helke J, Koka MR, Kaplan EL. Pitfalls of intraoperative quick parathyroid hormone monitoring and gamma probe localization in surgery for primary hyperparathyroidism. Arch Surg. 2002; 137: 659-669.

Johnson, NA. Tublin ME, Ogilvie JB. Parathyroid imaging: Technique and role in the preoperative evaluation of primary hyperparathyroidism. AJR, 2007; 188: 1706-1715.

Kaplan EL, Yahiro T, Salti G. Primary Hyperparathyroidism in the 1990s: Choice of surgical procedures for this disease. Ann. Surg., 1992; 300-317.

Keating FR. Diagnosis of primary hyperparathyroidism: Clinical and laboratory diagnosis. JAMA, 1961; 178: 547-555.

Kern KA, Shawker TH, Doppman JL, Miller DL, Marx SJ, Spiegel AM, Aurbach GD, Norton JA. The use of high-resolution ultrasound to locate parathyroid tumors during reoperations for primary hyperparathyroidism. World J. Surg., 1987; 11: 579-585.

Krausz Y, Bettman L, Guralnik L, Yosilevsky G, Keidar Z, Bar-Shalom R, Even-Sapir E, Chisin R, Isreal O. Technetium-99m-MIBI SPECT/CT in primary hyperparathyroidism. World J Surg, 2006; 30: 76–83.

Kukora JS, Zeiger MA. The American Association of Clinical Endocrinologists and The American Association of Endocrine Surgeons position statement on the diagnosis and management of primary hyperparathyroidism: AACE/AAES task force on primary hyperparathyroidism. Endocrine Practice, 2005; 11: 49-54.

Lorenz K, Nguyen-Thanh P, Dralle H. Unilateral open and minimally invasive procedures for primary hyperparathyroidism: a review of selective approaches. Langenbeck's Arch Surg, 2000; 385:106–117.

Low RA, Katz AD. Parathyroidectomy via bilateral cervical exploration: a retrospective review of 866 cases. Head Neck, 1998; 20: 583-587.

Lucas RJ, Welsh RJ, Glocer JL. Unilateral neck exploration for primary hyperparathyroidism. Arch Surg., 1990; 125: 982-985.

Lumachi F, Zucchetta P, Marzola MC, Boccagni P, Angelini F, Bui F, D'Amico DF, Favia G. Advantages of combined techneticum-99m-sestamibi scintigraphy and high-resolution ultrasonography in parathyroid localization: comparative study in 91 patients with primary hyperparathyroidism. European Journal of Endocrinology, 2000; 143: 755-760.

Lumachi F, Tregnaghi A, Zucchetta P, Marzola MC, Cecchin D, Marchesi P, Fallo F, Bui F. Technetium-99m sestamibi scintigraphy and helical CT together in patients with primary hyperparathyroidism: a prospective clinical study. BJR, 2004; 77: 100-103.

Mallette LE, Bilezikian JP, Heath DA, Aurbach GD. Primary hyperparathyroidism: Clinical and biochemical features. Medicine, 1974; 53: 127-146.

Miccoli P, Bendinelli C, Conte C, Pinchera A, Marcocci C. Endoscopic parathyroidectomy by a gasless approach. J Laparoendosc Adv Surg Tech A., 1998; 8: 189-194.

Mihai R, Simon D, Hellman P. Imaging for primary hyperparathyroidism—an evidence-based analysis. Langenbeck's Arch Surg, 2009; 394:765–784.

Moalem J, Guerrero M, Kebebew E. Bilateral exploration in primary hyperparathyroidism—When is it selected and how is it performed? World J Surg, 2009; 33:2282–2291.

Naitoh T, Gagner M, Garcia-Ruiz A, Heniford BT. Endoscopic endocrine surgery in the neck: An initial report of endoscopic subtotal parathyroidectomy. Surg Endosc, 1998; 12: 202–205.

Neumann, DR. Obuchowski NA. DiFilippo FP. Pre-operative $^{123}I/^{99m}Tc$-Sestamibi subtraction SPECT and SPECT/CT in primary hyperparathyroidism. Nucl Med 2008; 49:2012–2017.

Osamura RY, Hunt JL. Current practices in performing frozen sections for thyroid and parathyroid surgery. Virchow Arch, 2008; 453: 443-440.

Pyrah LN, Hodgkinson A, Anderson CK. Critical Review: Primary hyperparathyroidism. Brit J Surg, 1966; 53: 245-316.

Rohaizak M, Munchar MJJ, Meah FA, Jasmi AY. Prospective study comparing scrape cytology and frozen section in the intraoperative identification of parathyroid tissue. Asian J Surg, 2005; 28: 82–5.

Rubello D, Piotto A, Muzzio PC, Shapiro B, Pelizzo MR. Role of gamma probes in performing minimally invasive parathyroidectomy in patients with primary hyperparathyroidism: optimization of preoperative and intraoperative procedures. European Journal of Endocrinology, 2003; 149: 7-15.

Saaristo RA, Salmi JJO, Koobi T, Turjanmaa V, Sand JA, Nordback IH. Intraoperative localization of parathyroid glands with gamma counter probe in primary hyperparathyroidism: A prospective study. J Am Coll Surg, 2002; 195: 19–22.

Sacks BA, Pallotta JA, Cole A, Hurwitz J. Diagnosis of parathyroid adenomas: efficacy of measuring parathormone levels in needle aspirates of cervical masses. AJR, 1994; 163: 1223-1226.

Shaha AR, Sarkar S, Strashun A, Yeh S. Sestamibi scan for preoperative localization in primary hyperparathyroidism. Head Neck , 1997; 19: 87–91.

Smit PC, Rinkes IHMB, van Dalen A, van Vroonhoven TJVMV. Direct, minimally invasive adenomectomy for primary hyperparathyroidism: An alternative to conventional neck exploration? Ann. Surg., 2000; 231: 559-565.

Sosa JA, Powe NR, Levine MA, Udelsman R, Zeiger MA. Profile of a clinical practice: Thresholds for surgery and surgical outcomes for patients with primary hyperparathyroidism: A National survey of endocrine surgeons. J Clin Endocrinol Metab, 1998; 83: 2658-2665.

Stavrakis AI, Ituarte PHG, Ko CY, Yeh MW. Surgeon volume as a predictor of outcomes in inpatient and outpatient endocrine surgery. Surgery 2007; 142: 887-99.

Sywak MS, Knowlton ST, Pasieka JL, Parsons LL, Jones J. Do the National Institutes of Health consensus guidelines for parathyroidectomy predict symptom severity and surgical outcome in patients with primary hyperparathyroidism? Surgery, 2002; 132: 1013-1020.

Vignali E, Picone A, Materazzi G, Steffe S, Berti P, Cianferotti L, Ambrogini E, Miccoli P, Pinchera A, Marcocci A. A quick intraoperative parathyroid hormone assay in the surgical management of patients with primary hyperparathyroidism: a study of 206 consecutive cases. European Journal of Endocrinology, 2002; 146: 783-788.

Westra WH, Pritchett DD, Udelsman R. Intraoperative confirmation of parathyroid tissue during Parathyroid Exploration: A Retrospective Evaluation of the Frozen Section. The American Journal of Surgical Pathology, 1998; 22: 538-544.

Yang GP, Levine S, Weigel RJ. A spike in parathyroid hormone during neck exploration may cause a false-negative intraoperative assay result. Arch Surg. 2001; 136: 945-949.

Yeung GHC, Ng JWT. The technique of endoscopic exploration for parathyroid adenoma of the neck. Aust. N.Z. J. Surg., 1998; 68: 147-150.

Zollinger RM, Zollinger RM. Parathyroidectomy. In Zollinger RM, Zollinger RM. Zollinger's Atlas of Surgical Operations. 8th ed. Colombia: McGraw-Hill; 2003.

15

Synthetic and Plant Derived Thyroid Hormone Analogs

Suzana T. Cunha Lima[1], Travis L. Merrigan[2] and Edson D. Rodrigues[3]
[1]*Federal University of Bahia*
[2]*Community Colleges of Spokane*
[3]*Centro Universitário Estácio da Bahia*
[1,3]*Brazil*
[2]*USA*

1. Introduction

Nuclear receptors (NRs) are transcription factors that regulate gene expression in response to small signaling molecules. The NR family includes receptors for thyroid hormone (TH) (Yen, 2001), retinoids, vitamin D, steroid hormones, fatty acids, bile acids and cholesterol derivatives, a variety of xenobiotics and other ligands. Additionally, other members are called orphans and could either bind to ligands that have not yet been identified or modulate gene expression in a ligand independent fashion (Webb et al., 2002).

Since NR play important roles in development and disease, they are important candidates for pharmaceuticals. This family of proteins can be modulated by natural and synthetic ligands and are therefore promising targets for drug discovery. The natural ligands may include different kinds of plant molecules or even a combination of compounds present in raw extracts of medicinal plants.

1.1 Compounds that bind NR

Ligands that target NRs include TH, glucocorticoids, estrogens for hormone replacement therapy (HRT), the diabetes drug thiazolidinedione, synthetic retinoids, and many others. Though the list of possible targets is extensive, it is restricted by the fact that NR ligands have both beneficial and deleterious effects. For instance, TH improves overall lipid balance and promotes weight loss by increasing metabolism, but causes tachycardia that can be severe enough to lead to heart failure, muscle wasting and osteoporosis (Felig & Baxter, 1995; Braverman et al. 2000). Likewise, estrogen use in HRT alleviates symptoms of hot flashes and reverses bone loss, but increases the risk of breast and uterine cancers, and stroke (Gustafsson, 1998; McKenna & O´Mally, 2000; McDonnel & Norris, 2002).

1.2 Thyroid hormone receptor (TR) isoforms

Thyroid hormone signals are transduced by two related thyroid receptor subtypes, TR α and TR β (Figure 01.) which are encoded by different genes (Gauthier et al., 1999).

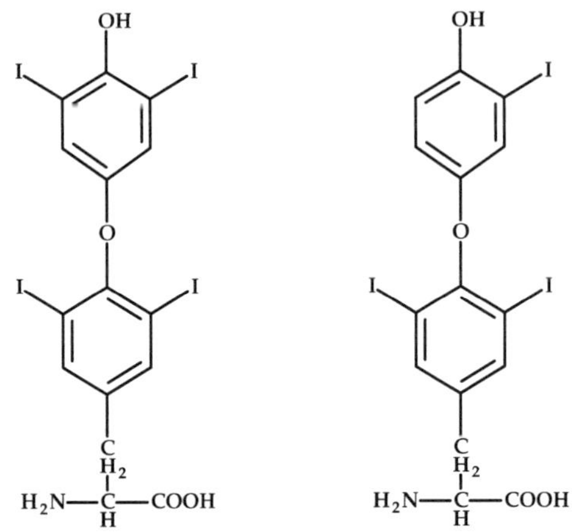

Thyroxine **Triiodothyronine**

Fig. 1. Chemical structures of thyroid hormones thyroxine (α) and triiodothyronine (β).

Studies of TR isoform-specific knockout mice and patients with resistance to thyroid hormone syndrome suggest that TR α mediates the effects of thyroid hormone on heart rate, whereas analogs that exclusively stimulate TR beta might have desirable effects without causing cardiac distress. Indeed, animal studies using thyroid receptor agonists with modest TR beta selectivity have validated this hypothesis (Taylor et al. 1997; Baxter et al., 2001; Grover et al., 2003). However, structure-based approaches to develop ligands with further improvements in isoform specificity are limited by the fact that the LBDs of TR alfa and TR beta are ~75% identical in amino acid sequence, and that the internal hydrophobic cavities that hold the hormone, called the pocket of the receptor, differ by just one amino acid (Ser-277 in TR alfa versus Asn-331 in TR beta). Therefore, it would be interesting to develop selective TR agonists that increase metabolism and improve lipid balance, but do not cause side effects on the heart. The first compound to show this property was GC-1 (Figure 02), an analog of T3 (Chiellini et al., 2002).

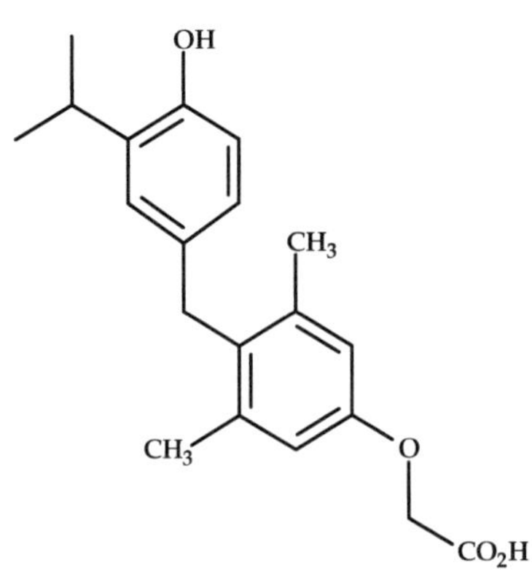

GC-1

Fig. 2. Chemical structure of the β-specific thyroid hormone receptor agonist GC1.

2. TR antagonists

2.1 First generation of synthetic ligands

TR antagonists would be useful for short-term relief from the symptoms of hyperthyroidism, and might even be used on a long term basis. The first generation of T3 antagonists, which include DIBRT, HY-4, and GC-14, used the "extension hypothesis" as a general guideline in hormone antagonist design (Baxter et al., 2002; Yashihara et al., 2001; Chiellini et al., 2002). This extension in the ligand structure blocks normal receptor function by occupying the pocket region where the hormone normally binds.

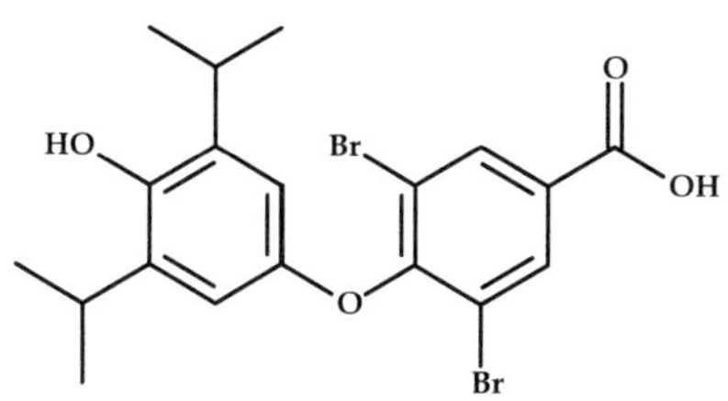

Thyroid hormone receptor antagonist DIBRT

Fig. 3. Chemical structure of thyroid hormone receptor antagonist DIBRT.

2.2 Novel series of antagonist compounds

Although the "extension hypothesis" is applicable to the design of nuclear receptor antagonists, the nature of chemical groups that convert agonist ligands to antagonists will likely depend on specific interactions between residues of the receptor and the ligand extension, to help stabilize the antagonist conformation. Following the first designed TR antagonists it was reported the design and synthesis of a novel series of compounds sharing the GC-1 halogen-free thyronine scaffold (second generation). One of them (NH-3) is a T3 antagonist with improved TR binding affinity and potency that allow for further characterization of its observed activity. One mechanism for antagonism appears to be the ability of NH-3 to block TR-coactivator interactions (Ngoc-Ha et al., 2002). NH-3 (Figure 04.) is the first T3 antagonist to exhibit potent antagonism in vivo and therefore may prove to be a generally useful tool for studying the effects of TR inactivation in a variety of animal models. Until now, such studies have been done primarily using TR-knockout mice because a pharmacological tool for inducing TR inactivation has not been available. TR inactivation was limited under previous ligands because they have only a modest affinity and potency for the thyroid hormone receptor (TR), which limits studies of their actions. T3 antagonists such as NH-3 may be useful therapeutic agents in the treatment of hyperthyroidism and other metabolic disorders.

3. Plant ligands of nuclear receptors

3.1 Estrogen analogs

Although modern research on drug discovery involves the design of hormone analogs based on the structure of the receptor, natural ligands can also be found in nature. Estrogen analogs are most common and have been discovered in a variety of plants. Ginsenosides (Figure 05.)

for instance, found in *Ginko biloba*, have demonstrated pharmacological effects on the central nervous, cardiovascular, and endocrine systems. Although no direct interaction of the compound with estrogen receptor seems to be necessary for estrogenic action, the author classified this plant ligand as a novel class of potent phytoestrogen (Chan et al., 2002).

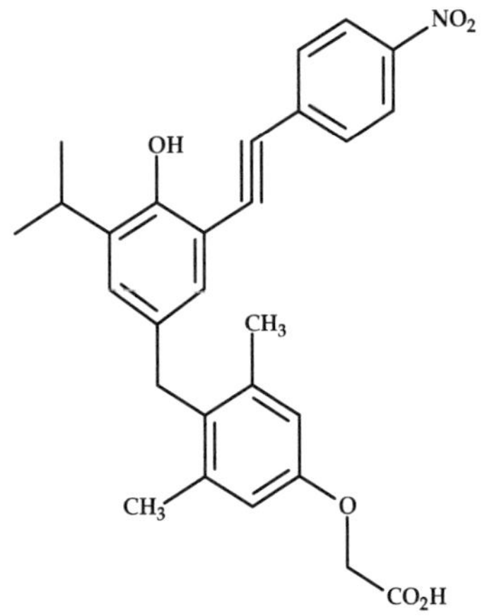

NH-3

Fig. 4. Chemical structure of the thyroid hormone receptor antagonist NH-3 (Lim et al. 2002), designed by the extension hypothesis from GC-1 compound.

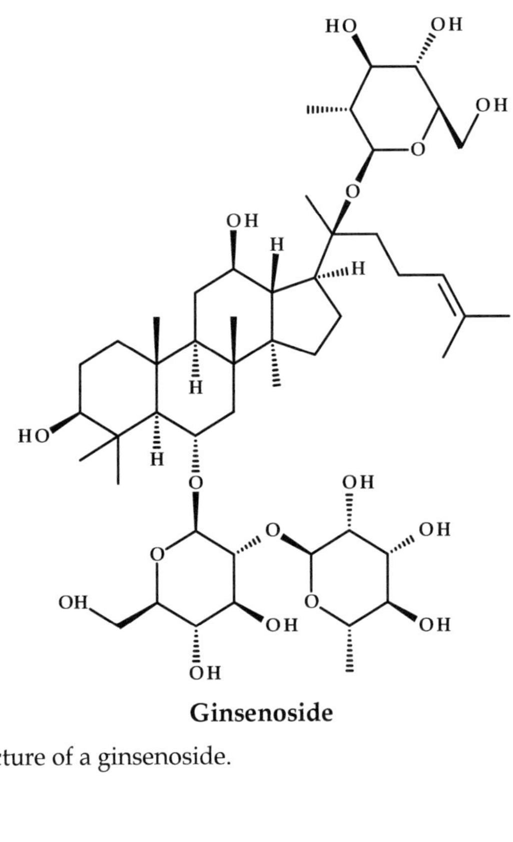

Ginsenoside

Fig. 5. Chemical structure of a ginsenoside.

Recently, *Tephrosia candida* (native to the tropical foothills of the Himalayas in India and introduced in South America) was reported to contain estrogenically active chemical constituents, which acted by binding to estrogen receptor ERα. Results were interpreted via virtual docking of isolated compounds to an ERα crystal structure (Hegazy et al., 2011). Also sesame ligands, from *Sesamum indicum* (flowering plant, native to Africa and widely naturalized in tropical regions around the world), and their metabolites have been evaluated for estrogenic activities (Pianjing et al., 2011). Two of them, enterodiol (Figure 06.) and enterolactone, have been indicated to have estrogenic/antiestrogenic properties on human breast cancer cells.

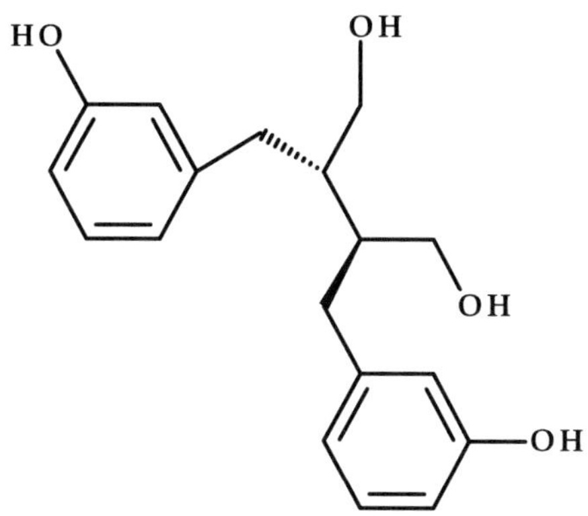

Enterodiol

Fig. 6. Chemical structure of an enterodiol

3.2 Androgen analogs

As compared to estrogen analogs, androgen-like compounds in the flora are less frequently referred in scientific literature. But a few chemicals have shown androgen-like activity. Andrographolide (Figure 07.), an herbal medicine, inhibits interleukin-6 expression and suppresses prostate cancer cell growth (Chun et al., 2010). According to the author, this phytochemical could be developed as a therapeutic agent to treat both androgen-stimulated and castration-resistant prostate cancer. Another compound, Isoangustone A, present in hexane/ethanol extract of *Glycyrrhiza uralensis*, induces apoptosis in DU145 human prostate cancer (Seon et al., 2010). This species, also known as Chinese liquorice, is a flowering plant native to Asia, which is used in traditional Chinese medicine.

3.2.1 Androgen ligands in the diet

Some studies have specifically demonstrated that consuming one or more portions of broccoli per week can reduce the incidence of prostate cancer, and also induce the progression from localized to aggressive forms of prostate cancer (Trakka, et al. 2008). The reduction in risk may be modulated by glutathione S-transferase mu 1 (GSTM1) genotype, with individuals who possess at least one GSTM1 allele (i.e. approximately 50% of the population) gaining more benefit than those who have a homozygous deletion of GSTM1, according to the author.

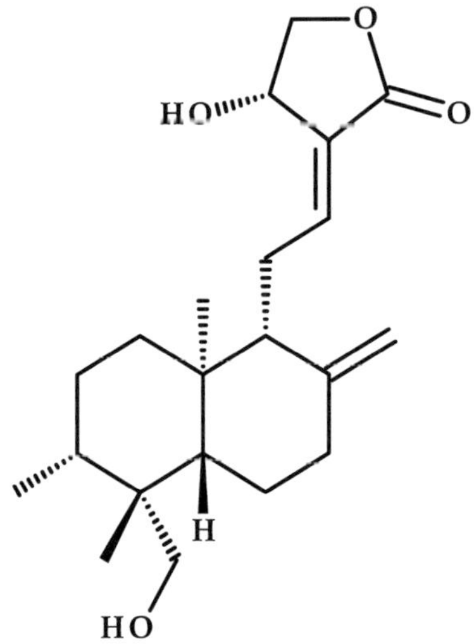

Andrographolide

Fig. 7. Chemical structure of an andrographolide.

From these studies, we can conclude that diet has a significant influence on the activity of the androgen receptors and possibly other types of nuclear receptor. If so, a wide range of diseases may be avoided by increasing intake of food that contains hormone analogs or other nuclear receptor modulators.

3.3 Plant thyroid hormone analogs

Concerning the thyroid hormone receptor, we find even fewer studies about thyroid hormone (T_3 and T_4) analogs in plants. In a work about patients where thyroid have been removed partially or totally due to thyroid cancer, the plant *R. rosea* was seen as a viable alternative treatment for the symptoms of short-term hypothyroidism in patients who require hormone withdrawal (Zubeldia et al., 2010). Some compounds of natural origin have also shown to affect the thyroid hormone feedback system by interfering with different components of this homeostatically regulated system: biosynthesis, secretion and metabolism, transport, distribution, and action of thyroid hormones, including the feedback mechanism.

Genistein (Figure 07.) and daidzein, the major components of soy, influence thyroid hormone synthesis by inhibition of the iodide oxidizing enzyme thyroperoxidase. This interferes with thyroid hormone transport proteins and 5'-deiodinase type I activities in peripheral tissues, leading to altered thyroid hormone action at the cellular level. Synthetic flavonoids, such as F21388, which is structurally similar to thyroxine, cross the placenta and also reach the fetal brain of animal models (Hamann et al. 2008).

The cruciferous family was also referred when we consider thyroid modulators in plant. In a study that examined the effects of both soy-foods and specific phytoestrogenic molecules on the development of thyroid cancer in humans it was demonstrated that intake of plants from that family decreases the risk of this kind of cancer (Horn-Ross et al., 2002). The compounds that may be associated with this effect are, according to the author, isoflavones, lignans and 2-hydroxyestrogens. Although anti-carcinogenic response was linked to those molecules, it was not explained how they may affect metabolism in humans or their physiological mechanism of action. Another compound, indole-3-carbinol, the most studied component of cruciferous vegetables, has been demonstrated to have chemopreventive activity in several different animal models of carcinogenesis, including mammary gland, but in another hand, the same compound has also been reported to exhibit adverse promoting effects, including liver and thyroid gland tumorigenesis (Murilo & Mehta, 2001).

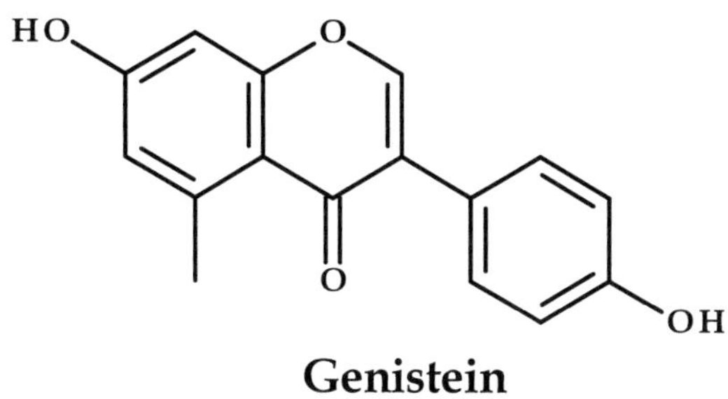

Fig. 8. Chemical structure of a Genistein.

It seems to have a cross talk between the thyroid hormone receptor and the estrogen receptor. Our recent results (Cunha Lima et al, not published) have shown that ligands originally referred for thyroid diseases have activated estrogen receptor in transient transfection assays. This could explain why phytoestrogens have caused responses in thyroid cancer and thyroid hormone analogs have also effect in breast cancer, for example.

3.4 Toxicity of thyroid hormone analogs

Considering medications used for thyroid hormone replacement, as sodic levothyroxine, aT_4 analog, the side effects referred (Cunha Lima , 2008) may include headache, chest pain, rapid or irregular heartbeat, shortness of breath, trembling, sweating, diarrhea and weight loss. The most severe responses are those related to the heart, which can lead to serious cardiopathies and are due to the α isoform of the receptor, as cited previously. A single base difference in the pocket of the protein can lead to these harmful responses. This means that we have a two step work on the search for new agonists and antagonists: they should mimesis the response caused by the thyroid hormone (or antagonize it, depending on the disease) and second, they should have a β specificity to avoid tachycardia and more serious heart problems.

In the other hand, some compounds that modulate TR may not be specific for this receptor, as it is very common with estrogen ligands. Since women hormone analogs may interfere with the function of the thyroid, as referred before with some flavonoids, they may have beneficial effects in cases of thyroid cancer. Nevertheless those compounds may influence thyroid actions at the cellular level and could cause side effects harmful for healthy individuals.

3.5 Ethnobotanical search for TR plant ligands

Since thyroid hormone analogs have much fewer discovered natural ligands, and most of those nuclear receptor ligands are found from plant sources, ethnobotanical surveys can be a good strategy to discover hormone analogs in nature. This approach has an increased probability of success in locations with higher biodiversity; because they contain a privileged number of candidate species. Along with botanical diversity, ethnobotanical surveys are likely to succeed where the population has an in depth knowledge of medicinal plants and systematically uses those plants to treat a range of metabolic disorders.

In a recent work (Cunha Lima et al., 2008) we investigated the medicinal flora used for the treatment of metabolic disorders in Salvador, Bahia, in Northeastern Brazil. The city has hot, tropical weather, with average daily highs reaching 17ºC in the winter and 38ºC in the summer. Northeastern Brazil is the economically poorest region of the country, 60% of the active population has an income under $100 per month, (Brazilian Institute of Statistics and Geography, 2003) and many residents depend on medicinal plants to treat multiple ailments and diseases.

The referred study analyzed the knowledge of the urban population of Bahia city on the use of potentially therapeutic plants for the treatment of Diabetes mellitus type 2 (DM2), thyroid diseases, obesity and cardiopathies. Questionnaires were applied to traditional healers as well as to patients of the thyroid disease and diabetes ambulatory in the Hospital from Federal University of Bahia (UFBA). Thirty-one cited species were collected, taxonomically classified, and stored in Alexandre Leal Costa Herbarium (ALCB) from UFBA. Leaves were most commonly used in preparations (87%), followed by the whole plant (10%), and fruits and seeds (3%). The majority of the preparation (88%) required decoction (boiling the plant tea for at least 5 minutes); the rest includes infusion (liquid preparation without boiling) and ingestion of the fresh plant. Among the plant parts used the leaves were more frequent (87%), followed by the whole plant (10%), seeds and fruits (3%). The families Asteraceae (17%), Lamiaceae (15%) and Myrtaceae (12%) were the most cited among plants referred.

This survey identified botanical families frequently cited in other surveys of medicinal plant use in Brazil. In two studies conducted in the state of Rio de Janeiro, one in Rio city (Azevedo & Silva) and one in the reservation of Mangaratiba (Medeiros et al., 2005), the Asteraceae and Lamiaceae family of plants were the most frequently cited, the same happening in Conceição Açú-MT (Pasa et al., 2005). Species from the Asteraceae family were also the most frequently noted for medicinal use in a survey done in Ingaí-MG (Botrel et al., 2006) and by a "quilombola"(community of people descended from former Brazilian slaves), among the plants with possible action in the central nervous system (Rodrigues & Carlini, 2004). These data suggest that the Asteraceae and Lamiaceae family have excellent pharmacological potential on different kinds of diseases and they are currently being investigate in many clinical studies.

In the survey performed by our group in Salvador (Cunha Lima, 2008), the plant most used for the treatment of DM2 belongs to the genus Bauhinia (pata-de-vaca). The most commonly cited species in this work, *B. forficate*, has the flavonoid Kaempferitrina, Kaempferol-3-O-α-Diraminoside and the steroid Sitosterol as the hypoglycemic active principle (da Silva & Cechinel Filho, 2002). *Terminalia catappa* was the second most cited species for the treatment of DM2. Ahmed et al. (2005) demonstrated that the extract from this plant also has hypoglycemic activity and improves general clinical conditions.

Among the plants used for obesity control, with probable effect on the metabolism, *Borreria verticillata* (carqueija or vassorinha-de-botão) was the species with the highest number of references in our survey. This plant, also used for the treatment of diabetes type 2, is found across Brazil. Phytochemical studies have demonstrated the presence of alcaloids and iridoids (Vieira et al., 1999) associated with their antipyretic and analgesic properties, although no active principle linked to obesity was confirmed. The leaves of *Bauhinia forficata*, *Costus spiralis* and *Theobroma cacao*, were used as teas in combination with the commercial medical prescriptions sibutramine (an oral anorexiant used for weight control) and niphedipine (a dihydropyridine calcium channel blocker used for high blood pressure) indicated by the physicians from the Diabetes Ambulatory of the Federal University of Bahia Hospital (HUPES). The teas of *Tragia volubilis* leaves and the seeds of *Ocimum gratissimum* were also used in combination with niphedipine and aspirin.

The problems related to the thyroid attended at the Hospital of Federal University of Bahia include throat itch, tachycardia, arm pain, chokings, dizziness and fainting. The most extreme side effects symptoms are associated with the T4 hormone replacement for patients whose thyroid was partially or completely removed. The doses used vary from 50 to 200mcg/day of sodic levotiroxine. In addition to the plants cited for treatment of thyroid problems, watercress (*Nasturtium officinale* R.Br.) and spring-green (*Brassica oleraceae* L.) were eaten as iodine source. Although the majority of the patients did not tell their doctors they were using those teas, there are no reported adverse side effects due to the combination of the plant products and the medications indicated, nor any reference in the literature about harmful effect of such interaction.

Ethnobotanical surveys are good source of information for drug candidates and offer a less expensive way of finding hormone analogs than the design of synthetic compounds. The cited information represents an important source of regional knowledge on plants with pharmacological potential and presents 31 candidates (Table 1) that might contain triiodothyronine (T3) and thyroxin (T4) analogs, including agonists, antagonists and other compounds able to modulate thyroid receptor that may act against metabolic disorders.

Brazil has more than 55.000 species of cataloged plants (Simões & Schenkel, 2002), a significant portion of which has some phytotherapic activity known by the local population. However, the number of patents on plant-based pharmaceuticals is very small. In particular, the capital of Bahia has numerous plants used by inhabitants to treat diseases and this use is part of the local culture, based in the Candomblé (religion of African origin which uses many plants in rituals and treatments). Traditionally, information about medicinal plants is shared orally. Therefore, it is necessary to scientifically systematize and analyze this phytotherapic knowledge so that those species can be identified and their pharmacological properties tested.

Table 2 lists the species referred in this survey that had their active principles identified and/or properties confirmed, and the bibliographic references where the data was obtained. These works include results from clinical and experimental studies aiming the confirmation of therapeutic properties.

	Vernacular Name	ALCB	Family	Species
1.	aroeira	76103	Anacardiaceae	*Schinus terebinthifolius* Raddi
2.	graviola	76101	Annonaceae	*Annona muricata* L.
3.	jaca-de-pobre	76154	Annonaceae	*Annona montana* Macfad
4.	carrapixo-de-agulha	76135	Asteraceae	*Bidens bipinnata* L.
5.	carrapixo-preto	76111	Asteraceae	*Bidens pilosa* L.
6.	chapéu-de-couro	76138	Asteraceae	*Zinnia elegans* Jacq.
7.	urucum	76100	Bixaceae	*Bixa orellana* L.
8.	cactus	78152	Cactaceae	*Cereus sp.* L.
9.	pata-de-vaca	76159	Caesalpiniaceae	*Bauhinia forficata* Link
10.	amendoeira	76096	Combretaceae	*Terminalia catappa* L.
11.	cana-de-macaco	76122	Costaceae	*Costus spiralis* (Jacq,) Roscoe
12.	mamona	76141	Euphorbiaceae	*Ricinus communis* (L.) Müll. Arg.
13.	urtiga	76108	Euphorbiaceae	*Tragia volubilis* (L.) Müll. Arg.
14.	alecrim ou alecrim-do-reino	76128	Lamiaceae	*Rosmarinus officinalis* L.
15.	hortelã-grosso	76110	Lamiaceae	*Plectranthus amboinicus* (Lour.) Spreng
16.	quiôiô	76112	Lamiaceae	*Ocimum gratissimum* L.
17.	canela	76099	Lauraceae	*Cinnamomum zeylanicum* Breyn
18.	erva-de-passarinho	76107	Loranthaceae	*Struthanthus flexicaulis* Mart.
19.	Murici	78150	Malpighiaceae	*Byrsonima sericea* DC.
20.	barbatimão	76158	Leguminosae	*Abarema cochliocarpum* (Gomez) Barnbey
21.	jamelão	76156	Myrtaceae	*Syzygium cumini* (L.) Skeels
22.	pitangueira	76163	Myrtaceae	*Eugenia uniflora* L.
23.	capim- cidreira ou capim-santo	75150	Poaceae	*Cymbopogon citratus* Stapf.
24.	roma	76162	Punicaceae	*Punica granatum* L.
25.	carqueija ou vassourinha-de-botão	76132	Rubiaceae	*Borreria verticillata* (l.) G.Mey
26.	laranjeira	76097	Rutaceae	*Citrus aurantium* L.
27.	vassourinha	76114	Scrophulariacea	*Scoparia dulcis* L.
28.	cacau	78148	Sterculiaceae	*Theobroma cacao* L.
29.	erva cidreira	76105	Verbenaceae	*Lippia alba* N.E.Brown
30.	melissa	76120	Verbenaceae	*Lippia alba* L..
31.	levante	76123	Zingiberaceae	*Alpinia nutans* Roscoe

Table 1. Medicinal plants candidates for thyroid hormone analogs according to ethnobotanical research in Salvador-Bahia, Brazil (Cunha Lima, 2008).

Species	Properties associated to the referred use	Reference
Bauhinia forficata	The flavonoids Kaempferitrin and Kaempferol-3-*O*-α-Diraminoside and the steroid Sitosterol found in the extract own hypoglycemic properties.	da Silva & Cechinel Filho (2002)
Terminalia catappa	Leaf extract prepared in different ways produced antidiabetic response with 1/5 of the lethal dose revealed by the lipid, creatine and urea profile as also serum alkaline phosphatase. The same dose caused anti-diabetic effects with fruit extracts.	Ahmed et al (2005) Nagappa et al (2003)
Rosmarinus officinalis	The anti-oxidants impair the mechanism of oxidation that occurs in cancer, heart disease , atherosclerosis and aging.	Ibanez et al (2000)
Cymbopogon citratus	Intense anti-oxidant activity due to the phenolic composition. The essential oil extracted from the leaf causes depression of the CNS in rats.	Prakash et al (2007); Negrelle (2007)
Bidens pilosa	Deposits of opaline silica in the leaves and extracts of the whole plant obtained with n- hexane demonstrated significant anti-cancer activity.	Parry (1986); Sundararajan et al (2006)
Lippia alba	Flavonoids found in this plant are active against different kinds of cancer including thyroid cancers.	Ren et al (2003)
Annona muricata	Graviola, a Brazilian fruit from the plant *Annona muricata* demonstrated anti-diabetic effect greater than the medication Clorpropamide, oral hypoglycemic from the sulphonilurea class.	Carvalho (2005)
Annona montana	The plant has kinase protein inhibitors that act creating obesity resistance and increasing insulin production.	Bialy et al (2005)
Syzygium cumini	The species presents anti-diabetic action in clinical and animal studies. Stem extracts stimulate the development of cells positive for insulin in the pancreatic epithelial duct.	Mentreddy (2007); Teixeira et al (2004); Schossler et al (2004)
Citrus aurantium	The combination of *C. aurantium* extract, caffeine and Saint John´s Herb (*Hypericum perforatum)* is safe and effective for weight lost and improvement of lipid levels in obese adults.	Colker et al (1999)
Alpinia nutans	The hidroalcoolic extract induces a dose-dependent decrease in artery pressure in rats and dogs.	Mendonça et al (1991)
Lippia alba	The aqueous extract of leaves from this plant, associated to the ones from *Melissa officinalis* and *Cymbopogon citratus* caused significant reduction in cardiac rhythm in rats, without changing the contractile strength.	Gazola et al (2004)

Species	Properties associated to the referred use	Reference
Bauhinia forficata	The rats treated with decoction of the plant leaves demonstrated significant reduction in serum and urine glucose. The results obtained with the purified extracts confirmed the therapeutic use for treatment of diabetes in clinical studies.	Pepato et al (2002); da Silva & Cechinel Filho (2002)
Eugenia uniflora	The empiric use of this plant is due to the hypotensive effect, mediated by vessel dilatation and weak diuretic effect that may be related to increased renal blood flow.	Consolini et al (1999)
Punica granatum	Flavonoid rich fractions obtained from fruit extracts demonstrated antiperoxidative effect. Malondialdehyde, hydroperoxide, and conjugated dienes were significantly decreased in the liver, while enzymatic activity of catalase, superoxide dismutase and glutathione reductase have shown significant increase.	Sudheesh (2005)
Scoparia dulcis	Plant extracts were effective on decreasing hyperglycemia and the susceptibility to free oxygen radicals in rats.	Latha & Pari (2004)

Table 2. Plant species referred in the survey that have their therapeutic properties confirmed or active principles isolated according to scientific publications.

4. Conclusion

Studying medicinal plants can be a less expensive way of finding treatments for hundreds of diseases. This can be an important factor in areas where a great part of the population lacks financial conditions of buying allopathic medication and, in the other hand, have a big incidence of metabolic disorders.

The search for hormone analogs in medicinal plants is extremely promising. Over 100 existing nuclear receptors have been identified, not counting the orphan NRs that lack known ligands. Since those transcription factors modulate almost all genetic activity and human physiology, they are important targets for drug discovery. Besides the ligands, usually hormones, other molecules can also modulate nuclear receptors, including cofactors (co-activators and co-repressors), responsive elements, and other ligands (not exclusively the hormone that naturally binds this receptor). According to that, the molecules found in plants do not have to be only analogs of hormones, but also compounds similar to all other complementary modulators of NRs.

Countries with higher biodiversity are good targets for discovery of plant molecules that can control the activity of thyroid receptor. Unfortunately there is not enough scientific knowledge about their medicinal plants or about patent procedures that would guarantee intellectual property of discoveries made by local scientists. In addition to that, the forests are being devastated very fast before important plant compounds can be found. Therefore, additional research needs to be done to identify new ligands and other molecules in the flora that can modulate TR and may be used in the treatment of diseases related to thyroid malfunction.

5. References

Ahmed, S.M., Vrushabendra, B.M., Dhanapal, P.G. & Chandrashekara, V.M. (2005). Anti-Diabetic activity of *Terminalia catappa* Linn. Leaf extracts in alloxan-induced diabetic rats. *Iranian Journal of Pharmacology & Therapeutics*, Vol. 4, No. 1, pp. 36-39. ISSN: 1735-2657.

Azevedo, S.K.S. & Silva, I.M. (2006). Plantas medicinais e de uso religioso comercializadas em mercados e feiras livres no Rio de Janeiro, RJ, Brasil. *Acta Botanica Brasílica*, Vol. 20, No. 1, pp.185-194. ISSN 0102-3306.

Baxter, J. D., Dillmann, W. H., West, B. L., Huber, R., Furlow, J. D., Fletterick, R. J., Webb, P., Apriletti, J. W. & Scanlan, T. S. (2001). Selective modulation of thyroid hormone receptor action. *Journal of Steroid Biochemistry and Molecular Biology*, Vol. 76, No.1-5, pp. 31–42. ISSN: 0960-0760.

Baxter, J.D., Goede, P., Apriletti, J.W., West, B.L. & Feng, W. (2002). Structure-Based Design and Synthesis of a Thyroid Hormone Receptor (TR) Antagonist. *Endocrinology*, Vol. 143, No. 2, pp. 517-524. ISSN: 1945-7170.

Botrel, R. T., Rodrigues, L. A., Gomes, L. J., Carvalho, D.A., & Fontes, M.A.L. (2006). Uso da vegetação nativa pela população local no município de Ingaí, MG, Brasil. *Acta Botanica Brasílica*, Vol. 20, No. 1, pp. 143-156. ISSN: 0102-3306.

Bialy, L., Waldmann, H., Chemie, A. (2005). Review. Inhibitors of protein tyrosine phosphatases: Next-generation drugs? *Angewandte Chemie International Edition*, Vol. 44, No. 25, pp. 3814-3839. ISSN: 1521-3773.

Braverman, E., Utiger, R.D. (2000). *Ingbar, S.H. & Werner, S.C. The Thyroid: A Fundamental and Clinical Text* (9th Edition), Lippincott Williams & Wilkins, Philadelphia. ISBN-10: 0781750474.

Carvalho, A.C.B., Diniz, M.F.F.M., Mukherjee, R. (2005). Hypoglycemic activity studies of some plants used in diabetes treatment in Brazilian traditional medicine. *Revista Brasileira de Farmácia*, Vol. 86, No 1, pp.11 16. ISSN. 2176-0667.

Chan, R.Y., Chen , W.F., Dong, A., Guo, D. & Wong, M.S. (2002). Estrogen-like activity of ginsenoside Rg1 derived from *Panax notoginseng*. *The Journal of Clinical Endocrinology & Metabolism*, Vol. 87, No. 8, pp. 3691-3695. ISSN: 1945-7197.

Chiellini, G., Nguyen, N. H., Apriletti, J.W., Baxter, J.D. & Scanlan, T.S. (2002). Synthesis and biological activity of novel thyroid hormone analogues: 5′-aryl substituted GC-1 derivatives. *Bioorganic & Medicinal Chemistry Letters*, Vol. 10, No. 2, pp. 333-346. ISSN: 0960-894X.

Chiellini, G., Nguyen, N., Apriletti, J. W., Baxter, J.D., Scanlan, T. S., Laudet V. & Gronemeyer, H. (2002). *The Nuclear Receptor Facts Book. Factsbook Series*, 1st ed., Academic Press, London. ISBN 10: 0124377356.

Chun , J.Y. , Tummala , R., Nadiminty, N., Lou, W., Liu, C., Yang, J., Evans, C.P., Zhou, Q. & Gao, A.C. (2010). Andrographolide, an herbal medicine, inhibits interleukin-6 expression and suppresses prostate cancer cell growth. *Genes Cancer*. Vol. 1, No. 8, pp. 868-876. ISSN: 1947-6019.

Colker, C.M., Kalman, D.S., Torina, G.C., Perlis, T., Street, C. (1999). Effects of *Citrus aurantium* extract, caffeine, and St. John's Wort on body fat loss, lipid levels, and mood states in overweight healthy adults. *Current Therapeutic Research*, Vol. 60, No. 3, pp.145-153. ISSN: 0011-393X.

Consolini, A.E., Baldini, O.A., Amat, A.G. (1999). Pharmacological basis for the empirical use of *Eugenia uniflora* L. (Myrtaceae) as antihypertensive. *Journal of Ethnopharmacology*, Vol. 66, No. 1, pp.33-39. ISSN: 0378-8741.

Cunha Lima, S.T., Rodrigues, E.D., Melo, T., Nascimento, A.F. Guedes, M.L.S., Cruz, T., Alves, C., Meyer, R., & Toralles, M.B (2008). Levantamento da flora medicinal usada no tratamento de doenças metabólicas em Salvador, BA- Brasil. *Revista Brasileira de Plantas Medicinais,* Vol. 10, No. 4, pp. 83-89. ISSN: 1516-0572.

da Silva, K.L. & Cechinel Filho, V. (2002). Plants of the genus Bauhinia: chemical composition and pharmacological potential. *Química Nova*, Vol. 25, No. 3, pp. 449-454.

Felig, P.F. & Baxter J.D. (1995). *The thyroid: physiology, thyrotoxicosis, hypothyroidism, and the painful thyroid.* Frohman (Eds.), *Endocrinology and Metabolism*, McGraw-Hill, New York. ISBN: 0070204489 / 0-07-020448-9.

Gauthier, K., Chassande, O., Plateroti., M., Roux, J.P., Legrand, C., Pain, B., Rousset, B., Weiss, R., Trouillas, J., Samarut, J. (1999). Different functions for the thyroid hormone receptors TRα and TRβ in the control of thyroid hormone production and post-natal development. *EMBO Journal*, Vol. 18, No. 3, 623 - 631. ISSN: 0261-4189.

Gazola, R., Machado, D., Ruggiero, C., Singi, G., Macedo Alexandre, M. (2004). *Lippia alba, Melissa officinalis* and *Cymbopogon citratus*: effects of the aqueous extracts on the isolated hearts of rats. *Pharmacological Research*, Vol. 50, No. 5, pp. 477-480. ISSN: 1096-1186.

Grover, G. J., Mellström, K., Ye, L., Malm, J., Li, Y. L., Bladh, L. G., Sleph, P. G., Smith, M. A., George, R. & Vennström, B., Mookhtiar, K., Horvath, R., Speelman, J., Egan, D. & Baxter, J.D. (2003). Selective thyroid hormone receptor-β activation: A strategy for reduction of weight, cholesterol, and lipoprotein (a) with reduced cardiovascular liability. *Proceedings of the National Academy of Science of the United States of America*, Vol. 100, No. 17, pp. 10067–10072. ISSN: 0027-8424.

Gustafsson, J.A. (1998). Therapeutic potential of selective estrogen receptor modulators. *Current Opinion in Chemical Biology*, Vol. 2, No. 4, pp. 508–511. ISSN: 1367-5931.

Hamann, I., Seidlova-Wuttke, D., Wuttke, W. & Köhrle, J. (2008). Environment and endocrinology: The case of thyroidology. *Annales d'Endocrinologie*, Vol. 69, No. 2, pp. 116-122. ISSN: 0003-4266.

Hegazy, M.E., Mohamed, A.E., El-Halawany, A.M., Djemgou, P.C., Shahat, A.A. & Pare´, P.W. (2011). Estrogenic Activity of Chemical Constituents from *Tephrosia candida*. *Journal of Natural Products*, Vol. 74, No. 5, pp 937–942. ISSN: 0163-3864.

Horn-Ross, P.L., Hoggatt, K.J. & Lee, M.M. (2002). Phytoestrogens and Thyroid Cancer Risk: The San Francisco Bay Area Thyroid Cancer Study. *Cancer Epidemiology Biomarkers Prevention*, Vol. 11, pp.42-49. ISSN: 1055-9965.

Ibañez , E., Cifuentes, A., Crego, A.L., Señoráns, F.J., Cavero, S. & Reglero, G. (2000). Combined use of supercritical fluid extraction, micellar electrokinetic chromatography, and reverse phase high performance liquid chromatography for the analysis of antioxidants from rosemary (*Rosmarinus officinalis* L.). *Journal of Agricultural and Food Chemistry*, Vol. 48, No. 9, pp. 4060-4065. ISSN: 0021-8561.

Latha, M. and PARI, L. (2004). Effect of an aqueous extract of *Scoparia dulcis* on blood glucose, plasma insulin and some polyol pathway enzymes in experimental rat diabetes. *Brazilian Journal of Medical and Biological Research*, Vol. 37, No. 4, pp. 577-586. ISSN: 1678-4510.

Lim ,W., Nguyen, N., Ha, Y. Y., Scanlan, T. S. & Furlow, J. D. (2002). A Thyroid Hormone Antagonist That Inhibits Thyroid Hormone Action *in Vivo*. *Journal of Biological Chemistry*, Vol. 277, No. 38, pp. 35664–35670. ISSN: 1083-351X.

McDonnell, D.P. & Norris, J.D. (2002). Connections and regulation of the human estrogen receptor, *Science*, Vol. 296, No. 5573, pp. 1642–1644. ISSN: 1095-9203.

McKenna, N.J. & O'Malley, B.W. (2000). An issue of tissues: divining the split personalities of selective estrogen receptor modulators. *Nature Medicine*, Vol. 6, pp. 960–962. ISSN: 1546-170X.

Medeiros, M.F.T., Fonseca, V.S. & Andreata, R.H.P. (2004). Plantas medicinais e seus usos pelos sitiantes da reserva do Rio das Pedras, Mangaratiba, RJ, Brasil. *Acta Botanica Brasílica*, Vol. 18, No. 2, pp. 391-399. ISSN: 0102-3306.

Mendonça, V.L.M., Oliveira, C.L.A., Craveiro, A.A., Rao, V.S., Fonteles, M.C. (1991). Pharmacological and toxicological evaluation of *Alpinia speciosa*. *Memórias do Instituto Oswaldo Cruz*, Vol. 86, No. 2, pp. 93-97. ISSN: 0074-0276.

Mentreddy, S.R. (2007). Medicinal plant species with potential antidiabetic properties. *Journal of the Science of Food and Agriculture*, Vol. 87, No. 5, pp.743-750. ISSN: 1097-0010.

Murillo, G. & Mehta, R.G. (2001). Cruciferous Vegetable and Cancer Prevention. *Nutrition and Cancer*, Vol. 41 (1-2), pp. 17-28. ISSN: 0163-5581.

Nagappa, A.N. , Thakurdesai, P.A. , Rao, N.V. & Singh, J. (2003). Antidiabetic activity of *Terminalia catappa* Linn fruits. *Journal of Ethnopharmacology*, Vol. 88, No. 1, pp. 45-50. ISSN: 0378-8741.

Negrelle, R.R.B. & Gomes, E.C. (2007). *Cymbopogon citrates* (DC.) Stapf.: chemical composition and biological activities. *Revista Brasileira de Plantas Medicinais*, Vol. 9, No. 1, pp. 80-92. ISSN: 1516-0572.

Ngoc-Ha, N., Apriletti, J.W., Cunha Lima, S.T., Webb, P., Baxter, J.D. & Scanlan, T. S. (2002). Rational Design and Synthesis of a Novel Thyroid Hormone Antagonist That Blocks Coactivator Recruitment. *Journal of Medicinal Chemistry*, Vol. 45, No. 15, pp. 3310-3320. ISSN: 0022-2623.

Parry, D.W., O'neill C. H., Hodson, M.J. (1986). Opaline silica deposits in the leaves of *Bidens pilosa* L. and their possible significance in cancer. *Annals of Botany*, Vol. 58, No. 5, pp. 641-647. ISSN: 1095-8290.

Pasa, M.C., Soares, J.J. & Germano, G.N. (2005). Estudo etnobotânico na comunidade de Conceição-Açú. *Acta Botanica Brasílica*, Vol. 19, No. 2, pp. 195-207. ISSN: 0102-3306.

Pepato, M.T., Keller, E.H., Baviera, A.M., Kettelhut, I.C., Vendramini, R.C., Brunetti, I.L. (2002). Anti-diabetic activity of *Bauhinia forficata* decoction in streptozotocin-diabetic rats. *Journal of Ethnopharmacology*, Vol. 81, No. 2, pp. 191-197. ISSN: 0378-8741.

Pianjing , P., Thiantanawat, A., Rangkadilok, N., Watcharasit, P., Mahidol, C.& Satayavivad J. (2011). Estrogenic activities of sesame lignans and their metabolites on human breast cancer cells. *The Journal of Agricultural and Food Chemistry*, Vol. 12, No. 1, pp. 212-221. ISSN: 0021-8561.

Prakash, D., Suri, S., Upadhyay, G. & Singh, B.N. (2007). Total phenol, antioxidant and free radical scavenging activities of some medicinal plants. *International Journal of Food Sciences and Nutrition*, Vol. 58, No. 1, pp. 18-28. ISSN: 0963-7486.

Ren, W., Qiao, Z., Wang, H., Zhu, L., Zhang, L. (2003). Flavonoids: Promising anticancer agents. *Medicinal Research Reviews*, Vol. 23, No. 4, pp. 519-534. ISSN: 0198-6325.

Rodrigues, E. & Carlini, E.A (2004). Plants used by a Quilombola group in Brazil with potential central nervous system effects. *Phytotherapy Research*, Vol. 18, No. 9, pp. 748- 53. ISSN: 0951-418X.

Schossler, D.R.C., Mazzanti, C.M., da Luz, S.C.A., Filappi, A., Prestes, D., da Silveira, A.F., Cecim, M. (2004). Syzygium cumini and the regeneration of insulin positive cells from the pancreatic duct. *Brazilian Journal of Veterinary Research and Animal Science*, Vol. 41, No. 4, pp. 236-239. ISSN: 1413-9596.

Seon , M.R., Lim , S.S., Choi, H.J., Park, S.Y., Cho, H.J., Kim, J.K., Kim, J., Kwon, D.Y. & Park, J.H. (2010). Isoangustone A present in hexane/ethanol extract of *Glycyrrhiza uralensis* induces apoptosis in DU145 human prostate cancer cells via the activation of DR4 and intrinsic apoptosis pathway. *Molecular Nutrition & Food Research*, Vol. 54, No. 9, pp. 1329-39. ISSN: 1613-4133.

Simões, C. M. O. & Schenkel, E. P. (2002). A pesquisa e a produção brasileira de medicamentos a partir de plantas medicinais: a necessária interação da indústria com a academia. *Revista Brasileira de Farmacognosia*. Vol. 2. No.1, PP. 35-40. ISSN 0102-695X.

Sudheesh, S., Vijayalakshmi, N.R. (2005). Flavonoids from *Punica granatum* - potential antiperoxidative agents. *Fitoterapia*, Vol. 76, No. 2, pp.181-186. ISSN: 0367-326X.

Sundararajan, P., Dey, A., Smith, A., Doss, A.G., Rajappan, M. & Natarajan, S. (2006). Studies of anticancer and antipyretic activity of *Bidens pilosa* whole plant (2006). *African Health Sciences*, Vol. 6, No. 1, pp. 27-30. ISSN: 1680-6905.

Taylor, A. H., Stephan, Z. F., Steele, R. E. & Wong, N. C. (1997). Beneficial Effects of a Novel Thyromimetic on Lipoprotein Metabolism. *Molecular Pharmacology*, Vol. 52, No. 3, pp. 542–547. ISSN: 0026-895X.

Teixeira, C.C., Weinert, L.S., Barbosa, D.C., Ricken, C., Esteves, J.F. & Fuchs F.D. (2004). *Syzygium cumini* (L.) Skeels in the treatment of type 2 diabetes: results of a randomized, double-blind, double-dummy, controlled trial. *Diabetes Care*, Vol. 27, No. 12, pp. 3019-3020. ISSN: 0149-5992.

Traka, M., Gasper, A.V., Melchini, A., Bacon, J.R., Needs, P.W., Frost, V., Chantry, A., Jones, A.M.E., Ortori, C.A., Barrett, D.A., Ball, R.Y., Mills, R.D., Mithen, R.F. (2008). Broccoli Consumption Interacts with GSTM1 to Perturb Oncogenic Signalling Pathways in the Prostate. *PLoS One*, Vol. 3, No. 7, pp. 1-14. ISSN: 1932-6203.

Vieira, I. J. C. , Mathias, L., Braz-Filho, R. & Schripsema, J.. (1999). .Iridoids from Borreria verticillata.*Organic Letters*, Vol.1, No.8, pp.1169-71. ISSN: 1523-7052.

Webb, P., Nguyen , N.H., Chiellini , G., Yoshihara, H.A., Cunha Lima, S.T., Apriletti, J.W., Ribeiro, R.C., Marimuthu, A., West, B.L., Goede, P., Mellstrom, K., Nilsson, S., Kushner, P.J., Fletterick, R.J., Scanlan, T.S. & Baxter, J.D. (2002). Design of thyroid hormone receptor antagonists from first principles. *Journal of Steroid Biochemistry and Molecular Biology*, Vol. 83, No. 1–5, pp. 59–73. ISSN: 0960-0760.

Yen, P.M. (2001). Physiological and molecular basis of thyroid hormone action. *Physiological Reviews*, Vol. 81, No. 3, pp. 1097–1142. ISSN: 0031-9333.

Yoshihara, H.A., Apriletti, J.W., Baxter, J.D. & Scanlan, T.S. (2001). A designed antagonist of the thyroid hormone receptor. *Bioorganic & Medicinal Chemistry Letters*, Vol. 11, No. 21, pp. 2821-2825. ISSN: 0960-894X.

Zubeldia, J.M., Nabi, H.A., Jiménez, D.R.M, & Genovese, J. (2010). Exploring new applications for *Rhodiola rosea*: can we improve the quality of life of patients with short-term hypothyroidism induced by hormone withdrawal? *Journal of Medicinal Food*, Vol. 13, No. 6, pp. 1287-1292. ISSN: 1096-620X.

Part 3

Psychiatric Disturbances Associated to Thyroid Diseases

16

Thyroid and Parathyroid Diseases and Psychiatric Disturbance

A. Lobo-Escolar[1,2], A. Campayo[2,3,4], C.H. Gómez-Biel[3] and A. Lobo[2,3,4]
[1]*Miguel Servet University Hospital (Department of Surgery)*
[2]*The University of Zaragoza*
[3]*Clínico University Hospital (Department of Psychiatry)*
[4]*Center for Biomedical Research in Mental Health Network (CIBERSAM)*
Institute of Health "Carlos III", Madrid
Spain

1. Introduction

Different factors have stimulated the interest on the relationships between psychiatric conditions and endocrine disturbances in general and thyroid disease in particular (Lishman, 1998). Historically, several authors have speculated about the role of hormones and endocrine disorders in relation to psychiatric conditions, and important attention has been devoted to the role of hormones in relation to control and feedback processes in neural structures (Carroll et al. 1981). Psychiatric syndromes have consistently been described or documented in endocrine diseases (Lishman, 1998; Kathol, 2002) and may pose a real clinical challenge for psychiatrists working in general hospitals (liaison or psychosomatic psychiatrists), but the evidence in the literature to support his or her intervention is limited, according to modern criteria. The purpose of this chapter is primarily to review available data in relation to the characteristics and frequency of specific psychiatric syndromes in primary thyroid and parathyroid disturbances; issues of diagnosis and differential diagnosis; mechanisms of production of psychiatric symptomatology; and treatment issues, including response of psychiatric syndromes to treatment of the endocrinopathy and to psychotropic medication.

2. General clinical and epidemiological aspects

The most severe psychiatric syndromes in endocrine diseases are not as frequent as in the past, due to improvements in diagnosis and treatment of the hormonal disorders (Kathol, 2002). Still, a high prevalence of psychiatric disturbances has been reported in most endocrine conditions, including thyroid and parathyroid diseases. Depression and anxiety together with cognitive disorders are the most common presentations (Table 1). As expected, lifetime prevalence is even higher in several reports (Eiber et al. 1997). Cognitive impairment is rather frequent in conditions such as hyperparathyroidism, particularly among the elderly, and dementia can also be found; delirium, but also psychosis in clear consciousness, including paranoid psychosis and mania may be seen in severe endocrine diseases. Methodological issues limit the value of the available data: case studies and case reports abound in this literature, research diagnostic criteria have rarely been used and comparison between studies is difficult due to wide differences in the samples selected and methods used. However, standardized research interviews were used in some studies reviewed here and standardized instruments in most. The emerging general picture suggests the clinical relevance of the documented psychopathology, including the depressive and anxiety syndromes, which may be very severe in diseases such as hyperthyroidism (Table 2).

	Hyperthyroidism	Hypothyroidism	Hyperpara-thyroidism	Hypopara-thyroidism
Any Disorder	53%-100%		23%-66%	
Depression	++ 30%-70%	++	++ 16%-36%	+
Apathy	"Apathetic hyperthyroidism"	+	+	
Delirium	+	+	++ 2%-5%	++
Impaired cognition	++	+++ Cretinism	++ 3%-12%	+
Dementia	Risk Factor DAT?	++	+	+/-
Others	• Overactivity • Irritability • Organic personality in the elderly	• Slowing/Lethargy • Mania (Treatment induced)	• Fatigue • Violent behaviour?	• Social withdrawl • "Neurotic" behaviour

DAT: Dementia, Alzheimer Type.
+/+++: Clinical relevance.
Brown et al., 1987; Bunevicius et al.; Casella et al., 2008; Eiber et al., 1997; Espiritu et al., 2010; Joborn et al., 1986; Kathol & Delahunt, 1986; Mooradian, 2008; Pérez- Echeverria, 1985; Velasco et al., 1999; Solin et al., 2009

Table 1. Psychiatric syndromes in thyroid and parathyroid disorders: prevalence and clinical relevance.

It was in this context that we completed a study in 100 consecutive patients admitted to the Endocrine Unit in our University hospital (Pérez-Echeverría, 1985; Lobo et al., 1988). Patients hospitalized in the Internal Medicine ward were used as a comparison group, as well as outpatient groups of both the internal medicine and the endocrine Departments. Standardized instruments, including the Clinical Interview Schedule (CIS) and the General Health Questionnaire-28 items (GHQ-28), were used throughout the study. In support of the relevance of psychiatric syndromes in these patients and specifically in hyperthyroid patients, the prevalence of disorder at the time of admission (first three days) was significantly higher than in all the comparison groups (Table 2). Similarly, according to standardized criteria, the severity of disorder was significantly higher in the endocrine inpatients (68% had "moderate" or "severe" syndromes) than in the control groups (26,6%, 16% and 40%, respectively).

	Prevalence of any Disorder		Comments
	Admission	Discharge	Severity of psychiatric disorders is significantly higher in endocrine in-patients (++); and decreases significantly at discharge (+++)
All patients (n=100)	91%	54%	
Controls			
I.M. in-patients (n=30)	53,3%		
I.M out-patients (n=100)	38%		
Endocrine out-patients (n=100)	70%		
Hyperthyroidism	100%	86%	Correlations biochemical variables (any)/ Irrtability, Psychastenia.

+ Significance p< 0,05; ++ p<0,01; +++ p<0,001.
* Pérez-Echeverría, 1985; Lobo et al., 1988.

Table 2. Psychiatric disorders in endocrine in-patients and in hyperthyroidism in- patients. Prevalence and correlation with biochemical variables.*

This epidemiological documentation may be important to identify the individuals at risk for specific psychiatric syndromes in liaison programs with endocrine departments; or to search for the syndromes when the psychiatrist consults in specific endocrine patients such as the individuals with thyroid or parathyroid conditions. Screening instruments such as the Hospital Anxiety and Depression Scale (HADS) (Lloyd et al., 2000) or the General Health Questionnaire-28 Items (Lobo et al., 1988) are considered to be appropriate in endocrine patients. The sections dedicated to specific endocrine diseases suggest when the search may be mandatory, such as in cases of hyperthyroidism, where anxiety, but also depressive syndromes may be severe or in cases of cognitive deficits in hypothyroid disease. Table 1 also summarizes the authors' judgement about the clinical relevance (+ to +++) of the psychiatric syndromes in these specific endocrine conditions, according to their frequency, severity and/or special characteristics.

Non-biological hypotheses have been formulated to explain depressive or anxiety syndromes when there is considerable stress and psychosocial difficulties associated with conditions such as hyperthyroidism. However, the authors suggest that the "organic", endocrine origin of the psychiatric syndromes in these patients is most important. The following data support this contention: studies documenting a higher prevalence of psychiatric disturbance than in comparable general population samples (Mayou et al., 1991) and, in particular, in medical samples of comparable severity of the medical disorder (Pérez-Echeverría, 1985); both clinical practice and studies documenting that the prevalence of psychiatric disorder and/or its severity decreases after successful treatment of the endocrine condition (Pérez-Echeverría, 1985). Although some reports are discrepant (Joborn et al., 1988), special support comes from studies documenting statistically significant correlations between severity of psychiatric symptoms/syndromes and hormonal levels or biological parameters (Table 2) (Pérez-Echeverría, 1985; Lobo et al., 1988; Linder et al., 1988).

In relation to diagnosis the dictum of experienced, anonymous liaison psychiatrists seem to be quite appropriate here: "In the general hospital, every psychiatric symptom is "organic"...unless you can document otherwise". In taking the history of rather atypical psychiatric presentations, the clinical psychiatrist should include questions related to the thyroid or parathyroid disorder, particularly when there are signs and /or symptoms suggesting the endocrine abnormality (table 3). If the suggestions are well founded, he or she should also perform at least focal physical examinations to document the presence or absence of endocrine signs. In these cases, but not routinely, he or she should also indicate tests of endocrine function.

Endocrinopathy	Symptoms	Signs
Hyperthyroidism	Diaphoresis Heat intolerance Oligomenorrhea	Exophthalmos Tachycardia Arrytmia (in elderly) Tremor
Hypothyroidism	Cold intolerance Menorrhagia	Goiter Slow relaxing reflexes Myxedema
Hyperparathyroidism	Nausea Muscular weakness (proximal) Abdominal pain	Hypertension
Hypoparathyroidism	Muscle spams Paresthesias	Choreiform movements Chvostek´s sign Trousseau´s sign

Table 3. Somatic symptoms and signs suggesting a thyroid disease.

According to the International Classification of Diseases (10th edition or ICD-10), the diagnosis of an "organic" psychiatric syndrome of thyroid or parathyroid origin in a given patient should be considered when the presenting syndrome is known to be associated with the specific endocrine disease, and is supported by the absence of suggestive evidence of an alternative cause of the mental syndrome. Specifically, the "organic" psychiatric syndrome in cases of thyroid or parathyroid disease is supported when: a) the psychiatric symptoms, the course of illness and/or the age of presentation are atypical for a primary psychiatric disorder; b) there is no family or personal history of the psychiatric condition; c) no precipitating stress is known; d) there is a temporal relationship between the onset of the psychiatric and the endocrine symptoms. The challenge for the consulting psychiatrist is to make explicit the diagnosis of the endocrine origin of the psychiatric syndrome early in the procedure, before his or her diagnosis is confirmed after observing that the syndrome disappears following the removal or improvement of the underlying endocrine disorder.

Most psychiatric syndromes in endocrine patients resolve with standard treatment of the endocrine disease, and this applies to thyroid and parathyroid disorders. However, when symptoms are particularly severe or life-threatening; or when they last longer than reasonably expected (table 4), good clinical sense suggests the importance of psychiatric treatment. Well-controlled studies are lacking, but syndrome specific medication is usually recommended, as well as supportive psychotherapy and, recently, cognitive-behavioural psychotherapy in cases of abnormal illness behaviour. Relevant clinical factors, and exceptions to these general norms will now be discussed for the specific endocrine diseases.

Endocrinophaty	**Psychiatric syndromes**	**Treat if psychiatric syndromes persist after adequate endocrine treatment***
Hyperthyroidism	Anxiety (Depression)	>4 weeks or extreme severity
Hypothyroidism	Depression/ Anxiety	>4 weeks
Hyperparathyroidism		>4 weeks
Hypoparathyroidism	Depression	?

*Treatment should also be recommended when syndromes are very severe or life threatening.
Lobo et al., 2007.

Table 4. Treatment of psychiatric syndromes with psychotropic medications in endocrine patients.

3. Thyroid disease and the "clustering" of somatic and psychiatric morbidity

In relation to epidemiology, we have recently studied the role of thyroid disease in the clustering of somatic and psychiatric morbidity in the elderly population. Pioneer studies by authors such as Eastwood and Trevelyan found that psychiatric and somatic illnesses tend to "cluster" in a limited group of individuals in the general population. The first author speculated about vulnerability to illness, and research in this area was considered "the main task for epidemiology in the field of psychosomatic medicine". Since then, a considerable number of studies have approached this subject, and some authors argued that the association between somatic and psychiatric morbidity is well established. However, previous research was conducted primarily in clinical samples, and not in representative, general population samples (Scott et al., 2007). Furthermore, Eastwood's statement (Eastwood, 1989) suggesting that the association of general psychiatric and somatic morbidity has not been convincingly shown in the elderly population is still valid. Given the relationships between comorbidity and frailty described in the elderly, as well as the negative consequences (Slaets, 2006), studies in the older population were considered to be a research priority.

The study we conducted was part of the ZARADEMP Project, an epidemiological enquiry to document in the elderly community the prevalence, incidence and risk factors of dementia, depression and psychiatric morbidity, as well as their association with somatic morbidity (Lobo et al., 2005). The main objective in this specific study was to try to confirm in the elderly population the tendency of general psychiatric morbidity to cluster with general somatic morbidity. In view of the considerable prevalence of thyroid disease in the elderly and the documented association between thyroid disturbances and psychopathology, we also set as an objective to study the role of thyroid disease in the clustering.

The site of the study was Zaragoza, a capital concentrating 622,371 inhabitants (fifth city in Spain) or 51% the population of the historical kingdom of Aragón. The objectives and general methodology of the ZARADEMP Project have been previously described (Lobo et al., 2005). It is a longitudinal, epidemiological study with four waves, and Wave I (*ZARADEMP I*) was relevant for this report (Figure 1). It was the baseline, cross-sectional study, intended to document the prevalence and distribution of somatic and psychiatric morbidity and of comorbidity. Participating individuals have been followed up in Waves II, III and IV (or *ZARADEMP II, III* and *IV*) to eventually study the influence of hypothesized risk factors for incident cases.

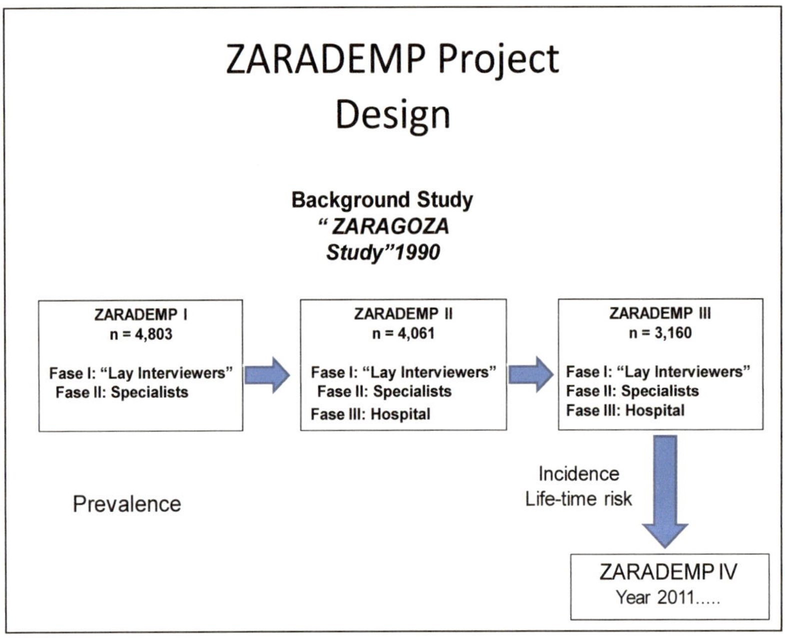

Fig. 1.

A stratified, random sample of 4,803 individuals aged 55 and over was selected for the baseline study. The elderly were assessed with standardized, Spanish versions of instruments, including the Geriatric Mental State (GMS)-AGECAT (Lobo et al, 2005). The GMS is a semistructured standardized clinical interview used for assessing the mental state of elderly people. A computerized diagnostic program, *AGECAT* is available to be applied to it. This interview is also a syndrome case finding instrument, the *GMS-B* threshold scores discriminating between "non-cases", "subcases" and "cases". We also used the *History and Aetiology Schedule (HAS)*, a standardized method of collecting history and etiology data from an informant, or directly from the respondent when he or she was judged to be reliable. Psychiatric cases were diagnosed according to GMS-AGECAT criteria, and somatic morbidity, and specifically thyroid disease was documented with the EURODEM Risk Factors Questionnaire.

	Cases (*n*)	Prevalence (%)	95% CI
55 - 64 years (*n*=1088)	29	2,7	1.8 - 3,8
65 - 74 years (*n*=1702)	66	3,9	3.0 - 4,9
75 - 84 years (*n*=1097)	34	3,1	2.2 - 4,3
≥85 years	21	2,3	1,4 - 3,5

Table 5. Prevalence of thyroid disease in community-dwelling individuals aged ≥ 55 years (distribution by age group).

The relevant results for this chapter may be summarized as follows. As expected, the prevalence of somatic disease tended to increase with age in most categories (Table 4). However, it decreased after the age of 84 in several categories, including thyroid disease. General comorbidity clustered in 19.9% of the elderly when hypertension was removed from the somatic conditions category, 33.5% of the sample remaining free of both somatic and psychiatric illness. General comorbidity was associated with age, female sex and limited education, but did not increase systematically with age. The frequency of psychiatric illness was higher among the somatic cases than among non-cases, and the frequency of somatic morbidity among the psychiatric cases was higher than among non-cases. This association between somatic and psychiatric morbidity remained statistically significant after controlling for age, sex and education (OR= 1.61, IC 1.38-1.88). Most somatic categories were associated with psychiatric illness but, adjusting for demographic variables and individual somatic illnesses, the association remained statistically significant only for cerebro-vascular accidents, CVA's (OR= 1,47, CI 1,09-1,98) and thyroid disease OR= 1,67, CI 1,10-2,54).

	Without psychiatric morbidity (*n*=2211)		
	Cases (*n*)	**Prevalence (%)**	**95% CI**
Thyroid disease	46	2,1	1,5 - 2,8
	Psychiatric morbidity (*n*=2592)		
Thyroid disease	**Cases (*n*)**	**Prevalence (%)**	**95% CI**
	104	4.0	3,3 - 4,8

Table 6. Prevalence of thyroid disease in patients with or without psychiatric morbidity in community-dwelling individuals aged ≥ 55 years.

This was the first study documenting in the (predominantly) elderly population that there is a positive and statistically significant association of general somatic and general psychiatric morbidity. Furthermore, in support of the initial hypothesis our results suggest that thyroid disease may have more weight in this association.

4. Hyperthyroidism

Hyperthyroidism is usually accompanied by physiological symptoms such as sweating, heat intolerance and muscle weakness. However, also common symptoms such as nervousness, fatigue or weight lost may be confounded for primary psychiatric symptoms. Graves´ disease, an autosomal disorder, is the most frequent cause of hyperthyroidism or thyrotoxicosis. While proponents of psychosomatic theories suggested in the last century that an important etiological factor for hyperthyroidism was the presence of psychological conflicts, there is very slight evidence to support the theory. Clinicians in Europe, certainly do not support this conjecture, as shown in the E.C.L.W. study (Huyse et al, 2000). No cases of this endocrine condition were referred for psychiatric consult among 15,000 medical inpatients seen in psychosomatic psychiatry services because of psychopathological reasons (Lobo et al , 1992). However, there is some evidence to support the idea that stress can precipitate the hyperthyroidism (Santos et al, 2002) or complicate the clinical course (Fukao et al , 2003).

The study by Pérez- Echeverría was one of the early investigations reporting the prevalence of psychiatric disturbance among hyperthyroid patients. Only few more studies have reported prevalence data since then. (Trzepacz et al., 1988; Bunevicius et al., 2005). The study by Stern conducted in members of a patients` foundation documented, as expected, that anxiety (72%) and irritability (78%) were the commonest symptoms (Stern et al., 1996).

Psychological disturbance of some degree is universal in Graves` disease (Pérez-Echeverría et al., 1986; Stern et al., 1996), and may delay the diagnosis of the hormonal disorder. Anxiety is most frequently reported, but also depressive syndromes. Rather unusual symptoms may accompany these psychopathological syndromes such as overactivity and restlessness or hyperacuity of perception and increased reaction to noise stimulus. It is the unusual presentation of anxiety (or depression) that may help the physician to differentiate the endocrine disorder from primary affective disturbance. Emotional lability may also be apparent, and both anxiety and irritability may be quite severe and stimulate relatively understandable behavior such as impatience and intolerance of frustration. While depression is not so common, it may be quite prominent and be accompanied by weakness, fatigue and other somatic symptoms. Psychomotor retardation is rare, the exception being the subgroup of elderly patients. "Apathetic hyperthyroidism" has been described in this age group (Mooradian & Arshg, 2008), and some of these cases may progress to stupor and coma.

Classical studies suggested that up to 20% of Graves` disease patients might have some kind of psychosis. However, as discussed by Lishman , there was probably a selection bias (Lishman, 1998). Delirium-type, acute organic syndromes are now rare because of advances in medical treatment. However, delirium in such cases may be a medical emergency. Affective psychoses have been described (Brownlie et al., 2000; Marian et al, 2009), but also schizophrenia-type psychoses, most commonly with paranoid ideation. Organic personality disorder has been described, particularly among the apathetic elderly. Distraibility and over-arousal have also been reported, sometimes leading to persistent cognitive impairment, which may continue even after the patient is euthyroid (Stern et al, 1996). Specific cognitive difficulties in hyperthyroid patient have been described, such as deterioration of memory, concentration or visuomotor speed (MacCrimmon et al., 1979; Álvarez et al., 1983).

The possibility that subclinical hyperthyroidism in the elderly increases the risk of Alzheimer´s disease has been suggested (Kalmijn, 2001) and we are now involved in a large longitudinal study to assess specific risks of dementia, including thyroid disease, in a 15-year follow-up study ingrained in the ZARADEMP project. (Lobo, 2005).

The initial symptoms in hyperthyroidism may be quite similar to anxiety disorders, but the described, unusual symptoms of anxiety may alert the clinicians (Kathol et al., 1986). Other symptoms that should alert the physicians are the preference for cold and intolerance to heat, or loss of weight coupled with increased appetite. A careful medical history and examination are mandatory in such cases and the laboratory test would usually give unequivocal answers to the diagnostic difficulties. An accelerated pulse during sleep or cognitive difficulties are also considered to suggest the diagnosis of hyperthyroidism in such cases (Hall et al., 1979; Mackenzie,1988). To help in the differential diagnosis some specific scales have been developed (Iacovides et al, 2000). Transient thyroid hormone elevations, usually mild, may occur in approximately 10% of psychiatric inpatients, but should not be diagnosed of hyperthyroidism. Thyroid abnormalities have also been documented in some studies in primary affective disorders (Oomen et al., 1996). However, later studies did not replicate the findings (Engum et al., 2002) and the possibility of factors of confusion such as the use of psychotropic medication has been considered. Other clinical situations may mimic the thyroid condition before the laboratory results are available, such as abuse of stimulants or drug intoxications. However, the nervousness and emotional lability in hyperthyroid patients may be wrongly diagnosed as alcohol abuse or abstinence.

Subclinical hyperthyroidism has also stirred interest in recent studies. The clinical interest derives from the fact that it has been associated with cognitive deterioration and dementia in the elderly (Kalmijn,2000;Ceresini,2009), both in cross-sectional and longitudinal studies.

While the clinical and epidemiological studies reviewed support the association of hyperthyroid function with psychopathological disturbance, the causal mechanisms are not clear (Bunevicius et al., 2006). One study suggested that the active thyroid hormone (T3) influenced mental performance in healthy subjects (Kathmann et al., 1994). The individuals overestimated time intervals and increased their word fluency, but no other cognitive problems were detected. Pérez-Echeverría (1985) and Lobo et al (1988) documented direct, convincing correlations between abnormal levels of thyroid hormones and psychopathology. The abnormal psychological phenomenon seemed to be directly related to the endocrine disturbance, since non-endocrine medical patients in the same ward, and with similar levels of illness severity had lower levels of psychopathology. Furthermore, in support of the direct effect of thyroid hormones elevation on the psychopathology, anxiety, depression and related phenomenon improved with "treatment as usual", when hormonal levels returned to normal, at the time of hospital discharge.

In general, there is a good resolution of anxiety and depression with antithyroid treatment alone, unless there is previous psychiatric history (Kathol et al., 1986). Beta-blockers such as propanolol are also considered to be effective in cases of anxiety (Trzepacz et al, 1988). However, recovery may be slow and reduced psychological well-being has been reported in a considerable proportion of "remitted" hyperthyroidism (Pérez-Echeverría, 1985). Bunevicius also reported persistent mood and anxiety symptoms in treated hyperthyroidism (Bunevicius et al., 2005). Psychosis may occur or be exacerbated by antithyroid medication. Low potency neuroleptics such as haloperidol and perphenazine have been reported, including symptoms resembling thyroid storm and malignant neuroleptic syndrome. There is a limited clinical experience with the new generation of neuroleptics. Finally, treatment of depression is recommended if psychopathological symptoms are severe or persistent.

5. Hypothyroidism

Classical symptoms of hypothyroidism include fatigue and weakness, somnolence, weight gain, constipation and cold intolerance. However, other common symptoms may suggest primary psychiatric disease and include lethargy, progressive slowing, diminished initiative and impaired concentration and memory. (Kornstein et al., 2000).

Congenital hypothyroidism is also well known, and usually occurs as the consequence of thyroid dysgenesis, and more rarely as the result of inherited defects in the synthesis of thyroid hormone. The cretinism syndrome emerges if hypothyroidism is untreated. This syndrome is characterized by mental retardation, aside from the classical somatic and neurological signs. Screening programs for hypothyroidism at birth are now mandatory to prevent this severe condition. (American Academy of Pediatrics, 2006), since early treatment should lead to normal intellectual development. The most frequent cause of adult hypothyroidism is Hashimoto´s thyroiditis or autoimmune thyroiditis. Treatment of Grave´s disease with radioactive iodine may also lead to hypothyroidism, but an important iatrogenic cause in psychiatric patients is the side effect of lithium, particularly in vulnerable individuals such as women or rapid cyclers.

There are no good prevalence studies of psychiatric disturbance in hypothyroid patients, but the main psychiatric syndromes have been described in case reports and/or clinical samples. Depression and, to a lesser extent anxiety (Sait Gönen et al., 2004), occur rather frequently, even with moderate hormonal deficits, and could be observed as early as few weeks after the onset of the condition. Previous history of affective disorder is considered to increase the risk. The depressive syndromes may mimic primary affective disorder, particularly in old women, and may need the checking of hormonal levels for the differential diagnosis. The initial symptoms of hypothyroidism mimic the somatic symptoms of depression, and may include low energy, fatigue, apathy, low appetite and sleep disturbance. Marked irritability and labiliy of mood may alert to the presence of atypical syndromes, suggesting an organic condition. Thyroid replacement is required in such cases and is usually effective, although depression persists in a proportion of patients

A special emphasis should be placed in subclinical hypothyroidism. In this controversial condition, which is sometimes classified as grade 2 and grade 3 hypothyroidism, there may be minimal clinical, traditional symptoms, and thyroid levels may be normal, but with increased TSH. The relevance of subclinical hypothyroidism is derived from the fact that depression is common and may severely affect quality of life. (Haggerty et al., 1993; Dermatini et al., 2010). In the study by Chueire et al. (2003), using standardized instruments and psychiatric diagnostic citeria, they found depression among 49% of subclinical hypothyroid, elderly patients. The same authors have recently reported that depression in such patients is more frequent than among patients with overt hyperthyroidism (Chueire et al., 2007). Furthermore, they conclude that subclinical hypothyroidism increases more than four times the risk of depression, and highlight the relevance of thyroid screening tests in the elderly. Treatment of depression in such cases is recommended (Carvalho et al., 2009), but may be frustrating (Hendrick et al., 1998). It has been suggested that subclinical hypothyroidism is rather common in the general population, particularly in the adult and elderly women, but may go undetected and untreated. Screening tests of hormonal levels may be crucial in doubtful cases.

Delirium has been observed in approximately 10% of severe cases of hypothyroidism, and organic delusional syndromes have been documented in some case reports. "Mixedema madness", a psychosis in untreated cases of hypothyroidism was described before the standard use of thyroid function tests (Kudrjavcev, 1978), but is quite rare now. Some authors have called "Hashimoto`s encephalopathy" the clinical picture of delirium with focal neurological signs and seizures. It has been considered to be associated with high levels of serum antithyroid antibodies, but the psychopathological symptoms probably overlap with delirium of different etiologies (Schiess & Pardo, 2008).

Longstanding hypothyroidism may end up in a marked dementia syndrome. Before, cognitive disturbance may be apparent (Samuels et al, 2008). Memory deterioration is common, but may be accompanied by impairment of other cognitive functions. While some cognitive difficulties may be associated with the depressive syndromes, some authors have reported independent, cognitive difficulties (Burmeister et al.,2001). Mild hypothyroidism has also been associated with mild cognitive difficulties (Bunevicius et al, 1999; Miller et al, 2007). While most cases of cognitive disturbance improve with hormonal treatment, some studies reported negative results (Walsh et al., 2003). Hypothyroidism used to be considered one example of reversible dementia with appropriate hormonal treatment (Cummings et al., 1980). However, most authors doubt about its effectiveness in well established cases of dementia (Clarnette & Patterson, 1994; Lobo et al., 2010).

Present knowledge about the effects of thyroid hormones in the central nervous system suggests the critical influence in brain development, and probably a direct role in adult brain homeostasis. Multiple isolated effects have been described, including a modulation of noradrenergic, serotonergic, and dopaminergic receptor function, and an influence on second messenger, calcium homeostasis, axonal transport mechanisms, and morphology. However, both the biochemical mechanisms and the physiological relevance are poorly understood.

Even minor changes in thyroid hormone may induce important affective changes (Bauer et al., 1990). However, the connections between this hormone and primary affective disorder remain controversial .Some authors conclude that depressed patients are basically euthyroid (Baumgartner, 1993). Thyroid autoimmunity has been reported in bipolar disorder (Kupka et al., 2002) but the finding needs replication. Special consideration merit the cases of hypothyroidism seen in 10% of patients treated with lithium. Disregulation in the hypothalamic-pituitary-thyroid axis is commonly linked to primary affective disorders (Hendrick, 1998; Engum et al., 2002). Close to 50% of depressive patients with major depression have a positive, blunted TSH response to TRH. While these findings support the connection between thyroid disorder and primary affective disorder (Stipcevic et al., 2008), other authors conclude that depressed patients are basically euthyroid (Baumgartner et al., 1993). New studies are considered to be needed to clarify this relationship.

The neuropsychiatric symptoms of hypothyroidism maybe the first to recover, probably in few days, with adequate hormonal replacement. Slow correction is usually recommended, particularly in the elderly, because the risk of cardiac or psychiatric dysfunction. Short periods of mania or hypomania may occur during the treatment, but will typically subside during the replacement. Moderate doses of neuroleptics are usually well tolerated in cases of psychosis, but these cases may not recover totally.

6. Hyperparathyroidism

Primary hyperparathyroidism is often caused by parathyroid adenomas (Bresler et al., 2002). It is characterized by the presence of elevated parathyroid hormone, elevated calcium and hypophosphatemia. Hyperparathyroidism may lead to renal calculus and bone disease. Classical symptoms of hypercalcemia, such as anorexia, lethargy or fatigue, may be attributed to primary psychiatric disease. The symptoms may be insidious, but gradually increase and may lead to coma. The early recognition of hyperparathyroidism is now more common, due to the use of routine biochemical screening.

The prevalence of hyperparathyroidism is considered to be around 0.1%, and increases both in women and with age. Radiation of head and neck may produce this condition, but is also a known consequence of lithium therapy in psychiatric patients (Kingsbury & Salzman, 1993). The common use of lithium in long term treatment of affective disorders should alert physicians about side effects, since hyperparathyroidism symptoms may be confounded for affective psychopathology. The determination of serum calcium levels may be considered in the protocol of atypical psychiatric presentations of cognitive difficulties or affective symptoms, particularly depression. Calcium levels may also be monitored in patients in lithium treatment, since hypercalcemia as a secondary affect has been reported and may be confounded with the relapse of affective symptoms (Pieri-Balandraud et al., 2001).The EEG is an important diagnostic tool in such cases, since the slow activity accompanied by frontal delta paroxysms are quite suggestive of hypercalcemia.

Lithium is considered to alter the feedback inhibition, and the set point of the parathyroid gland. It also stimulates hormone secretion. The lower incidence of stones in lithium-induced hypercalcemia, contrary to what is observed in primary hyperparathyroidism, has been considered to be the effect of interference of lithium in cAMP production (Kingsburg et al 1993). Hypercalcemia should be considered in the differential diagnosis of bipolar, lithium-treated patients with unusual psychopathological symptoms and/or resistance to treatment. Mild calcium elevations may be managed medically. However, cessation of lithium frequently does not correct the hyperparathyrodism and the parathyroidectomy may be necessary.

Psychopathological symptoms are considered to be quite common in hyperparathyroidism (Brown et al 1987). However, most studies are derived from case reports or were completed in short samples and standardized methods of assessment were rarely used (White et al 1996). Depressive and anxiety syndromes have been most frequently described (Joborn et al., 1986; Birder, 1988). Nevertheless, the preponderance of symptoms such as apathy, fatigue, irritability or neuro-vegetative symptoms should alert the physician. Cognitive symptoms of depression are usually not as severe as in primary affective disorder, the exception being the elderly patients (Linder et al 1988). Overt delirium has frequently been observed when hypercalcemia is high (above 16 mg/dl), and coma has been reported with serum levels above 19 mg/dl (Petersen 1968). In the elderly, cognitive disorders and eventually dementing syndromes may occur if the endocrine disorder persists (Joborn et al.,

1986). Psychosis has rarely been described, but Joborn et al reported paranoid ideas and hallucinations in their study and Bresler et al (2000) reported violent behavior, included attempted mass murder in a case of paranoid ideation in clear consciousness. More chronic cases, aside from cognitive disorder, have been associated with personality changes leading to withdrawn behavior and seclusion.

The pathogenesis of psychiatric syndromes in hyperparathyroidism may be explained by the hipercalcemia itself, since similar symptoms have been reported in different etiologies. The calcium ions are considered to be crucial in normal neurotransmission. High calcium levels have been associated with abnormal CSF concentrations of monoamine metabolites, such as 5-hydroxy-indoleacetic acid (5-HIAA) found in primary hyperparathyroid patients. Calcium levels correlated with depressive symptoms and returned to normal after parathyroid surgery (Joborn et al 1988). Affective symptoms in primary hyperparathyroidism have also been reported to correlate with abnormal levels of both cortisol and melatonin, which improve after successful surgery (Linder et al 1988). Nevertheless, other studies did not find a correlation of psychopathology and calcium levels. (Joborn et al 1988; White et al., 1996). The influence of hypomagnesemia and hypophosphoremia, as well as the parathormone itself and vitamin B have also been hypothesized to influence the pathogenesis of psychiatric symptoms in hyperparathyroidism.

Most studies suggest that psychiatric symptoms in hyperparathyroidism significantly improve or disappear after successful surgical treatment, unless the endocrine disorder is chronic. (Roman and Sosa 2007, Casella et al., 2008, Espiritu, 2010). Joborn reported that improvement may be observed in few days, and the same authors have shown that approximately half the patients significantly improved in a follow-up period of several years (Joborn et al., 1988). Wilheim et al 2004 observed that both depression and quality of life improved in a similar proportion of patients. However, Chiang (Chiang et al .,2005), did not find significant differences in neuropsychological performance between patients undergoing parathyroidectomy and the controls. On the basis of significant improvement in depressive symptoms and quality of life in patients with mild hypercalcemia, parathyroidectomy has been suggested in the management of asymptomatic hyperparathyroidism (Wilheim et al., 2004). However, in view of rather conflicting results, we have previously recommended a conservative treatment in asymptomatic cases or cases with mild symptoms (Lobo et al.,1992).

7. Hypoparathyroidism

Hypoparathyroidism can occur as a primary form with inadequate parathyroid hormone secretion, but the commonest cause is the removal of, or interference with blood supply in the parathyroid gland during neck surgery. The affected patients present with hypocalcemia, which causes neuromuscular irritability.

Muscle cramps and paresthesias are typical symptoms, but facial grimacing and seizures may occur, suggesting a neuro-psychiatric condition. In a classical study, Denko & Kaelbing (1962) and similarly other authors (Velasco et al., 1999), reported a high frequency of cognitive disorder, but a considerable proportion of patients had psychotic symptoms, including hallucinations and catatonic stupor. However, the systematic study of psychiatric symptoms in hyperparathyroid patients is sparse. Reviews of this subject have concluded that approximately half the cases due to surgery had psychopathological symptoms, and the frequency might be even higher in idiopathic cases (Lishman 1998). Delirium has been commonly reported in the post-surgery period, as might be expected in relation to abrupt biochemical disturbances.

In non-acute idiopathic hypoparathyroidism, emotional lability and anxious syndromes have been described, and also depressive syndromes. Cognitive difficulties and even dementia syndromes have also been reported in these patients. The emotional lability may coincide with fluctuating, neurotic kind of minor symptoms and behavior. Irritability, nervousness and socially inadequate behavior are among the symptoms most often described. On the contrary the reviews suggest that psychotic syndromes in clear conscientious are uncommon. Chronic cases of hypoparathyroidism may eventually lead to neurological and cognitive deficits. They are considered to be related to intracranial calcification, and in such cases they are irreversible (Kowdley et al., 1999).

Hypoparathyroidism is also frequent in the velocardiofacial syndrome (22q.11.2 deletion syndrome), in wich attentional and behavioral disorders are common among children, and schizophreniform and bipolar disorders are common in adults. (Jolin et al., 2009). In the pathogenesis of this condition, the hypocalcemia itself is considered to be the main agent. Patients with calcium levels in the lower limit of normal may be relatively asymptomatic ("partial parathyroid insufficiency"), but psychopathological symptoms such as depression and anxiety may appear episodically, precipitated by calcium deprivation. In an early study, Fourman et al (1967) reported the efficacy of calcium versus placebo in a double blind clinical trial to improve the psychopathological symptoms.

An important issue, similarly to other endocrine disorders, is the failure to detect and diagnose this condition. This is particularly relevant in cases of anxiety resistant to treatment. Since anxiety can provoke hyperventilation, tetany in hypoparathyroid patients may be precipitated (Fourman et al., 1967). In doubtful cases, calcium and phosphorus levels should be monitored, especially in patients operated in the neck. The presenting signs of hypoparathyroidism may be an epileptic crisis or an abnormal EEG.

Psychiatric syndromes in non-chronic hypoparathyroidism patients are treatable with calcium supplements and vitamin D. (Velasco et al., 1999). Depressive and anxiety syndromes have a good response, unless they are severe. The benzodiazepines are considered to be effective in cases of anxiety. Improvement in cognitive syndromes has also been reported in a considerable proportion of patients, the exception being the severe cases and the dementia syndromes. There is some report about the susceptibility of these patients to the parkinsonian side effects of neuroleptics. However, Pratty et al (1986) did not confirm this unwanted side effect.

8. Conclusions

This chapter reviews available data in relation to the characteristics and frequency of psychiatric syndromes in primary thyroid and parathyroid disturbances, including the contributions of the authors. It also reviews issues of diagnosis and differential diagnosis; mechanisms of production of psychiatric symptomatology; and treatment issues, including response of psychiatric syndromes to treatment of the endocrinopathy and to psychotropic medication. The most severe psychiatric syndromes in endocrine diseases are not as frequent as in the past, due to improvements in diagnosis and treatment of the hormonal disorders, but still, a high prevalence of psychiatric disturbances has been reported in both thyroid and parathyroid diseases. Depression and anxiety together with cognitive disorders are the most common presentations. Cognitive impairment is frequent among the elderly, and dementia can also be found; delirium, but also psychosis in clear consciousness, including paranoid psychosis and mania may be seen in severe endocrinopaties. Methodological issues limit the value of the available data. However, standardized research interviews were used in some studies reviewed here and standardized instruments in most. The emerging general picture suggests the clinical relevance of the documented psychopathology, which may be very severe in some cases. The authors review their contribution in two relevant, epidemiological type of studies. In the first one, neat correlations were documented between hormonal disturbances and psychopathology in patients hospitalized because of hyperthyroid conditions. In the second study, during the ZARADEMP project, the clustering of somatic and psychiatric morbidity was documented in a large, community sample of individuals aged 55 years or more, and thyroid disease was considered to have specific weight in this association.

9. Acknowledgements

Supported by Grants:

- 94-1562, 97-1321E, 98-0103, 01-0255, 03-0815, G03/128 from the Fondo de Investiugación Sanitaria, and the Spanish Ministry of Health, Instituto de Salud Carlos III. Madrid Spain.
- CIBERSAM PI10/01132 from the Instituto de Salud Carlos III

10. References

Alvarez Ma, Gomez A, Alavez E, et al: Attention disturbance in Grave´s disease. Psychoneuroendocrinology 8:451-454,1983

American Academy of Pediatrics, Section on Endocrinology an Committee on Genetics: Update of newborn screening and therapy for congenital hytpothyroidism. Pediatrics 117:2290-2303,2006

Bauer, M.S. and Whybrow, P.C. (1990). Rapid cycling bipolar affective disorder. II. Treatment of refractory rapid cycling with high-dose levothyroxine: a preliminary study. *Arch Gen Psychiatry.* 47, 435-440.

Baumgartner, A. (1993). Thyroid hormones and depressive disorders--critical overview and perspectives. Part 1: Clinical aspects. *Nervenarzt.* 64, 1-10.

Bresler, S.A., Logan, W.S. and Washington, D. (2000). Hyperparathyroidism and psychosis: possible prelude to murder. *J Forensic Sci.* 45, 728-730.

Brown, G.G., Preisman, R.C. and Kleerekoper, M. (1987). Neurobehavioral symptoms in mild primary hyperparathyroidism: related to hypercalcemia but not improved by parathyroidectomy. *Henry Ford Hosp Med J.* 35, 211-215.

Brownlie, BE., Rae, AM., Walshe, JW.,et al: Psychoses association-thytoxicosis-"thytotoxic psychosis": a report of with statistical analysis of incidence. Eur J End 142:438-444,2000

Bunevicius R, Prange AJ, Jr. Psychiatric manifestations of Graves' hyperthyroidism: pathophysiology and treatment options. CNS Drugs2006;20(11):897-909.

Burmeister LA, Ganguli M, Dodge HH, Toczek T, DeKosky ST, Nebes RD. Hypothyroidism and cognition: preliminary evidence for a specific defect in memory. Thyroid2001 Dec;11(12):1177-85.

Carroll, B.J., Feinberg, M., Greden, J.F., Tarika, J., Albala, A.A., Haskett, R.F., James, N.M., Kronfol, Z., Lohr, N., Steiner, M., de Vigne, J.P. and Young, E. (1981). A specific laboratory test for the diagnosis of melancholia. Standardization, validation, and clinical utility. *Arch Gen Psychiatry.* 38, 15-22.

Carvalho GA, Bahls SC, Boeving A, Graf H. Effects of selective serotonin reuptake inhibitors on thyroid function in depressed patients with primary hypothyroidism or normal thyroid function. Thyroid2009 Jul;19(7):691-7.

Casella C, Pata G, Di Betta E, Nascimbeni R. [Neurological and psychiatric disorders in primary hyperparathyroidism: the role of parathyroidectomy]. Ann Ital Chir2008 May-Jun;79(3):157-61; discussion 61-3.

Ceresini G, Lauretani F, Maggio M, Ceda GP, Morganti S, Usberti E, et al. Thyroid function abnormalities and cognitive impairment in elderly people: results of the Invecchiare in Chianti study. J Am Geriatr Soc2009 Jan;57(1):89-93.

Chiang, C. Y., D. G. Andrewes, D. Anderson, M. Devere, I. Schweitzer and J. D. Zajac. 2005. "A controlled, prospective study of neuropsychological outcomes post parathyroidectomy in primary hyperparathyroid patients." Clin Endocrinol (Oxf) 62(1):99-104.

Chueire VB, Romaldini JH, Ward LS. Subclinical hypothyroidism increases the risk for depression in the elderly. Arch Gerontol Geriatr. 2007 Jan-Feb;44 (1):21-8.

Chueire VB, Silva ET, Perotta E, Romaldini JH, Ward LS. High serum TSH levels are associated with depression in the elderly. Arch Gerontol Geriatr. 2003 May-Jun;36(3):281-8.

Clarnette RM, Patterson CJ. Hypothyroidism: does treatment cure dementia? J Geriatr Psychiatry Neurol1994 Jan-Mar;7(1):23-7.

Cummings, J., D. F. Benson and S. LoVerme, Jr. 1980. "Reversible dementia. Illustrative cases, definition, and review." JAMA 243(23):2434-2439.

Demartini, B., Masu, A., Scarone, S., Pontiroli, AE., & Gambini, O. Prevalence of depression in patients affected by subclinical hypothyroidism. Panminerva Med Dec;52(4):277-82.

Denko, J. D. and R. Kaelbling. 1962. "The psychiatric aspects of hypoparathyroidism." Acta Psychiatr Scand Suppl 38(164):1-70.

Eastwood R. Relationship between physical and psychological morbidity. In: Williams P, Wilkinson G, Rawnsley, K. editors The scope of epidemiological psuchiatry. London: Routledge, 1989. pp.210-21

Eiber, R., Berlin, I., Grimaldi, A. and Bisserbe, J.C. (1997). Insulin-dependent diabetes and psychiatric pathology: general clinical and epidemiologic review. *Encephale.* 23, 351-357.

Engum, A., Bjoro, T., Mykletun, A. and Dahl, A.A. (2002). An association between depression, anxiety and thyroid function--a clinical fact or an artefact? *Acta Psychiatr Scand.* 106, 27-34.

Espiritu RP, Kearns AE, Vickers KS, Grant C, Ryu E, Wermers RA. Depression in Primary Hyperparathyroidism: Prevalence and Benefit of Surgery. J Clin Endocrinol Metab Sep 14.

Fourman, P., Rawnsley, K., Davis, R.H., Jones, K.H. and Morgan, D.B. (1967). Effect of calcium on mental symptoms in partial parathyroid insufficiency. *Lancet.* 2, 914-915.

Fukao A, Takamatsu J, Murakami Y, Sakane S, Miyauchi A, Kuma K, et al.(2003) The relationship of psychological factors to the prognosis of hyperthyroidism in antithyroid drug-treated patients with Graves' disease. Clin Endocrinol (Oxf)2003 May;58(5):550-5.

Haggerty JJ, Jr., Stern RA, Mason GA, Beckwith J, Morey CE, Prange AJ, Jr. Subclinical hypothyroidism: a modifiable risk factor for depression? Am J Psychiatry1993 Mar;150(3):508-10.

Hall RC, Gruzenski WP, Popkin MK. Differential diagnosis of somatopsychic disorders. Psychosomatics1979 Jun;20(6):381-5, 8-9.

Hendrick V, Altshuler L, Whybrow P. Psychoneuroendocrinology of mood disorders. The hypothalamic-pituitary-thyroid axis. Psychiatr Clin North Am1998 Jun;21(2):277-92.

Huyse FJ, Herzog T, Lobo A, Malt UF, Opmeer BC, Stein B, Creed F, Crespo MD, Cardoso G, Guimaraes-Lopes R, Mayou R, van Moffaert M, Rigatelli M, Sakkas P, Tienari P. European Consultation Liaison Psychiatric Services: the ECLW collaborative study. *Acta Psychiatrica Scandinavica* 2000; 101(5): 360-366.

Iacovides A, Fountoulakis KN, Grammaticos P, Ierodiakonou C. Difference in symptom profile between generalized anxiety disorder and anxiety secondary to hyperthyroidism. Int J Psychiatry Med2000;30(1):71-81.

Joborn, C., Hetta, J., Palmer, M., Akerstrom, G. and Ljunghall, S. (1986). Psychiatric symptomatology in patients with primary hyperparathyroidism. *Ups J Med Sci.* 91, 77-87.

Joborn, C., Hetta, J., Rastad, J., Agren, H., Akerstrom, G. and Ljunghall, S. (1988). Psychiatric symptoms and cerebrospinal fluid monoamine metabolites in primary hyperparathyroidism. *Biol Psychiatry.* 23, 149-158.

Jolin, E. M., R. A. Weller and E. B. Weller. 2009. "Psychosis in children with velocardiofacial syndrome (22q11.2 deletion syndrome)." Curr Psychiatry Rep 11(2):99-105.

Kalmijn, S., Mehta, K.M., Pols, H.A., Hofman, A., Drexhage, H.A. and Breteler, M.M. (2000). Subclinical hyperthyroidism and the risk of dementia. The Rotterdam study. *Clin Endocrinol (Oxf).* 53, 733-737.

Kathmann N, Kuisle U, Bommer M, Naber D, Muller OA, Engel RR. Effects of elevated triiodothyronine on cognitive performance and mood in healthy subjects. Neuropsychobiology1994;29(3):136-42.

Kathol R.G. (2002). Endocrine Disorders. In *The American Psychiatric Publishing textbook of consultation-liaison psychiatry psychiatry in the medically ill,* ed., M.G. Wise and J.R. Rundell, 2nd edn, pp. 563-567. Washington, DC: American Psychiatric Pub.

Kathol, R.G. and Delahunt, J.W. (1986). The relationship of anxiety and depression to symptoms of hyperthyroidism using operational criteria. *Gen Hosp Psychiatry.* 8, 23-28.

Kathol, R.G., Turner, R. and Delahunt, J. (1986). Depression and anxiety associated with hyperthyroidism: response to antithyroid therapy. *Psychosomatics* 27, 501-505.

Kingsbury SJ, Salzman C. Lithium's role in hyperparathyroidism and hypercalcemia. Hosp Community Psychiatry1993 Nov,44(11):1017-8.

Kowdley, K. V., B. M. Coull and E. S. Orwoll. 1999. "Cognitive impairment and intracranial calcification in chronic hypoparathyroidism." Am J Med Sci 317(5):273-277.

Kornstein SG, Sholar EF, Gardner DG: Endocrine disorders, in Psychiatric Care of the Medical Patient, 2nd Edition. Edited by Stoudemire A, Fogel BS, Grennberg D. New York, Oxford University Press,2000, pp 801-819

Kupka, R.W., Nolen, W.A., Post, R.M., McElroy, S.L., Altshuler, L.L., Denicoff, K.D., Frye.M.A.,Keck, P.E. Jr, Leverich, G.S., Rush, A.J., Suppes, T., Pollio, C. and Drexhage, H.A. (2002). High rate of autoimmune thyroiditis in bipolar disorder: lack of association with lithium exposure. *Biol Psychiatry.* 51, 305-311.

Kudrjavcev T. Neurologic complications of thyroid dysfunction. Adv Neurol1978;19:619-36.

Linder, J., Brimar, K., Granberg, P.O., Wetterberg, L. and Werner, S. (1988). Characteristic changes in psychiatric symptoms, cortisol and melatonin but not prolactin in primary hyperparathyroidism. *Acta Psychiatr Scand.* 78, 32-40.

Lishman´s, W.A. (2009). Endocrine diseases and metabolic disorders. In Organic Psychiatry, 4th edn. Wiley-Blackwell.

Lishman, W.A. (1998). Endocrine Diseases and Metabolic Disorders. In *Organic psychiatry the psychological consequences of cerebral disorder* , 3rd edn, pp. 507-69. Oxford: Blackwell Science.

Lloyd, C.E., Dyer, P.H. and Barnett, A.H. (2000). Prevalence of symptoms of depression and anxiety in a diabetes clinic population. *Diabet Med.* 17, 198-202.

Lobo, A, Campos R, Marcos G, García-Campayo J, Campayo A, Lopez-Antón R & Pérez-Echeverría MJ.(2007). Somatic and psychiatric co-morbidity in Primary Care patients in Spain. Eur J Psychiat 2007; 21(1): 71-8.

Lobo, A., Saz, P., Marcos G, Dia JL, De-la-Camara, C., & Ventura T. Prevalence of dementia in a southern European population in two different time periods: the ZARADEMP Project. Acta Psychiatr Scand2007 Oct;116(4):299-307.

Lobo, A., Saz, P. Marcos, C. Día, JL. De la Cámara, C. Ventura, T. (2005). The ZARADEMP Project on the Incidence, Prevalence and Risk Factors of Dementia (and Depression) in the Elderly Community: ll. Methods an First Results. Eur J Psychiatry 2005;19-40-54

Lobo, A, Huyse, F., Herzog, T., Malt, V.F. and E.C.L.W. (1992). Profiles of psychiatric and physical co-morbidity. Paper read before the E.C.L.W. Health Service Study Conference: Amsterdam

Lobo, A., Perez-Echeverria, M.J., Jimenez-Aznarez, A. and Sancho, M.A. (1988). Emotional disturbances in endocrine patients. Validity of the scaled version of the General Health Questionnaire (GHQ-28). *Br J Psychiatry.* 152, 807-812.

Lobo-Escolar A, Saz P, Marcos G, Quintanilla MA, Campayo A, Lobo A. Somatic and psychiatric comorbidity in the general elderly population: results from the ZARADEMP Project. J Psychosom Res2008 Oct;65(4):347-55.

Lobo A, Saz P, Quintanilla MA. Dementia. In: Levenson JL, editor. Textbook of Psychosomatic Medicine. Washington: American Psychiatric Press (2010, in press)

MacCrimmon DJ, Wallace JE, Goldberg WM, et al: Emotional disturbance and cognitive deficits in hyperthyroidism. Psychosom Med 41:331-340, 1979

Mackenzie AH. Differential diagnosis of rheumatoid arthritis. Am J Med1988 Oct 14;85(4A):2-11.

Marian G, Nica EA, Ionescu BE, Ghinea D. Hyperthyroidism--cause of depression and psychosis: a case report. J Med Life2009 Oct-Dec;2(4):440-2.

Mayou, R., Peveler, R., Davies, B., Mann, J. and Fairburn, C. (1991). Psychiatric morbidity in young adults with insulin-dependent diabetes mellitus. *Psychol Med.* 21, 639-645.

Miller KJ, Parsons TD, Whybrow PC, Van Herle K, Rasgon N, Van Herle A, et al.(2007) Verbal memory retrieval deficits associated with untreated hypothyroidism. J Neuropsychiatry Clin Neurosci2007 Spring;19(2):132-6.

Miller KJ, Parsons TD, Whybrow PC, van Herle K, Rasgon N, van Herle A, et al. Memory improvement with treatment of hypothyroidism. Int J Neurosci2006 Aug;116(8):895-906.

Mooradian AD. Asymptomatic hyperthyroidism in older adults: is it a distinct clinical and laboratory entity? Drugs Aging2008;25(5):371-80.

Oomen, H.A., Schipperijn, A.J. and Drexhage, H.A. (1996). The prevalence of affective disorder and in particular of a rapid cycling of bipolar disorder in patients with abnormal thyroid function tests. *Clin Endocrinol (Oxf).* 45, 215-223.

Pérez-Echeverría, M.J. (1985). Correlaciones entre trastornos endocrinológicos, niveles hormonales en sangre, variables de personalidad y alteraciones psicopatológicas. *Doctoral Thesis,* Universidad de Zaragoza.

Petersen, P. (1968). Psychiatric disorders in primary hyperparathyroidism. *J Clin Endocrinol Metab.* 28, 1491-1495.

Pieri-Balandraud N, Hugueny P, Henry JF, Tournebise H, Dupont C. [Hyperparathyroidism induced by lithium. A new case]. Rev Med Interne2001 May;22(5):460-4

Pratty, J.S. , Ananth, J. and O'Brien, J.E. (1986). Relationship between dystonia and serum calcium levels. *J Clin Psychiatry.* 47, 418-419.

Roman S, Sosa JA. Psychiatric and cognitive aspects of primary hyperparathyroidism. Curr Opin Oncol2007 Jan;19(1):1-5.

Sait Gönen M, Kisakol G, Savas Cilli A, Dikbas O, Gungor K, Inal A, et al. Assessment of anxiety in subclinical thyroid disorders. Endocr J2004 Jun;51(3):311-5.

Samuels MH. Cognitive function in untreated hypothyroidism and hyperthyroidism. Curr Opin Endocrinol Diabetes Obes2008 Oct;15(5):429-33.

Santos AM, Nobre EL, Garcia e acosta:Graves´s disease and stress.ActaMed Port 15:423-427,2002

Schiess N, Pardo CA: Hashimoto´s encephalopathy. Ann New York academy Science 1142:254-265, 2008.

Scott KM, Bruffaerts R, Tsang A, Ormel J, Alonso J, Angermeyer MC, et al.(2007) Depression-anxiety relationships with chronic physical conditions: results from the World Mental Health Surveys. J Affect Disord2007 Nov;103(1-3):113-20.

Slaets JP. Vulnerability in the elderly: frailty. Med Clin North Am2006 Jul;90(4):593-601.

Stern RA, Robinson B, Thorner AR, et al: A survery study of neuropsychiatric complaints in patients with Grave´s disease. J Neupsychiatry Clin Neurosci 8:181,1996

Stipcevic T, Pivac N, Kozaric-Kovacic D, Muck-Seler D. Thyroid activity in patients with major depression. Coll Antropol2008 Sep;32(3):973-6.

Trzepacz, P.T., McCue, M., Klein, I., Levey, G.S. and Greenhouse, J. (1988). A psychiatric and neuropsychological study of patients with untreated Graves' disease. *Gen Hosp Psychiatry*. 10, 49-55.

Velasco PJ, Manshadi M, Breen K, Lippmann S. Psychiatric aspects of parathyroid disease. Psychosomatics1999 Nov-Dec;40(6):486-90.

Walsh JP, Shiels L, Lim EM, Bhagat CI, Ward LC, Stuckey BG, et al. Combined thyroxine/liothyronine treatment does not improve well-being, quality of life, or cognitive function compared to thyroxine alone: a randomized controlled trial in patients with primary hypothyroidism. J Clin Endocrinol Metab2003 Oct;88(10):4543-50.

White, R.E., Pickering, A. and Spathis, G.S. (1996). Mood disorder and chronic hypercalcemia. *J Psychosom Res*. 41, 343-347.

Wilhelm SM, Lee J, Prinz RA. Major depression due to primary hyperparathyroidism: a frequent and correctable disorder. Am Surg2004 Feb;70(2):175-9; discussion 9-80.

17

Depressive Disorders and Thyroid Function

A. Verónica Araya[1], Teresa Massardo[2], Jenny Fiedler[3], Luis Risco[4], Juan C. Quintana[5] and Claudio Liberman[1]
[1]*Endocrinology Section, Clinical Hospital of the University of Chile*
[2]*Nuclear Medicine Section, Clinical Hospital of the University of Chile*
[3]*Faculty of Chemical and Pharmaceutical Sciences, University of Chile*
[4]*Psychiatric Clinic of the Clinical Hospital of the University of Chile*
[5]*Department of Radiology, School of Medicine, Pontificia Universidad Católica de Chile*
Chile

1. Introduction

The complex relationship of thyroid hormones (TH) with brain function is known since a century. The TH mediate important effects on central nervous system (CNS) during development and throughout life (Bauer et al., 2002a; Smith et al., 2002). Is well known that hyper and hypothyroidism are frequently associated with subtle behavioral and psychiatric symptoms. By the other side, patients with mood disorders show alterations in thyroid-stimulating hormone (TSH) release under thyrotropin-releasing hormone (TRH) stimulation although, circulating TH: triiodothyronine (T3) and thyroxine (T4) are usually in the normal range (Linkowski et al., 1981; Loosen, 1985; Larsen et al., 2004; Risco et al., 2003). Animal studies have provided considerable data on the reciprocal interactions between TH and neurotransmitter systems related with the pathogenesis of mood disorders (Bauer et al., 2002a). These studies provide the basis for several hypotheses, which propose that the modulatory effects of TH on mood are mediated by their actions on different neurotransmitter as norepinephrine and serotonin (Belmaker&Agam, 1998). There is also experimental evidence that some antidepressant drugs have some effects on brain TH concentration and T3 generation through a modulatory effect on deiodinases. Many trials have demonstrated that under certain conditions the use of TH can enhance or accelerate the therapeutic effects of antidepressants (Kirkegaard & Faber, 1998).

Considering that major depression is currently viewed as a serious public health problem with significant social and economic consequences, we found interesting to review how thyroid function and brain could interact in depressive disorders and how some new aspects as evaluation of some polymorphism of deiodinases and neuroimaging, can help in identifying depressive subjects susceptible to be treat with TH.

2. Thyroid hormones and brain

Thyroid hormones participate in the normal neurological development increasing the rate of neuronal proliferation in the cerebellum, acting as the "time clock" to end neuronal proliferation, differentiation and also stimulating the development of neuronal processes, axons and dendrites. As well TH mediate effects on CNS occur throughout life (Bauer et al., 2002a; Smith et al., 2002). Different studies have demonstrated the presence of thyroid receptors in rat CNS with a particular distribution during development and adulthood (Bradley et al., 1992; Bradley et al., 1989). Thus, TH regulate the expression of genes implicated in myelination, neuronal and glial cell differentiation (Bernal, 2005; Bernal & Nunez, 1995) and neuronal viability and function (Smith et al., 2002). These hormones are able to modify cell morphology by acting on cytoskeleton machinery required for neuronal migration and outgrowth (Aniello et al., 1991; Morte et al., 2010). Additionally, TH are present in noradrenergic nuclei of CNS (Rozanov & Dratman, 1996) probably acting as neuromodulator or co-neurotransmitter (Dratman & Gordon, 1996). In line with this, TH increase β-adrenergic receptors levels (Ghosh & Das, 2007; Whybrow & Prange, 1981) and improve both cholinergic (Smith et al., 2002) and serotonin neurotransmission in animals (Bauer et al., 2002a). The effect of TH on serotonin (5 HT) has been explained by a desensitization of 5HT1A autoreceptor in the raphe nuclei which probably results in enhancement of firing and release of serotonin from raphe neurons (Heal & Smith, 1988). Furthermore, these hormones can stimulate the expression of neuronal growth factor (NGF) suggesting certain trophic actions on CNS (Walker et al., 1979; Walker et al., 1981).

In mice models, maternal hypo and hyperthyroidism cause some malformation and developmental defects in the cerebellar and cerebral cortex of their newborns. Concomitantly, there is some degeneration, deformation and severe growth retardation in neurons of these regions in both groups (El-Bakry et al., 2010). Therefore, TH play an important role in brain development, neuronal migration and axonal projection to target cells. *In vitro* and *in vivo* studies have shown that TH exert a non genomic action over the actin citoskeleton development in astrocytes and neurons. The lack of TH impaire cell growth, granule cells migration and explain those defects in the hypothyroid brain (Farwell et al., 2006; Leonard&Farwell, 1997; Farwell&Dubord, 1996).

Moreover, both acute and chronic Thyroxine treatment in rats increases the cognitive function, probably through an enhancement in cholinergic neurotransmission (Smith et al., 2002).

In humans, TH deficiency during the fetal and postnatal periods may cause irreversible mental retardation, neurological and behavioral deficits, and long lasting, irreversible motor dysfunctions. In adulthood, hypothyroidism may also determine profound behavioral consequences such as depressive symptoms, impaired memory, impairment in learning, verbal fluency, and spatial tasks (Miller et al., 2007; Samuels et al., 2007). Probably these alterations are due to neurotransmission impairment in brain areas related to learning and memory, such as hippocampus. Thus, the reduction of TH levels in CNS, can promote an altered neurotransmission activity contributing to some mood disorders like major depression.

The biologically active thyroid hormone T3 exerts its effects by interacting with their specific nuclear thyroid receptors (TRs) that are positively regulated by its own ligand, acting as transcription factors. TRs are encoded for two different genes: TRβ located on chromosome 3, encodes three isoforms: β1, β2 and β3, and TRα located on chromosome 17, encodes the isoforms α1, α2 and α3. TRα1 is expressed early in the embryonic development and TRβ is expressed at later stages of development. By the other hand, the expression of these isoforms is tissue dependent; in the brain, the main isoforms of TRs are: TRα1, TRα2, TRβ1 and TRβ2. TRα1 and α2 accounting for most of TRs in the organ, whereas TRβ1 and β2 are detected in only a few areas as retina, cochlea, anterior pituitary and hypothalamus. In mice in which TRα or TRβ were inactivated, different phenotypes are observed indicating that TRs isoforms mediate specific functions but also, they can substitute each other to mediate some actions of T3 (Jones et al., 2007; Forrest et al., 1996a; Forrest et al., 1996b; Wikström et al., 1998; Fraichard et al., 1997; Göthe et al., 1999).

Some studies have reported, in propylthiouracyl-induced hypothyroidal adult rats, a decreased expression of TRα1 and TRβ in the hippocampus, associated with an increase in β-amyloid peptides in the same area. Hypoactivity of the thyroid signaling in the hippocampus could induce modifications in the amiloydogenic pathway and this could be related with a greater vulnerability of developing Alzheimer disease in hypothyroidal subjects (Ghenimi et al., 2010).

2.1 T3 generation in the central nervous system: The importance of deiodinases

Although both forms of TH (T4, T3) are present in the circulating blood, some studies have demonstrated that T4 is transported into the brain much more efficiently than T3 (Hagen & Solberg, 1974). In contrast to peripheral tissue, in the brain T4 and T3 are in equimolar range indicating mechanisms for an efficient transformation into biological active hormone.

TH production is regulated by the HPT axis, while its biological activity is mainly regulated by three selenodeiodinasas coded by different genes (D1, D2, D3). Deiodinases act at prereceptor level influencing both, extracellular and intracellular TH levels and its action. Whether it activates or inactivates it, will depend on the level where deiodination occurs (5 or 5` position on the iodothyronine molecule). In the periphery, in the kidney and liver, D1 isoform is responsible for the production of most of the circulating T3 (Bianco et al., 2002).

In the CNS, the most important isoforms are D2 and D3. In the brain, T3 is produced locally by the action of D2 which is also expressed in pituitary, thyroid, brown adipose tissue, skeletal muscle, and aortic smooth muscle cell, in humans. D2 activity varies extensively in different brain regions, with the highest levels found in cortical areas and lesser activity in the midbrain, pons, hypothalamus and brainstem (Bianco et al., 2002; Gouveia et al., 2005; Zavacki et al., 2005). It has been described in adult rats, that approximately 80% of T3 bound to nuclear receptors is produced locally by D2 activity (Crantz et al., 1982). Moreover, inactivation of TH is mainly carried out by D3 as well as glucoronosyltransferase and sulfotransferases. D3 is highly expressed within the CNS, with low peripheral expression. D3 degrades T_4 to rT_3 and T_3 to 3,3'-diiodothyronine (T2) therefore preventing or finishing actions of T3. Thus, combined actions of D2 and D3 can locally increase or decrease thyroid hormone signaling in a tissue -and a temporal- fashion, and more importantly in a way independent of thyroid hormone plasma levels. In addition, increasing evidences pointed out that deiodinase expression can be modulated by a wide variety of endogenous signaling molecules, suggesting a local modulation of T3 production in the brain (Gereben et al., 2008a, Gereben et al., 2008b). D2 enzymatic activity is increased also in hypothyroidism and decreased in hyperthyroidism (Kirkegaard & Faber, 1998).

2.2 Association between deionidase polymorphisms and thyroid hormone metabolism

Genetic variations in deionidade genes may impact significantly thyroid function and TH levels in euthyroid subjects (Hansen et al., 2007; Peeters et al., 2007; Peeters et al., 2006; Peeters et al., 2003). The effect of two polymorphisms in D1 gene, D1-rs11206244 (D1-C785T) and D1-rs12095080 (D1-A1814G) on thyroid hormone metabolism has been evaluated in randomly selected subjects (Peeters et al., 2003). The allele T of D1-rs11206244 was associated with high levels of rT3 and high rT3/T4 ratio and a low T3/rT3 in plasma; whereas the G allele of D1-A1814G was associated with a high T3/rT3 (de Jong et al., 2007; Peeters et al., 2003). These results suggest a lower activity in T carriers of rs11206244 than G carriers (Peeters et al., 2003).

Of special interest is the common polymorphism in humans: D2 rs225014 (D2-Thr92Ala), characterized by a threonine (Thr) change to alanine (Ala) at codon 92 (D2 Thr92Ala). It is associated with insulin resistance in different populations, suggesting that D2-generated T3 in skeletal muscle plays a role in insulin sensitivity (Mentuccia et al., 2002, Canani et al., 2005). The minor allele (G) is associated with a low D2 activity in thyroid samples obtained from patients (Canani et al., 2005). In accordance, G allele seems to predict the need for higher T4 intake in thyroidectomized patients (Torlontano et al., 2008). Nonetheless, it has been observed that GG subjects show a delayed serum T3 rise in response to TRH-mediated TSH secretion consistent with decreased D2 activity (Butler et al., 2010). Some studies have described a naturally occurring polymorphism located in 5'-untranslated region of the D2 gene (Coppotelli et al., 2006). In healthy blood donors, the minor allele of this polymorphism (D2-ORFa-Asp variant, rs12885300) is associated with an increase in circulating T3/T4 ratio but not with plasma T3 and TSH levels, suggesting an increased D2 gene expression (Peeters et al., 2005). In agreement, *in vitro* studies suggested that D2-rs1288530 polymorphism leads to higher activity of D2 at the pituitary level (Coppotelli et al., 2006). In a long case-control Chinese study, the haplotypes ORFa-3Asp-92Ala and ORFa-3Gly-92Ala indicated higher susceptibility for bipolar disorders, while ORFa-3Asp-92Thr probably played a protective role (He et al., 2009). According to this evidence, it is feasible that variants of D2 gene can produce "brain hypothyroidism" limiting T3 action on CNS affecting brain neurotransmission.

3. Thyroid and depression

The similarity and overlapping between symptoms of depression and thyroid disorders has been the theoretical base for the hypothesis regarding a possible relationship between both entities. As we mention above, hypothyroidism could induce cognitive dysfunction and depressive symptoms besides psychological distress in a very similar way to primary depression (Constant et al., 2005; Bould et al., 2011; Mowla et al., 2011). Likewise, TH effect as augmentation therapy in refractory depression, and thyroid disorders as risk factors for rapid-cycling in bipolar disorder sustain a possible association between both types of diseases.

The involvement of HPT axis in the pathogenesis of depression is supported by multiple data. There are few studies that show normal range TH levels during a depressive episode; however most of them demonstrate diverse changes in different hormones associated with this axis. Concerning TSH levels, data are contradictory, some authors have reported a decrease in basal TSH values as well as in those observed in response to exogenous TRH

(Forman-Hoffman & Philibert, 2006; Stipcević et al., 2008) and other studies showed TSH elevation in bipolar depression (Brouwer et al., 2005; Saxena et al., 2000).

In reference to T3 levels, results are more conclusive, showing a trend to decrease in the presence of depression, as well as an association with high risk of long term relapse. In addition there seems to be a more pronounced T3 decrease in direct relation with the severity of depression (Stipcević et al, 2008; Saxena et al., 2000). Reported T4 levels in depression are also contradictory, since there is evidence showing a rise as well as a decrease of T4 during depressive episodes. (Saxena et al., 2000; Kirkegaard&Faber, 1998). In a study, with more than 6,000 subjects, it was shown that a low TSH and a high T4 levels were associated with depression specially in young men but, in women only a higher T4 levels correlated with current depression syndrome (Forman-Hoffman&Philibert, 2006). It is possible that these findings could be explained by a diversity of factors, such as differences in phenotypes of depressive patients, severity and duration of the disease, difficulties in isolating drugs effects in TH levels (antidepressants and mood stabilizers) and probably, gender and other differences.

Overt thyroid disease is infrequent among depressive patients. Nevertheless, many authors have seen that a subgroup of depressive patients manifest a subclinical hypothyroidism and this might be a negative prognostic factor (Fountoulakis et al., 2006). On the other side, some antidepressants as lithium inhibits TH secretion and could increase antithyroid antibodies, promoting hypothyroidism in susceptible subjects (Emerson et al., 1972; Myers et al., 1985).

There is still no hypothesis that can satisfactory integrate these data. Interactions between TH and neurotransmitters, gene expression and neurohormonal receptors are not clear yet. For instance, 5 HT seems to inhibit TRH secretion and somatostatin TSH secretion (Kirkegaard&Faber, 1998); both of them are reduced in cerebro spinal fluid (CSF) in patients with psychiatric illness and affective disorders (Gerner&Yamada, 1982, Roy-Birne et al., 1983; Rubinow et al., 1983). Otherwise, T3 influx to intracellular level in the brain is determined by many factors, including T3 and T4 circulating levels, protein transporters, and deiodinase activity.

About a 25% of major depressed patients show a reduction in TSH release under TRH stimulation (Loosen 1985, Risco et al, 2003). It has been proposed that in them exist a blunted response due to the raise of circulating cortisol, associated to hypothalamic-pituitary-adrenal axis hyperactivity. This response has also been observed in bipolar disorders (Linkowsky et al., 1981). On the other hand, in rapid cycling depressives, TSH hypersecretion is observed in response to TRH (20% of basal TSH levels above the normal range) (Szabadi, 1991, Larsen et al., 2004).

Nevertheless, as we mentioned before, the mechanism by which TH affect the adult brain is not completely clear, because the complex interactions between neurotransmitters and thyroid. One hypothesis is that TH modulate the number of post-synaptic β-adrenergic receptors in the cerebral cortex and cerebellum This could be relevant considering the influence of catecholamines deficit, mainly norepinephrine as a cause of depression (Atterwill et al., 1984). Another possible mechanism is the modulation of 5 HT and its receptors. It has been suggested that TH inhibit the impulse rate of neurons present at the raphe and reducing the release of 5HT. T3 administration to mice attenuates the function of 5HT1A and 5HT1B receptors, increasing the cortical and hippocampus synthesis and turnover of 5-HT. Administration of T3 plus electroconvulsive shock markedly potentiated its actions on 5-HT2-mediated responses. (Heal&Smith, 1988). These findings provide evidences for possible antidepressant effects of T3 and/or potentiating therapy by TH. This issue is relevant in patients suffering depressive disorders, related with reduction in mono amine neurotransmission such as serotonin (reviewed in Belmaker&Agam 2008).

A positive correlation between serotonin levels and circulating T3 has been described in humans. Indirect evidences showed that brain serotonin is increased in hyperthyroidism and decreased in hypothyroidism (Singhal et al., 1975). In the last situation, this is reversed with TH replacement (Bauer et al., 2002b, Strawn et al., 2004). In depressed subjects, the decrease in serotoninergic tone could be related to lower brain T3 levels, perhaps due to a reduction of deiodinases activity. Furthermore, an imbalance in T3 conversion could account for depressive disorder and/or clinical outcome to antidepressants therapy. It has been suggested that in depression, T3 may favor the release of cortical 5-HT and thus synergize the response to antidepressants. Administration of desipramine a selective serotonergic reuptake inhibitor (SSRI) in rats, induces an increase of D2 activity and T3 concentration in cortical tissue. Interestingly, T4 concentrations were significantly lowered after administration of the antidepressant but, serum T3 levels were significantly reduced only after toxic dosis of desipramine. Other commonly used SSRI, fluoxetine also decreases D3 activity (Eravci et al., 2000). Based on these data, one might suggest that depression occurs by the inhibition of D2, determining decreased T3 levels and secondarily, reduced levels of brain 5HT.

The efficacy of T3 as a supplement of sertraline therapy, another SSRI, was studied recently in relation D1 polymorphism (Cooper-Kazaz et al., 2009). Patients carrying the T allele of D1-rs11206244 showed a significant response to 8 week of antidepressant treatment in comparison with non-carriers of the allele. Additionally, there was no effect of T allele on sertraline response, suggesting that the polymorphism is not associated to antidepressant effect (Cooper-Kazaz et al., 2009). As we mentioned, the T allele of D1-rs11206244 showed lower T3 and higher rT3 than non-T carriers (de Jong et al., 2007; Peeters et al., 2003). Thus, it seems that patients genetically characterized by poor conversion of T4 to T3, are better responders to T3-antidepressant co-treatment (Cooper-Kazaz et al., 2007; 2008). Another study evaluated whether baseline thyroid function and D2 rs225014 (D2-Thr92Ala) predict response to paroxetine. It showed that high TSH levels predict the response, and heterozygous patients showed lower TSH levels than the wild-type allele (A) (Brouwer et al., 2006). However, up to date there is no study evaluating the influence of T3 and D2 polymorphisms on antidepressant response.

Based on these observations, we evaluated the presence of D2 polymorphism related with a lower activity of the enzyme: D2-Thr92Ala (T/C). The polymorphism was analyzed in 61 euthyroid patients with depression and 48 subjects of a population sample using the PCR-RFLP method. Clinical response to fluoxetine was evaluated before and after 8 weeks of treatment, using Hamilton Scale for Depression (HAM-D). We found that the CC genotype of Thr92Ala polymorphism was more frequent in depressed subjects and in non-responders patients (unpublished data). We concluded that Thr92Ala polymorphism of D2 gene could be considered a predictive marker of clinical response to fluoxetine, and hence of pharmacological therapy, but more studies are needed to confirm this preliminary results.

The presence of these polymorphisms could influence basal activity of type 2 deiodinase, and therefore of T3 bioavailability in the brain.

4. Use of thyroid hormone in depression

Several studies using thyroid hormones in the management of patients with mood disorders have been reported since the early seventies. TH have been used in euthyroid depressed patients to enhance the effects of antidepressants. In patients receiving electroconvulsive therapy, those treated with T3 required less sessions and presented less memory loss compared with placebo treated group (Stern et al., 1991). T3 has been employed in initial combination therapy, and T3 or T4 in refractary depression or non responder patients.

T3 in doses of 20 to 50 μg is able to enhance the effect of tricyclic antidepressants and shorten the depression period but, many studies have not demonstrated differences in the number of patients recovered (Prange et al., 1969; Wilson et al., 1970; Coppen et al., 1972; Wheatley, 1972). A meta-analysis showed that when T3 was used in refractary depression in addition to tricyclic antidepressant therapy, patients treated with it were twice as likely to respond as controls, decreasing depression severity scores (Aronson et al., 1996). However, samples size were small and deserve more evidence. Other studies, using T3 augmentation to SSRI-resistant depression, observed an improvement in mood scores (Agid&Lerer, 2003, Iosifescu et al., 2005, Abraham et al., 2006). Some authors found that patients who responded to T3 had higher serum TSH levels than non-responders and T3 appears to be less effective in men than in women (Agid&Lerer, 2003). Other authors reported that patients with atypical depression experienced significantly greater clinical improvement in final HAM-D with higher rates of treatment response and remission compared to subjects with non-atypical major depressive disorder (Iosifescu et al., 2005). All those cases were treated mainly with fluoxetine in a daily dose of 20 to 40 mg/ and 25-50 μg of T3, with few side effects.

L-thyroxine (T4) added to antidepressants has been used less frequently than T3. Some authors have suggested that T4 augmentation is less effective than T3 (Joffe&Singer, 1990) and that supra physiological doses (250-600 ug/day) are needed, as has been demonstrated in patients with resistant major depression or refractary uni and bipolar disorders (Baumgartner et al., 1994, Bauer et al., 1998, 2002). These results support the theory of a reduced deiodination of T4 compatible with an inhibition of the D2 or a stimulation of the D3 in brain tissues resulting in reduced local T3 concentration.

Nevertheless, the addition of T4 (100 ug /day during 4 weeks) to serotoninergic antidepressants obtained remission in 11 of 12 female patients with a resistant depressive episode but, these results did not show association with T3, T4 or TSH levels (Łojko & Rybakowski, 2007).

To date, the use of TH in mood disorders is controversial and the rationale for this therapy is still not completely clear. Main limitations of the studies are: small number of cases, lack of a placebo group, heterogeneity in diagnosis criteria, differences in observational period and in antidepressant therapy. For example, lithium has a known inhibitory effect on TH secretion; fluoxetine has a stimulatory effect over D2 as well as desipramine and both of them could induce deficit of T4.

In this line, we evaluated a group of euthyroidal adult female patients with major depression according to DSM IV-R criteria. All of them were free of antidepressants for at least for 6 month. We studied the effect of adding T3 in a dose of 50 ug per day (n=11) or placebo (n=10), to the standard antidepressant therapy with fluoxetine during 8 weeks. At the end of the observational period final HAM-D scores were similar in both groups. (See **Table 1**). Patients in T3 group showed significant T4, T3 and TSH changes; but they remain clinically euthyroid during the whole treatment period. Their body mass index , heart rate and other clinical parameters did not change. The placebo group showed a non significant increase of THS at the end of the observation time (See **Figure 1**, unpublished results).

	T3 Group		Placebo		p	
Age (y.o.)	40±12		36±10		ns	
	Initial	2m	Initial	2m	Initial vs 2m	Groups
HAM-D	24±4	8±4	26±6	7±4	<0.0001	ns

Table 1. Age and Hamilton score (HAM-D) with 21 items, in the groups with T3 addition or placebo. Both initial and 2 months means±SD were similar (using non paired t student test). The difference between initial and 2 month was highly significant in both groups (using paired t tests).

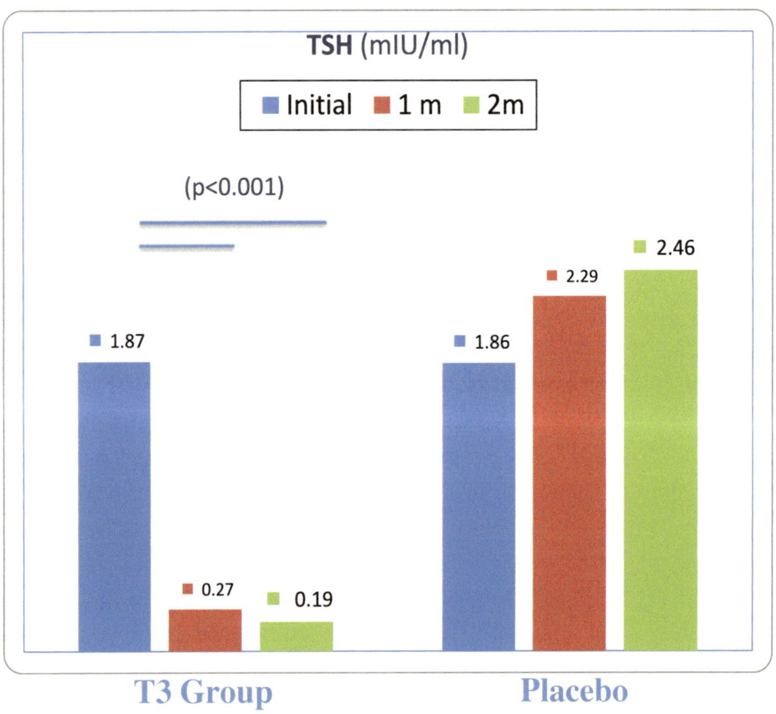

Fig. 1. TSH changes after addition of T3 or placebo in both groups. Measurements of TSH are shown at baseline, 1 month and 2 months using similar SSRI therapy. T3 hormone induced significant decreased TSH levels. No significant change was observed in placebo group.

Summarizing, our results suggest that TH addition to SSRI therapy in euthyroid depressed patients is safe and has not deleterious clinical effects in spite of TSH changes during treatment. Although, we could not demonstrated in this particular group, a significant antidepressant effect.

5. Hypothyroidism, depression and brain imaging

Single-photon tomography (SPECT), positron emission tomography (PET) and functional magnetic resonance imaging (fMRI) are able to capture physiological events linked to underlying neuronal activity. They have been employed to image and quantify brain perfusion, flow and metabolism in several conditions as well as the radionuclide techniques have been used to map neurotransmissors, receptors, drug actions and many metabolic pathways. Functional imaging in mood disorders may show abnormalities at different brain levels that could normalize with therapy. Several serotonin and adrenergic markers have also been employed to study negative emotional stimuli response in mood disorders. For instance: thalamic activity was increased by reboxetine, whereas citalopram primarily affected ventrolateral prefrontal regions. It would be interesting to have a method able to predict therapy responses to either noradrenergic or serotoninergic antidepressants (Carey et al., 2004; Navarro et al., 2004; Zobel et al., 2005; Kohn et al., 2007; MacQueen, 2009; Brühl et al., 2011).

It is also known that even mild hypothyroidism may produce changes in brain regions modulating attention, motor speed, memory and visual-spatial processing. In severe hypothyroidism induced by thyroidectomy in cancer patients, it have been reported a clear parietal and partial occipital lobe hypoperfusion, measured with SPECT; the abnormalities improved after reaching normal thyroid function, in some subjects. However, fluorodeoxyglucose (FDG) and oxygen-15-labeled water studies, in similar patients, showed lower global brain glucose metabolism and flow. Hypothyroidal patients were also significantly more depressed, anxious and psychomotor slowered than euthyroidal subjects (Nagamachi et al., 2004; Constant et al., 2001).

Brain metabolism and flow are usually decreased in major depression and bipolar disease being metabolism inversely associated with the severity of depression. Changes are variable and as we mentioned earlier, could reverse with adequate therapy. Subgenual prefrontal cortex presents abnormal blood flow and metabolism in the depressed state. Prefrontal cortex and limbic structures are involved in emotion regulation and amygdale is involved in emotional memory formation (Buchsbaum et al., 1997; Kennedy et al., 2007; Chen et al., 2011). In major depression patients, glucose metabolism in orbitofrontal and inferior frontal cortex correlates with therapy response; responders have a significant decrease in the orbitofrontal and ventrolateral regions compared with non-responders, implicating ventral prefrontal subcortical circuits in response to specific therapy with SSRI. In major depression and bipolar patients, FDG has shown an inverse correlation between brain metabolism and circulating TSH (Brody et al., 1999; Marangell et al., 1997; Milak et al., 2005).

Cerebral fMRI has been reported to be helpful in major depression intending to predict therapy response using brain activation. Morphometric studies have evaluated hippocampus volume association with response to treatment. Patients who remit have larger pretreatment hippocampus volumes bilaterally compared with those who do not remit. There are similar preliminary findings for the anterior cingulate cortex. A recent work demonstrated a significantly thinner posterior cingulate cortex in non-remitters than in remitters, and also significant decrease in perfusion in frontal lobes and anterior cingulate cortex in non-remitters compared with healthy controls, at baseline (MacQueen, 2009; Järnum et al., 2011).

There are reports with increased perfusion in anterior cingulate and prefrontal medial cortex when using SSRI or amesergide. Responders and non-responders to cognitive behavior therapy versus antidepressive pharmacotherapy and deep brain stimulation could also be differentiated using brain perfusion SPECT or glucose metabolism with PET (Vlassenko et al., 2004; Kennedy et al., 2007; Richieri et al., 2011).

Another work with fMRI demonstrated also that successful paroxetine treatment decreases amygdala activation, presumably by improved frontolimbic control, in line with SSRI, induced increased functional connectivity between pregenual anterior cingulated cortex, prefrontal cortex, and amygdala. Changes in amygdala activation when processing negative faces expressions might serve as an indicator for improved frontolimbic control required for clinical response (Ruhé, 2011).

We recently studied a group of major depression middle age patients using brain perfusion SPECT, all in their first episode of major depression and /or without any specific therapy for at least six months. Their initial HAM-D scores corresponded to 24±4.8; all of them received standard SSRI therapy. Ninety-three percent were responders at 2 months (HAM-D decrease >50%) and 59% were remitters (HAM-D score ≤5). There was association of decreased perfusion in diverse brain areas with HAM-D changes in the whole group using Statistical Parametric Analysis (SPM) as covariate (See Figure 2). We did not observe significant neocortical perfusion change after 2 months of standard dose of fluoxetine therapy. However, there was a bilateral decrease in parahippocampal gyrus, thalamus and striatum as well as in anterior cingulate gyrus (Brodmann 32 area) after SSRI therapy. No significant difference was observed between remitters and non-remitters.

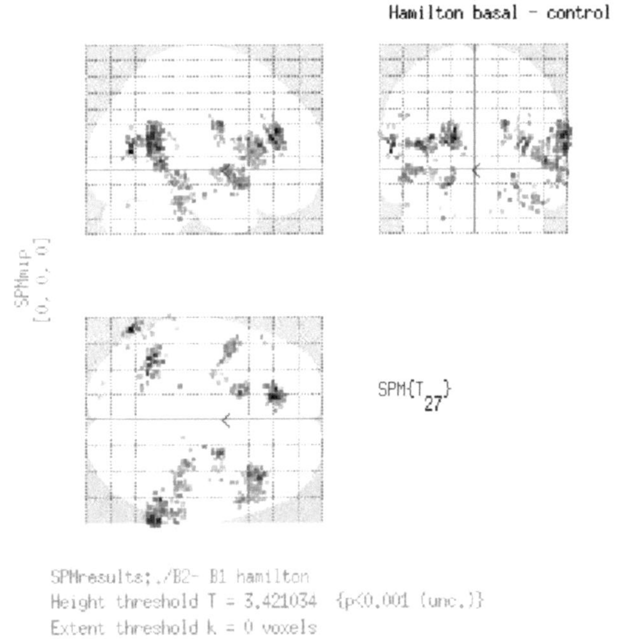

Fig. 2. In the whole group, SPM8 analysis demonstrated association between decreased perfusion and HAM-D scores considered as a covariate, at baseline and after 2 months of therapy (non corrected p <0.001): -at left: in amygdala, anterior cingulate, globus pallidum, putamen and Brodmann area 9 (mid frontal gyrus) -bilaterally: both hyppocampal gyrus, mid and superior temporal and insulas and cerebellar hemispheres -at right: in central and supramarginal gyrus

As we mentioned before, a half of the women in our group received T3 in addition of SSRI and the other half a placebo instead of T3. Our results showed no evidence that adding T3 to SSRI therapy in unipolar major depression females produces significant change in regional cerebral blood flow at neocortical level (See Figure 3). Only a small difference was found at deep structure level that could imply diverse brain mechanism involved [data not published].

These findings are in agreement with other reports showing relative normalization of perfusion and metabolism that were abnormally increased at baseline in patients with mood disorders. Some of these regional metabolism changes are correlated with emotional behavior. The amygdala and limbic structures have been associated with face recognition and emotional processing. It is well known that there is increased perfusion and metabolism in specific brain areas, reflecting molecular abnormalities in neurotransmitter systems. The development of new molecular imaging methods could help in the individualization of antidepressant therapies (Chen et al., 2011).

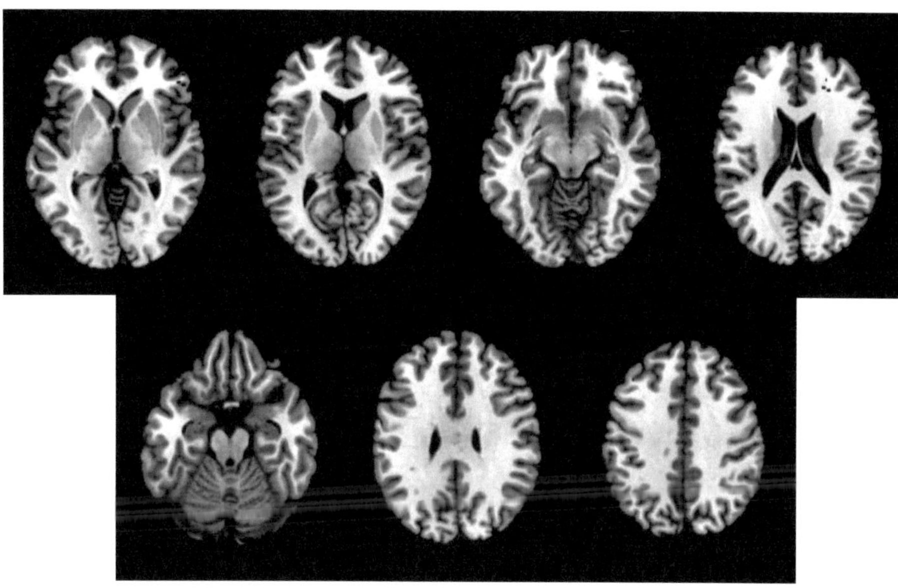

Fig. 3. Absence of regional cerebral blood flow change after SSRI therapy in T3 group, using Statistical Parametric Analysis (SPM8) with significant level <0.001; uncorrected p value.

6. Conclusions

Depressive and thyroid disorders are important public health problems. There is strong experimental evidence showing thyroid involvement on early stages of CNS development and on metabolic function of the mature brain. It is also accepted that overt hyper or hypothyroidism are not found frequently among mood disorders patients except in those with bipolar disorders, indicating that in most cases the underlying abnormality is at cellular or molecular levels. Although there is a prolific literature on the relationship between thyroid function and depressive disorders, clear results in humans on the role of TH in antidepressant therapy are still lacking. There are no randomized controlled trials, and the number of patients included in existing studies is too small. On the other hand, more research is needed in order to define the importance of genetic variants in deiodinases and the role of neuroimaging into the complex interactions between HPT function and mood disorders and in clinical response to treatments.

Therefore, considering the available evidence and our own experience, we can recommend this strategy only as an alternative treatment in major depression patients who have failed to respond to other measures.

7. Acknowledgments

The work described in this chapter was partially financed by the grant "Líneas de Investigación Prioritarias" #240/07 HCUCH from the Clinical Hospital of the University of Chile, Santiago, Chile.

The authors thank Dr. Rodrigo Jaimovich (Department of Radiology, School of Medicine, Pontificia Universidad Católica de Chile) who processed and analyzed all SPECT data; Dr. Tamara Galleguillos (Psychiatric Clinic of the Clinical Hospital of the University of Chile) by her collaboration in patient´s recruitment, selection and follow up; Mr. Egardo Caamaño for his technical laboratory support and Ms. Clara Menares who performed the molecular biology studies.

8. References

Abraham, G.; Milev, R. & Stuart Lawson, J. (2006). T3 augmentation of SSRI resistant depression. *Journal of Affective Disorders*, Vol.91, No.2-3 (April 2006), pp. 211–215.

Agid, O. & Lerer, B. (2003). Algorithm-based treatment of major depression in an outpatient clinic: clinical correlates of response to a specific serotonin reuptake inhibitor and to triiodothyronine augmentation. *International Journal of Neuropsychopharmacology*, Vol.6, No.1 (March 2003), pp.41-49.

Altshuler, L.L.; Bauer, M.; Frye, M.A.; Gitlin, M.J.; Mintz, J., Szuba, M.P., Leight, K.L. & Whybrow, P.C. (2001). Does thyroid supplementation accelerate tricyclic antidepressant response? A review and meta-analysis of the literature. *American Journal of Psychiatry*, Vol.158, No.10 (October 2001), pp. 1617-1622.

Aniello, F.; Couchie, D.; Bridoux, A.M.; Gripois, D. & Nunez, J. (1991). Splicing of juvenile and adult tau mRNA variants is regulated by thyroid hormone. *Proceedings of National Academic of Sciences*, Vol. 88, No.9 (May 1991), pp. 4035-4039.

Aronson, R.; Offman, HJ.; Joffe, RT. & Naylor, CD. (1996). Triiodothyronine augmentation in the treatment of refractory depression. A meta-analysis. *Archives General of Psychiatry*, Vol. 53, No.9 (September 1996), pp. 842-848.

Atterwill, C.K, Bunn S.J., Atkinson, D.J., Smith, S.L., Heal. D.J. Effects of thyroid status on presynaptic alpha 2-adrenoceptor function and beta-adrenoceptor binding in the rat brain. *Journal of Neural Transmission*, Vol. 59, N°1, (1984), pp.43-55.

Bauer, M., Heinz, A., Whybrow, P.C. (2002a). Thyroid hormones, serotonin and mood: of synergy and significance in the adult brain. *Molecular Psychiatry*, Vol.7, N° 2,(2002a) pp.140-156.

Bauer, M.; Berghöfer, A.; Bschor, T.; Baumgartner, A.; Kiesslinger, U.; Hellweg, R.; Adli, M.; Baethge, C. & Müller-Oerlinghausen, B. (2002b). Supraphysiological doses of L-

Thyroxine in the maintenance treatment of prophylaxis-resistant affective disorders. *Neuropsychopharmacology*, Vol.27, No.4 (October 2002), pp. 620–628.

Bauer, M.; Hellweg, R.; Gräf, KJ. & Baumgartner, A. (1998). Treatment of refractory depression with high-dose thyroxine. *Neuropsychopharmacology*, Vol.18, No.6 (June 1998), pp. 444-455.

Baumgartner, A.; Bauer, M. & Hellweg, R. (1994). Treatment of intractable non-rapid cycling bipolar affective disorder with high-dose thyroxine: An open trial. *Neuropsychopharmacology*, Vol.10, No.3 (May 1994), pp. 183–189.

Belmaker, RH. & Agam, G. (2008). Mechanisms of Disease: Major Depressive Disorder. *New England Journal of Medicine*, Vol.358, No.1 (January 2008), pp. 55-68.

Bernal, J. & Nunez, J. (1995). Thyroid hormones and brain development. *European Journal of Endocrinology*, Vol.133, No.4 (October 1995), pp. 390-398.

Bernal, J. (2005). Thyroid hormones and brain development. *Vitamines and Hormones*, Vol. 71, pp. 95-122.

Bianco, A.C.; Salvatore, D.; Gereben, B.; Berry, M.J. & Larsen, P.R. (2002). Biochemistry, cellular and molecular biology, and physiological roles of the iodothyronine selenodeiodinases. *Endocrine Reviews*, Vol.23, No. 1 (February 2002), pp. 38-89.

Bould, H., Panicker, V., Kessler, D., Durant, C., Lewis, G., Dayan, C., Evans, J. (2011). Investigation of thyroid dysfunction in general practice is more likely in patients with high psychological morbidity. *Family Practice* (September 2011) [Epub ahead of print]

Bradley, D.J.; Towle, H.C. & Young, W.S., 3rd. (1992). Spatial and temporal expression of alpha- and beta-thyroid hormone receptor mRNAs, including the beta 2-subtype, in the developing mammalian nervous system. *Journal of Neurosciences*, Vol.12, No.6 (June 1992), pp. 2288-2302.

Bradley, D.J.; Young, W.S. 3rd & Weinberger, C. (1989). Differential expression of alpha and beta thyroid hormone receptor genes in rat brain and pituitary. *Proceedings of National Academy of Sciences U S A*, Vol.86, No.18 (September 1989), pp. 7250-7254.

Breteler, M.M., (2007). The association of polymorphisms in the type 1 and 2 deiodinase genes with circulating thyroid hormone parameters and atrophy of the medial temporal lobe. *Journal of Clinical Endocrinology and Metabolism*, Vol.92, N°2, (February 2007), pp.636-640.

Brody, A.L., Saxena,S., Silverman, D.H., Alborzian, S., Fairbanks, L.A., Phelps, M.E., Huang, S.C., Wu, H.M., Maidment, K., Baxter, L.R. Jr. (1999). Brain metabolic changes in major depressive disorder from pre- to post-treatment with paroxetine. *Psychiatry Research*, (October 1999), Vol 91, N°.3 91, pp.127-139.

Brouwer, J.P., Appelhof, B.C., Hoogendijk, W.J., Huyser, J., Endert, E., Zuketto, C., Schene, A.H., Tijssen. J.G., Van Dyck, R., Wiersinga, W.M., Fliers, E. Thyroid and adrenal axis in major depression: a controlled study in outpatients. *European Journal of Endocrinology*, Vol.152, N°2, (February 2005) pp.185-191.

Brouwer, J.P.; Appelhof, B.C.; Peeters, R.P.; Hoogendijk, W.J.; Huyser, J.; Schene, A.H.; Tijssen, J.G.; Van Dyck, R.; Visser, T.J.; Wiersinga, W.M. & Fliers, E. (2006). Thyrotropin, but not a polymorphism in type II deiodinase, predicts response to paroxetine in major depression. *European Journal of Endocrinology*, Vol.154, No.6 (June 2006), pp. 819-825.

Brühl, A.B., Jäncke, L., Herwig, U. (2011). Differential modulation of emotion processing brain regions by noradrenergic and serotonergic antidepressants. *Psychopharmacology (Berlin)*, (August 2011), Vol. 216. N°3, pp.389-399.

Buchsbaum, M.S., Wu, J., Siegel, B.V., Hackett, E., Trenary, M., Abel, L., Reynolds, C. (1997). Effect of sertraline on regional metabolic rate in patients with affective disorder. *Biological Psychiatry*, Vol. 41, N°1. (January 1997), pp.15-22.

Butler, P.W.; Smith, S.M.; Linderman, J.D.; Brychta, R.J.; Alberobello, A.T.; Dubaz, O.M.; Luzon, J.A.; Skarulis, M.C.; Cochran, C.S.; Wesley, R.A.; Pucino, F. & Celi, F.S. (2010). The Thr92Ala 5' type 2 deiodinase gene polymorphism is associated with a delayed triiodothyronine secretion in response to the thyrotropin-releasing hormone-stimulation test: a pharmacogenomic study. *Thyroid,* Vol.20, No.12 (December 2010), pp. 1407-1412.

Campos-Barros, A., Meinhold, H., Kohler, R., Muller, F., Eravci, M., Baumgartner, A., (1995). The effects of desipramine on thyroid hormone concentrations in rat brain. *Naunyn Schmiedebergs Archives of Pharmacology,* Vol.351, N°5, (May 1995), pp.469-474.

Canani, L.H., Capp, C., Dora, J.M., Meyer, E.L., Wagner, M.S., Harney, J.W., Larsen, P.R., Gross, J.L., Bianco, A.C., Maia, A.L., (2005). The type 2 deiodinase A/G (Thr92Ala) polymorphism is associated with decreased enzyme velocity and increased insulin resistance in patients with type 2 diabetes mellitus. *Journal of Clinical Endocrinology and Metabolism,* Vol.90, N°6, (June 2005). pp.3472-3478.

Carey, P.D., Warwick, J., Niehaus, D.J., van der Linden, G., van Heerden, B.B., Harvey, B.H., Seedat, S., Stein, D.J. (2004). Single photon emission computed tomography (SPECT) of anxiety disorders before and after treatment with citalopram. *BMC Psychiatry,* (October 2004) 14;4:30.

Chen, Q., Liu, W., Li, H., Zhang, H., Tian, M. (2011). Molecular imaging in patients with mood disorders: a review of PET findings. *European Journal of Nuclear Medicine and Molecular Imaging,* Vol. 38, N°7, (July 2011), pp. 1367-1380

Constant, E.L., Adam, S., Seron, X., Bruyer, R., Seghers, A., Daumerie, C. (2005). Anxiety and depression, attention, and executive functions in hypothyroidism, *Journal of the International Neuropsychological Society,* (2005), Vol.11, N°5, (September 2005), pp.535–544.

Constant, E.L., de Volder, A.G., Ivanoiu, A., Bol, A., Labar, D., Seghers, A., Cosnard, G., Melin, J., Daumerie, C. (2001). Cerebral blood flow and glucose metabolism in hypothyroidism: a positron emission tomography study. *Journal of Clinical Endocrinology and Metabolism,* Vol 86, N° 8, (August 2001), pp.3864-3870.

Cooper-Kazaz, R., Apter, J.T., Cohen, R., Karagichev, L., Muhammed-Moussa, S., Grupper, D., Drori, T., Newman, M.E., Sackeim, H.A., Glaser, B., Lerer, B.(2007). Combined treatment with sertraline and liothyronine in major depression: a randomized, double-blind, placebo-controlled trial. *Archives of General Psychiatry,* Vol.64, N°6, (June 2007), pp. 679-688.

Cooper-Kazaz, R., van der Deure, W.M., Medici, M., Visser, T.J., Alkelai, A., Glaser, B., Peeters, R.P., Lerer, B. (2009). Preliminary evidence that a functional polymorphism in type 1 deiodinase is associated with enhanced potentiation of the antidepressant effect of sertraline by triiodothyronine. *Journal of Affective Disorders,* (July 2009), Vol.116, N°1-2, pp.113-116.

Cooper-Kazaz, R.Lerer, B. (2008). Efficacy and safety of triiodothyronine supplementation in patients with major depressive disorder treated with specific serotonin reuptake inhibitors. *International Journal of Neuropsychopharmacology,* Vol.11, N°5, (August 2008), pp. 685-699.

Coppen, A.; Whyborw, PC.; Noguera, R.; Maggs, R. & Prange, Jr AJ. (1972). The comparative antidepressant value of L-tryptophan and imipramine with and without attempted potentiation by liothyronine. *Archives of General Psychiatry*, Vol. 26, No.3 (March 1972), pp. 234-241.

Coppotelli, G., Summers, A., Chidakel, A., Ross, J.M., Celi, F.S. (2006). Functional characterization of the 258 A/G (D2-ORFa-Gly3Asp) human type-2 deiodinase polymorphism: a naturally occurring variant increases the enzymatic activity by removing a putative repressor site in the 5' UTR of the gene. *Thyroid*, (July 2006),Vol.16, N°7, pp. 625-632.

Crantz, F.R., Silva, J.E., Larsen, P.R. (1982). An analysis of the sources and quantity of 3,5,3'-triiodothyronine specifically bound to nuclear receptors in rat cerebral cortex and cerebellum. *Endocrinology*, Vol.110, N°2, (February 1982) pp.367-375.

de Jong, F.J., Peeters, R.P., den Heijer, T., van der Deure, W.M., Hofman, A., Uitterlinden, A.G., Visser, T.J., T.J. & Breteler M.M. (2007). The association of polimorphisms in the type 1 and 2 deidinase genes with circulating thyroid hormone parameters and atrophy of the medial temporal lobe. *Journal of Clinical Endocrinology and Metabolism*, Vol.92,No 2 (February 2007), pp. 636-640.

Dratman, M.B. & Gordon, J.T. (1996). Thyroid hormones as neurotransmitters. *Thyroid*, Vol.6; N°6 (December 1996) pp.639-647.

Dussault, JH. & Ruel, J. (1987). Thyroid hormones and brain development. *Annual Review of Physiology*, Vol.49, No. 3 (March 1987), pp. 321-334.

El-Bakry, A.M., El-Gareib, A.W., Ahmed, R.G. (2010). Comparative study of the effects of experimentally induced hypothyroidism and hyperthyroidism in some brain regions in albino rats. *Journal of Developmental Neuroscience*, Vol.28, No.5 (August 2010), pp. 371-389.

Emerson, CH.; Dyson, WL. & Utiger, RD. (1973). Serum thyrotropin and thyroxine concentrations in patients receiving lithium carbonate. *Journal of Clinical Endocrinology and Metabolism*, Vol. 36, No.2 (February 1972), pp. 338-346.

Eravci, M., Pinna, G., Meinhold, H., Baumgartner, A. (2000). Effects of pharmacological and nonpharmacological treatments on thyroid hormone metabolism and concentrations in rat brain. *Endocrinology*, Vol.141, N° 3, (March 2000) pp.1027-1040.

Farwell, A.P., Dubord, S.A. (1996) Thyroid hormone regulates neurite outgrowth and neuronal migration onto laminin. *Thyroid*, Vol.6, (Suppl 1) (1996) pp.S-6

Farwell, AP.; Dubord-Tomasetti, SA.; Pietrzykowski, AZ. & Leonard, JL. (2006). Dynamic nongenomic actions of thyroid hormone in the developing rat brain. *Endocrinology*, Vol.147, No.5 (May 2006), pp. 2567-2574.

Forman-Hoffman, V., Philibert, R.A. (2006). Lower TSH and higher T4 levels are associated with current depressive syndrome in young adults. *Acta Psychiatrica Scandinava*, Vol. 114, N°2, (August 2006) pp.132-139

Forrest, D.; Erway, LC.; Ng, L.; Altschuler, R. & Curran, T. (1996a). Thyroid hormone receptor beta is essential for development of auditory function. *Nature Genetics*, Vol.13, No.3 (July 1996), pp. 354-357.

Forrest, D.; Hanebuth, E.; Smeyne, RJ.; Everds, N.; Stewart, CL.; Wehner, JM. & Curran, T. (1996b). Recessive resistance to thyroid hormone in mice lacking thyroid hormone receptor beta: evidence for tissue-specific modulation of receptor function. *The EMBO Journal*, Vol.15, No.12 (June 1996), pp. 3006-3015.

Fountoulakis, K., Kantartzis, S., Siamouli, M., Panagiotidis, P., Kaprinis, S., Iacovides, A., Kaprinis, G. (2006). Peripheral thyroid dysfunction in depression. *The World Journal of Biological Psychiatry*, Vol.7, N°3, (2006), pp.131-137.

Fraichard, A.; Chassande, O.; Plateroti, M. Roux, JP.; Trouillas, J.; Dehay, C.; Legrand, C.; Gauthier, K.; Kedinger, M.; Malaval, L.; Rousset, B. & Samarut, J. (1997). The T3R alpha gene encoding a thyroid hormone receptor is essential for post-natal development and thyroid hormone production. *The EMBO Journal*, Vol.16, No.14 (July 1997), pp. 4412–4420.

Gereben, B., Zavacki, A.M., Ribich, S., Kim, B.W., Huang, S.A., Simonides, W.S., Zeold, A., Bianco, A.C., (2008a). Cellular and molecular basis of deiodinase-regulated thyroid hormone signaling. *Endocrinology Review* Vol.29, N° 7, (December 2008) pp. 898-938.

Gereben B, Zeöld A, Dentice M, Salvatore D, Bianco AC. (2008b). Activation and inactivation of thyroid hormone by deiodinases: local action with general consequences. *Cellular and Molecular Life Sciences*, Vol. 65, N°4, (February 2008), pp.570-590.

Gerner, RH. & Yamada, T. (1982). Altered neuropeptide concentrations in cerebrospinal fluid of psychiatric patients. *Brain Research*, Vol.238, No.1 (April 1982), pp. 298–302.

Ghenimi, N.; Alfos, S.; Redonnet, A.; Higueret, P.; Pallet, V. & Enderlin, V. (2010). Adult-onset hypothyroidism induces the amyloidogenic pathway of amyloid precursor protein processing in the rat hippocampus. *Journal of Neuroendocrinology*, Vol.22, No.8 (August 2010), pp. 951–959.

Ghosh, M. , Das, S. (2007). Increased beta(2)-adrenergic receptor activity by thyroid hormone possibly leads to differentiation and maturation of astrocytes in culture. *Cellular and Molecular Neurobiology*, Vol.27, N°8, (December 2007), pp.1007-1021.

Göthe, S.; Wang, Z.; Ng, L.; Kindblom, JM.; Barros, AC.; Ohlsson, C.; Vennström, B. & Forrest, D. (1999). Mice devoid of all known thyroid hormone receptors are viable but exhibit disorders of the pituitary-thyroid axis, growth, and bone maturation. *Genes & Development* , Vol.13, No.10 (May 1999), pp. 1329–1341.

Gouveia, C.H., Christoffolete, M.A., Zaitune, C.R., Dora, J.M., Harney, J.W., Maia, A.L., Bianco, A.C. (2005). Type 2 iodothyronine selenodeiodinase is expressed throughout the mouse skeleton and in the MC3T3-E1 mouse osteoblastic cell line during differentiation. *Endocrinology*, Vol.146, N°.1, (January 2005), pp. 195-200.

Hagen, G.A.Solberg, L.A., Jr. (1974). Brain and cerebrospinal fluid permeability to intravenous thyroid hormones. *Endocrinology*, Vol. 95, N°.5, (November 1974), pp.1398-1410.

Hansen, P.S., van der Deure, W.M., Peeters, R.P., Iachine, I., Fenger, M., Sorensen, T.I., Kyvik, K.O., Visser, T.J., Hegedus, L. (2007). The impact of a TSH receptor gene polymorphism on thyroid-related phenotypes in a healthy Danish twin population. *Clinical Endocrinology (Oxf)*, Vol.66, N°6, (June 2007), pp. 827-832.

He, B.; Li, J.; Wang, G.; Ju, W.; Lu, Y.; Shi, Y.; He, L. & Zhong, N. (2009). Association of genetic polymorphisms in the type II deiodinase gene with bipolar disorder in a subset of Chinese population. *Progress in Neuropsychopharmacology & Biological Psychiatry*, Vol. 33, No.6 (August 2009), pp. 986-990.

Heal, D.J., Smith, S.L. (1988). The effects of acute and repeated administration of T3 to mice on 5-HT1 and 5-HT2 function in the brain and its influence on the actions of repeated electroconvulsive shock. *Neuropharmacology*, Vol.27, N°.12, (December 1988), pp.1239-1248.

Iosifescu, DV.; Nierenberg, AA.; Mischoulon, D.; Perlis, RH.; Papakostas, GI.; Ryan, JL.; Alpert, JE. & Fava, M. (2005). An open study of triiodothyronine augmentation of selective serotonin reuptake inhibitors in treatment-resistant major depressive disorder. *Journal of Clinical Psychiatry*, Vol.66, No.8 (August 2005), pp. 1038-1042.

Järnum, H., Eskildsen, S.F., Steffensen, E.G., Lundbye-Christensen, S., Simonsen, C.W., Thomsen, I.S., Fründ, E.T., Théberge, J., Larsson, E.M. (2011). Longitudinal MRI study of cortical thickness, perfusion, and metabolite levels in major depressive disorder. *Acta Psychiatrica Scandinavica,* (September 2011)16. doi: 10.1111/j.1600-0447.2011.01766.x. [Epub ahead of print]

Joffe, RT. & Singer, W. (1990). A comparison of triiodotironine and thyroxine in the potentiation of tricyclic antidepressants. *Psychiatry Research*, Vol.32, No.3 (June 1990), pp. 241-251.

Jones, I.; Ng, L., Liu, H. & Forrest, D. (2007). An intron control region differentially regulates expression of thyroid hormone receptor beta2 in the cochlea, pituitary, and cone photoreceptors. *Molecular Endocrinology*, Vol.21, No.5 (May 2007), pp. 1108–1119.

Kennedy, S.H., Konarski, J.Z., Segal, Z.V., Lau, M.A., Bieling, P.J., McIntyre, R.S., Mayberg, H.S. (2007). Differences in brain glucose metabolism between responders to CBT and Venlafaxine in a 16-week randomized controlled trial. *American Journal of Psychiatry*, Vol.164, N°5. (May 2007), pp.778–788

Kirkegaard, C., Faber, J. (1998). The role of thyroid hormones in depression. *European Journal of Endocrinology,* (January1998), Vol.138, N°1, pp.1-9.

Kohn, Y., Freedman, N., Lester, H., Krausz, Y., Chisin, R., Lerer, B., Bonne, O. (2007). 99mTc-HMPAO SPECT study of cerebral perfusion after treatment with medication and electroconvulsive therapy in major depression. *Journal of Nuclear Medicine*, Vol. 48, N°8, (August 2007) pp. 1273-1278

Larsen, JK.; Faber, J.; Christensen, EM.; Bendsen, BB.; Solstad, K.; Gjerris, A. & Siersbaek-Nielsen, K. (2004). Relationship between mood and TSH response to TRH stimulation in bipolar affective disorder. *Psychoneuroendocrinology*, Vol.29, No.7 (August 2004), pp. 917–924.

Leonard, JL. & Farwell, AP. (1997). Thyroid hormone-regulated actin polymerization in brain. *Thyroid*, Vol.7, No.1 (February 1997), pp. 147–151.

Lifschytz, T., Segman, R., Shalom, G., Lerer, B., Gur, E., Golzer, T., Newman, M.E. (2006). Basic mechanisms of augmentation of antidepressant effects with thyroid hormone. *Current Drug Targets*, Vol.7, N°2, (February 2006), pp. 203-210.

Linkowski, P.; Brauman, H. & Mendlewicz, J. (1981). Thyrotrophin response to thyrotrophin-releasing hormone in unipolar and bipolar affective illness. *Journal of Affective Disorders*, Vol. 3, No.1 (March 1981), pp. 9–16.

Łojko, D. Rybakowski, JK. (2007). L-thyroxine augmentation of serotonergic antidepressants in female patients with refractory depression. *Journal of Affective Disorders*, Vol. 103, No. 1-3 (November 2007), pp. 253-256.

Loosen, PT. (1985). The TRH-induced TSH response in psychiatric patients: a possible neuroendocrine marker. *Psychoneuroendocrinology*, Vol.10, No.3, pp. 237–260.

MacQueen, G.M. (2009) Magnetic resonance imaging and prediction of outcome in patients with major depressive disorder. *Journal of Psychiatry & Neurosciences*, Vol. 34, N°5, (September 2009) pp.343-349.

Marangell, L.B., Ketter, T.A., George. M.S., Pazzaglia, P.J., Callahan, A.M., Parekh, P., Andreason, P.J., Horwitz, B., Herscovitch, P. & Post, R.M. (1997) Inverse relationship of peripheral thyrotropin-stimulating hormone levels to brain activity in mood disorders. *American Journal of Psychiatry*, Vol.154, N°2, (February 1997), pp.224-230,

Mentuccia, D., Proietti-Pannunzl, L., Tanncr, K., Bacci, V., Pollin, T.I., Poehlman, E.T., Shuldiner, A.R., Celi, F.S. (2002). Association between a novel variant of the human type 2 deiodinase gene Thr92Ala and insulin resistance: evidence of interaction with the Trp64Arg variant of the beta-3-adrenergic receptor. *Diabetes*, Vol.51, N°3, (March 2002), pp. 880-883.

Milak, M.S., Parsey, R.V., Keilp, J., Oquendo, M.A., Malone, K.M., Mann, J.J. (2005). Neuroanatomic correlates of psychopathologic components of major depressive disorder. *Archives of General Psychiatry*, Vol. 62, N°4, (April 2005), pp. 397-408,

Miller, K.J., Parsons, T.D., Whybrow, P.C., Van Herle, K., Rasgon, N., Van Herle, A., Martinez, D., Silverman, D.H., Bauer, M. (2007). Verbal memory retrieval deficits associated with untreated hypothyroidism. *Journal of Neuropsychiatry and Clinical Neurosciences*, Vol.19, N°2, (2007), pp. 132-136.

Morte, B., Diez, D., Auso, E., Belinchon, M.M., Gil-Ibanez, P., Grijota-Martinez, C., Navarro, D., de Escobar, G.M., Berbel, P., Bernal, J. (2010). Thyroid hormone regulation of gene expression in the developing rat fetal cerebral cortex: prominent role of the Ca2+/calmodulin-dependent protein kinase IV pathway. *Endocrinology*, Vol. 151,N°2, (February 2010), pp. 810-820.

Mowla, A., Kalantarhormozi, M.R., Khazraee, S. (2011) Clinical characteristics of patients with major depressive disorder with and without hypothyroidism: A comparative study. *Journal of Psychiatric Practice*, (January 2011), Vol 17, N°1, pp.67–71.

Myers, DH.; Carter, RA.; Burns, BH.; Armond, A.; Hussain, SB. & Chengapa, VK. (1985). A prospective study of the effects of lithium on thyroid function and on the prevalence of antithyroid antibodies. *Psychological Medicine*, Vol. 15, No.1 (February 1985), pp. 55–61.

Nagamachi, S., Jinnouchi, S., Nishii, R., Ishida, Y., Fujita, S., Futami, S., Kodama, T., Tamura, S., Kawai, K. (2004). Cerebral blood flow abnormalities induced by transient hypothyroidism after thyroidectomy-analysis by tc-99m-HMPAO and SPM96. *Annals of Nuclear Medicine*, Vol.18, N°6, (September 2004), pp. 469-77.

Navarro, V., Gasto, C., Lomena, F., Mateos, J.J., Portella, M.J., Massana, G., Bernardo, M., Marcos, T. (2004). Frontal cerebral perfusion after antidepressant drug treatment versus ECT in elderly patients with major depression: a 12-month follow-up control study *Journal of Clinical Psychiatry*, Vol. 65, N°5, (May 2004), pp. 656-661.

Peeters, R.P., van den Beld, A.W., Attalki, H., Toor, H., de Rijke, Y.B., Kuiper, G.G., Lamberts, S.W., Janssen, J.A., Uitterlinden, A.G., Visser, T.J. (2005). A new polymorphism in the type II deiodinase gene is associated with circulating thyroid hormone parameters. *American Journal of Physiology, Endocrinology and Metabolism*, Vol. 289, N°1, (July 2005), pp.E75-81.

Peeters, R.P., van der Deure, W.M., van den Beld, A.W., van Toor, H., Lamberts, S.W., Janssen, J.A., Uitterlinden, A.G., Visser, T.J. (2007). The Asp727Glu polymorphism in the TSH receptor is associated with insulin resistance in healthy elderly men. Clinical Endocrinology (Oxf), Vol. 66, N°6, (June 2007), pp. 808-815.

Peeters, R.P., van der Deure, W.M., Visser, T.J. (2006). Genetic variation in thyroid hormone pathway genes; polymorphisms in the TSH receptor and the iodothyronine deiodinases. *European Journal of Endocrinology* Vol.155, N°5, (November 2006), pp. 655-662.

Peeters, R.P., van Toor, H., Klootwijk, W., de Rijke, Y.B., Kuiper, G.G., Uitterlinden, A.G., Visser, T.J. (2003). Polymorphisms in thyroid hormone pathway genes are associated with plasma TSH and iodothyronine levels in healthy subjects. *Journal of Clinical Endocrinology and Metabolism*, Vol. 88, N°6, (June 2003), pp. 2880-2888.

Prange Jr, AJ.; Wilson, IC.; Rabon, AM. & Lipton, MA. (1969). Enhancement of imipramine antidepressant activity by thyroid hormone. *American Journal of Psychiatry*, Vol.126, No.4 (October 1969), pp. 457–469.

Richieri, R., Boyer. L., Farisse, J., Colavolpe, C., Mundler, O., Lancon, C., Guedj, E. (2011). Predictive value of brain perfusion SPECT for rTMS response in pharmacoresistant depression. *European Journal of Nuclear Medicine and Molecular Imaging*, Vol. 38, N°9, (September 2011), pp.1715-1722.

Risco, L., González, M., Garay, J., Arancibia, P., Nuñez, A., Hasler, G., Galleguillos, T. (2003). Evaluación funcional del eje hipotálamo-hipófisis-tiroides en episodio depresivo mayor único: ¿desregulación a nivel central?. *Revista de Neuro-Psiquiatría*, Vol.66, N°.4, (2003), pp. 320-328.

Roy-Byrne, P.; Post, RM.; Rubinow, DR.; Linnoila, M.; Savard, R. & Davis, D. (1983). CSF 5HIAA and personal and family history of suicide in affectively ill patients: a negative study. *Psychiatry Research*, Vol.10, No.4 (December 1983), pp. 263-274.

Rozanov, C.B.Dratman, M.B., (1996). Immunohistochemical mapping of brain triiodothyronine reveals prominent localization in central noradrenergic systems. *Neuroscience*, Vol. 74, N°3 (October, 1996), pp. 897-915.

Rubinow, DR.; Gold, PW.; Post, RM.; Ballenger, JC.; Cowdry, R.; Bollinger, J. & Reichlin, S. (1983). CSF somatostatin in affective illness. *Archives of General Psychiatry*, Vol.40, No.4 (April 1983), pp. 377–386.

Ruhé, H.G., Booij, J., Veltman, D.J., Michel, M.C., Schene, A. (2011). Successful pharmacologic treatment of major depressive disorder attenuates amygdala activation to negative facial expressions: a functional magnetic resonance imaging study. *Journal of Clinical Psychiatry*, (August 2011), [Epub ahead of print]

Samuels, M.H., Schuff, K.G., Carlson, N.E., Carello, P., Janowsky, J.S. (2007). Health status, mood, and cognition in experimentally induced subclinical hypothyroidism. *Journal of Clinical Endocrinology and Metabolism*, Vol. 92, N°7, (2007), pp.2545-2551.

Saxena, J., Singh, P.N., Srivastava, U., Siddiqui, A.Q. (2000). A study of thyroid hormones (T3, T4 & TSH) in patients of depression. *Indian Journal of Psychiatry*, Vol. 42, N°3, (July 2000) pp.243-246.

Singhal, R.L., Rastogi, R.B., Hrdina P.D. (1975) Brain biogenic amines and altered thyroid function. *Life Sciences*,Vol. 17, N°11, (December 1975),pp. 1617-1626.

Smith, J.W., Evans, A.T., Costall, B., Smythe, J.W. (2002). Thyroid hormones, brain function and cognition: a brief review. *Neurosciences and Biobehavioral Reviews*, Vol. 26, N°1, (January 2002), pp.45-60.

Stern, RA.; Nevels, CT.; Shelhorse, ME.; Prohaska, ML.; Mason, GA. & Prange Jr, AJ. (1991). Antidepressant and memory effects of combined thyroid hormone treatment and electroconvulsive therapy: Preliminary findings. *Biological Psychiatry*, Vol. 30, No.6 (September 1991), pp. 623–627.

Stipcević T, Pivac N, Kozarić-Kovacić D, Mück-Seler D. (2008) Thyroid activity in patients with major depression. *Collegium Antropologicum*, Vol. 32,No3 (September 2008),pp. 973-976.

Strawn, JR.; Ekhator, NN.; D'Souza, BB. & Geracioti Jr, TD. (2004). Pituitary-thyroid state correlates with central dopaminergic and serotonergic activity in healthy humans. *Neuropsychobiology*, Vol.49, No.2, pp. 84–87.

Szabadi, E. (1991). Thyroid dysfunction and affective illness. *British Medical Journal*, Vol.302, No. 6782 (April 1991), pp. 923–924.

Torlontano, M., Durante, C., Torrente, I., Crocetti, U., Augello, G., Ronga, G., Montesano, T., Travascio, L., Verrienti, A., Bruno, R., Santini, S., D'Arcangelo, P., Dallapiccola, B., Filetti, S., Trischitta, V. (2008). Type 2 deiodinase polymorphism (threonine 92 alanine) predicts L-thyroxine dose to achieve target thyrotropin levels in thyroidectomized patients. *Journal of Clinical Endocrinology and Metabolism*, Vol. 93, N°3, (March 2008) pp. 910-913.

Vlassenko, A., Sheline, Y.I., Fischer, K., Mintun, M.A. (2004). Cerebral perfusion response to successful treatment of depression with different serotoninergic agents. *Journal of Neuropsychiatry and Clinical Neurosciences*, Vol.16, N° 3, (Summer 2004), pp. 360-363.

Walker, P., Weichsel, M.E., Jr., Fisher, D.A., Guo, S.M. (1979). Thyroxine increases nerve growth factor concentration in adult mouse brain. *Science*, Vol. 204, N°4391, (April 1979), pp.427-429.

Walker, P., Weil, M.L., Weichsel, M.E., Jr., Fisher, D.A. (1981). Effect of thyroxine on nerve growth factor concentration in neonatal mouse brain. *Life Sciences*,Vol 28, N°15-16 (April 1981), pp. 1777-1787.

Wheatley, D. (1972). Potentiation of amitriptyline by thyroid hormone. *Archives of General Psychiatry*, Vol. 26, No.3 (March 1972), pp. 229–233.

Whybrow, P.C.Prange, A.J., Jr. (1981). A hypothesis of thyroid-catecholamine-receptor interaction. Its relevance to affective illness. *Archives of General Psychiatry*, Vol. 38, N°1, (1981), pp. 106-113.

Wikström, L.; Johansson, C.; Saltó, C.; Barlow, C.; Campos Barros, A.; Baas, F.; Forrest, D.; Thorén, P. & Vennström, B. (1998). Abnormal heart rate and body temperature in mice lacking thyroid hormone receptor alpha 1. *The EMBO Journal*, Vol.17, No.2 (January 1998), pp. 455–461.

Wilson, IC.; Prange Jr, AJ.; McClane, TK.; Rabon, AM. & Lipton, MA. (1970). Thyroid hormone enhancement of imipramine in nonretarded depressions. *New England Journal of Medicine*, Vol. 282, No.19 (May 1970), pp. 1063–1067.

Zavacki, A.M., Ying, H., Christoffolete, M.A., Aerts, G., So, E., Harney, J.W., Cheng, S.Y., Larsen, P.R., Bianco, A.C., (2005). Type 1 iodothyronine deiodinase is a sensitive marker of peripheral thyroid status in the mouse. *Endocrinology*, Vol.146, N°3, (March 2005)pp. 1568-1575.

Zobel, A., Joe, A., Freymann, N., Clusmann, H., Schramm, J., Reinhardt, M., Biersack, H.J, Maier, W., Broich, K. (2005). Changes in regional cerebral blood flow by therapeutic vagus nerve stimulation in depression: An exploratory approach *Psychiatry Research*, Vol. 139, N 3, (August 2005), pp. 165-179.

18

Psychosocial Factors in Patients with Thyroid Disease

Petra Mandincová
Tomas Bata University in Zlin
Czech Republic

1. Introduction

In the contemporary, or in endocrinological literature, there is still increasing interest in psychological or psychosocial aspects of thyreopathy (thyroid disease). Unfortunately, this theme is rather marginalized in the Czech Republic therefore we have begun to be interested in this topic (Janečková, 2007a, 2008a; Mandincová 2008a, 2008b, 2009a, 2009b, 2011a, 2011b).

We have delivered an overview of the research findings in journal Czechoslovak Psychology (Janečková, 2007b) and at conferences (Janečková, 2007c, 2008c). It is possible to trace down four main lines of the research abroad (see chap. 1.1 - 1.4).

1.1 Researches concerning stress

One part of the research aimed at the role of stress in pathogenesis of thyreopathies, within their process and prognosis, some of them also included research of modifying stress factors, but their importance has not been fully appreciated.

Although a lot of studies stated connection between stress and autoimmune disease, most of evidence is indirect and a mechanism, which the autoimmune disease is influenced by, is not fully recognised. Just the relation between Graves' disease origination and higher levels of stress is considered to be the best indirect proof of the thyroid autoimmune disease, though it is still the subject of discussions. Most of contemporary studies support hypothesis that stress effects origination and clinical course of Graves' disease. Stress influences immune system directly or indirectly through nervous and endocrine system. These immune modulators can lead to a development of autoimmune illness in genetically predisposed individuals (Mizokami et al. 2004; comp. Schreiber, 1985). Depression can be applied as an intervening variable between life stress and an outbreak of autoimmune disease, because evidence it modifies immune response is available (Harris, Creed, Brugha, 1992).

Anciently it was observed that hyperthyroidism was preceded by presence of life stresses. Even the latest study confirms the effect of stress on Graves' disease development. Patients with Graves' disease were researched exclusively. An exception is a research comprising also patients with non-autoimmune hyperthyroidism (Matos-Santos et al., 2001), which results can show the fact that stress contributes to origination of non-autoimmune hyperthyroidism, but less than with autoimmune Graves' disease. Recent studies looked into life events and observed more negative life events in patients with Graves' disease compared to a control group (Kung, 1995; Lee et al., 2003; Matos-Santos et al., 2001; Radosavljević et al., 1996; Sonino, et al., 1993; Winsa et al., 1991; Yoshiuchi et al., 1998a, 1998b). Some earlier studies rejected the relation between stressful events and hyperthyroidism origination. However, they had considerable methodological problems to which can be attributed the fact that a consistent coherence was not found. Most probably, a difference in Martin-du Pan's research was not proved due to the same reasons (1998, as cited in Mizokami et al., 2004), because he arguably created a control group. Some studies (Kung, 1995; Winsa et al., 1991; Yoshiuchi et al., 1998b) integrated modifying factors into the research - evaluation of coping and social support. Furthermore, Kung (1995) and Yoshiuchi et al. (1998b) realized that life events occur rarely and they cannot reflect total stress that an individual experiences and the source of distress can also be hassles or daily stresses and minor events.

Much less prospective studies dealing with the effect of stress on hyperthyroidism course were carried out, yet they denote that more important life events and daily hassles can be of a negative effect on Graves' disease course (Ferguson-Rayport, 1956, as cited in Whybrow, 1991; Fukao et al., 2003; Hobbs, 1992; Yoshiuchi et al., 1998a). Already Schreiber (1985) speaks about the fact as a psychological stress, difficult task from an environment and individual's reaction to it can exacerbate calmed hyperthyroidism, and even hypothyroidism.

It is difficult to evaluate stress influence on origination and course of another autoimmune disease - Hashimoto's thyroidism, because it is quite often developed inconspicuously, the stress influence could have been overlooked (Mizokami et al., 2004).

1.2 Researches concerning personality

Another group of surveys researched a personality of a sick. The research into a personality was very popular with researchers (Ham, Alexander and others), especially in 50s and 60s of 20th century, when specific personality traits predisposing to hyperthyroidism were sought. Later studies proved neither typical personality, nor found a specific conflict in childhood (in Whybrow, 1991; Rodewig, 1993; Kaplan, Sadock, Grebb, 1994). Robbins and Vinson (1960) also regard the result of their study as an evidence of the fact that the personality role was overestimated in hyperthyroidism. At present, these issues are getting into the background compared to other research topics.

Influence of the thyroid disease on a personality and relation between personality traits and thyreopathy is realised in a quite difficult way. It is difficult to make a decision what the cause and consequence is. Harineková (1976) describes specific personality characteristics in girls with eufunctional goitre. Similarly, Ma, Luo and Zeng (2002) found some personality characteristics in adult patients different from the control group. Jenšovský et al. (2000, 2002) did not prove changes of personality traits in individuals with subclinical hypothyroidism during T4 treatment in the Czech study. Caparevic et al. (2005) examined patients with nodular goitre with whom the occurrence of mental disorders was reduced after an operation. Yang and Zang (2001) indicate that the choice of coping strategy is influenced by the personality in the patients with Graves' disease. Fukao et al. (2003) carried out a prospective research in Japan and they realised that some personality traits worsen the prognosis of treated Graves' disease.

1.3 Psychological means usage with treatment of thyroid disease

Newly, works calling for usage of psychological means in the treatment of thyreopathies occasionally appear. Available resources discuss these issues, especially with hyperthyroidism treatment. Monographs provide only general recommendations concerning suitability of psychotherapy (e.g. Baštecký et al., 1993; Kaplan et al., 1994; Markalous & Gregorová, 2007). A few works confirm successful treatment of patients with hyperthyroidism with a combination of conventional medicine and psychological means (Fukao et al., 2000, as cited in Fukao et al., 2003; Zeng et al., 2003; comp. Brown et al., 2010).

In a British study Lincoln et al. (2000) realised that patients with hyperthyroidism do not have enough knowledge concerning this disease. Likewise, treated patients with hypothyroidism were not satisfied with insufficient or misleading information that was provided by the doctors on the disease and its treatment (Mc Millan et al., 2004). Air et al. (2006, 2007) state that it is not possible to rely on the Internet as a tool of patients' education, because the information concerning thyroid carcinoma on the web sites was quite often incomplete and outdated. Roberts et al. (2008) surveyed which information would be necessary for the patients with the carcinoma. Sawka et al. (2011) have developed a computerized educational tool (called a decision aid) to inform patients about available treatment options and have been utilized in oncologic decision-making. Huang et al. (2004) rightfully assume that a big potential is hidden in nurses' care (comp. Filická & Hadačová, 2006; Olosová & Filická, 2006).

We are informed on a range of organisations that help patients in thyroid disease or they associate them, and on a big amount of information materials for these patients (more detailed Janečková, 2008b; Mandincová, 2010). On the other hand, a lot of Czech patients have very little quality information and educational materials on the disease and its consequences, diagnostics and treatment. More or less, there is only one web site created by a female patient after a thyroid operation (available at www.stitnazlaza.estranky.cz dated 04/09/2011). As well as, special organisations supporting or associating patients, self-supporting groups are still missing. Practically, the situation in the Czech Republic has not change within the last two years.

We suppose if the mental disorder was not diagnosed in the patient with thyreopathy, the role of psychological and psychosocial means and psychotherapy itself has not been fully appreciated in their treatment (comp. Sinclair, 2006). Austrian researchers (König et al., 2007), among others, point out the importance of psychological and psychosocial methods introduction into the healthcare system with these patients. Ponto and Kahaly (2010) recommend psychosomatic treatment also in the ills with orbitopathy, as well as Hirsch et al. (2009) and Lee et al. (2010) in patients with carcinoma.

1.4 Researches concerning quality of life and perception of health status

The recent studies especially deal with examining health status and/or quality of life that often include examining of mental condition and cognitive functioning.

Measuring quality of life has become a key part in the evaluation of the disease impact and treatment or intervention effect (Razvi, McMillan, Weaver, 2005). Residual symptoms can often persist with the patient even after adequate treatment. Psychiatric symptoms usually subside with a suitable treatment nevertheless long-lasting disorders can contain a degree of disease process irreversibility and provoke highly individual affective response according to psychological losses and gains of individual patients. The quality of life can be seriously endangered even in case that the patient should be well (at least from the hormonal viewpoint). Therefore the contradiction in health perception among the patients, their partners and doctors is often emphasized in the quality of life research. The emphasis is often placed on laboratory measurements 'hard' data, but 'soft' data gained with reliable methods for quality of life evaluation are underestimated (Sonino, Fava, 1998). To assess seriousness of the disease and response to treatment it is necessary, except for biochemical test, to observe the symptoms, health status and quality of life with the help of suitable methods. The relation between physiological and clinical evaluation and consequences that are given by the patient is in fact moderate and rather changeable (Razvi, McMillan, Weaver, 2005). The results of many studies dealing with the health status measurement, alternatively quality of life, often signal their independence on the thyroid functioning (Biondi et al., 2000; Elberling et al., 2004; Wekking et al, 2005). Also König et al. (2007) realised that the evaluation of subjective and objective health status in the ills with thyroid have considerably differed, before the treatment and even after it.

The patients with non-treated thyreopathy independently of the type of disease suffer from a whole range of symptoms and their health status, alternatively quality of life, is considerably disrupted in most aspects. Moreover, it shows that this disruption persists in many patients for a long time, even if they are treated. Substantial part of patients with thyreopathy experience limitations in their common activities, they feel worsen health status and disruption of social and emotional areas. Cognitive ailments and tiredness are also frequent. Cosmetic problems are also usual. Long-term consequences of the treated by thyreopathies are very frequent. Approximately 1/2 of patients have stated total deterioration of the health status, alternatively quality of life, limitation in usual activities, as well as social and emotional problems. Two thirds feel tiredness and approximately one third is anxious, they have cognitive and sexual problems. Moreover, the patients with earlier hyperthyroidism very often suffer from classic symptoms of hypothyroidism and, vice versa, symptoms of hyperthyroidism persist approximately in one third. Patients with eufunctional goitre have been examined the least, there does not exist a study which would indicate that such patients suffer from cognitive ailments (Watt et al., 2006).

But insufficient defining the sample of patients (i.e. type of thyreopathy) and confusion or incorrect usage of basic notions is quite typical for current studies dealing with patients in thyreopathy. Only a few studies research patients' quality of life in the true sense of the word (Abraham-Nordling, 2005; Dow, Ferrell, Anello, 1997; Huang et al., 2004; McMillan et al., 2004, 2005; Terwee 1998, 1999, 2002). A lot of works confuse the evaluation of the quality of life for the measurement of symptoms non/presence, health status, psychical status, eventually mental well-being are often incorrectly described as the quality of life. People, whose health is bad, do not have to necessarily feel worsen quality of life. Incorrect understanding of the notions leads to the fact that the results of these studies can be incorrect or misleading, because a method for evaluation of one variable is used for measurement of something else. Moreover, available specific tools lack convincing data on validity, the exceptions are GO-QOL, ThyDQoL and ThyTSQ, which are of good psychometric characteristics. A disadvantage of the tools is that they only focus on a specific type of thyroid disease therefore they are not applicable across different thyreopathies. For a long time there has not been created a questionnaire that would cover all the relevant aspects of thyreopathies in longitudinal studies, when there can happen changes of hormonal status based on the character of the disease or treatment. (Razvi, Mc Millan, Weaver, 2005; Watt et al., 2006). According to available data we were the first who tried to create such method (Janečková 2001, 2006). Currently ThyPRO is being developed with promising psychometric characteristics focused on patients with any benign thyroid disorders (Watt et al., 2009).

1.4.1 Researches in hypothyroidism

There are studies which prove that despite the treatment of hypothyroidism with hormone T4 substitution, a lot of patients quote more or less vague complaints and feel worsened quality of life (Mc Millan et al., 2004, 2005, 2008; Saravanan et al., 2002; Wekking et al., 2005).

Researches of alternative therapy - treatment with hormone T4 and T3 combined substitution have been carried out. Based on Grozinsky-Glasberg et al.'s (2006) meta-analysis and Ma et al.'s (2009) systematic review it can be summed up that combined T4 and T3 treatment does not improve well-being, cognitive function, or health status compared with T4 itself. This is proved with works by Appelhof et al., 2005; Clyde et al., 2003; Joffe et al., 2004; Meng et al., 2004; Nygaard et al., 2009; Regalbuto et al., 2007; Saravanan et al., 2005; Sawka et al., 2003; Siegmund et al., 2004; Valizadeh et al., 2009; Walsh et al., 2003 and others. Whereas first works signalled differences in favour of combined T4 and T3 (Bunevičius et al., 1999, 2002; Bunevičius & Prange, 2000).

Hormonal therapy is considered as a very successful for reduction of morbidity and mortality. On the other hand, there are also real deficiencies that we have to be aware of - it is always dealt with imitation of normal hormone secretion. Additionally, it is difficult to quantify the effect of hormones on the level of tissues. Being aware of hormonal therapy deficiencies we can avoid incorrect marking of patients' complaints. In fact, it is probable that deficiencies of biological therapy partially participate in the complaints. On the contrary, it is important to strive for this treatment further improvement, because we contribute to creation a "chronic endocrine patient" (Kaplan, Sarne, Schneider, 2003; Lamberts, Romijn, Wiersinga, 2003; Romijn, Smit, Lamberts, 2003). There are several proofs that patients do not follow sufficient treatment that can be indicative of their dissatisfaction with the treatment (McMillan et al., 2004). There are a lot of organisations abroad associating patients with thyroid disease, especially those dissatisfied patients create a big stress on professional public, they have reservations about the diagnostics and therapy (they criticise laboratory testing as a diagnostic criteria, or they prefer dried pork thyroid to synthetic hormone substitution).

1.4.2 Researches in hyperthyroidism

A study realising that in patients with Graves' disease persists worsen health status in some aspects even after reaching the euthyreosis has been carried out (Elberling et al., 2004). Abraham-Nordling et al. (2005) have concluded similar results, but they have not found dependence of the health status on the way of therapy (surgical, drug, radioiodine). According to Watt et al. (2005) specialists and patients' opinions on the most important aspects of the quality of life with Graves' disease are significantly different. According to the patients, it is higher tiredness, perception of heart beating and internal restlessness, according to the endocrinologists it is dealt with hand shake, increased perspiration and weight loss.

Persistence of worsened health status even after the hyperthyroidism treatment has been proved by Fahrenfort, Wilterdink and Van-der-Veen (2000). Paschke et al.'s (1990, as cited in Rodewig, 1993) study indicates that higher anxiety appears in patients with hyperthyroidism in euthyroid status.

Studies of the quality of life are also focused on the patients with orbitopathy connected with Graves' disease. Orbitopathy (even in a moderate form) significantly influences patients' quality of life (Egle et al., 1999; Kahaly et al., 2002, 2005), and this negative influence is not in accordance with usual clinical evaluation (Gerding et al., 1997) and it often persists even many years after the treatment (Terwee et al., 2002). Other surveys have been devoted to the development of specific GO-QOL method that measures psychosocial consequences of a changed look and the consequences of diplopia (double vision) and worsen sharpness in common sight functioning (Terwee et al., 1998, 1999, 2001; Wiersinga et al., 2004). An interesting qualitative study in patients with orbitopathy has been carried out (Estcourt et al., 2008).

1.4.3 Researches in thyroid carcinoma

Evaluation of the quality of life and health status is especially important in the patients with thyroid carcinoma because they can experience changes of hormone statuses within the treatment - from long-term use of supra-physiological doses of T4 hormone (subclinical hyperthyroidism) to short-term time-limited period of T4 discontinuation (hypothyroidism) that is required by the preparation for diagnostics or radioiodine therapy.

Available studies are identical that there is a significant deterioration of patient's health status with short T4 discontinuation (Botella-Carretero et al., 2003; Pacini et al., 2006; Schroeder et al., 2006; Tagay et al., 2005). Due to the fact that T4 discontinuation is of a significant effect on patient's health status, other methods or preparation for diagnostics or radioiodine therapy have been sought. Usage of rhTSH (recombinant human thyrotropin hormone) is considered as a suitable method instead of the previous one what leads to improvement of patient's compliance and maintenance of patient's common daily routine and productivity (Duntas, Biondi, 2007).

Concerning the patients undergoing long-term usage of supra-physiological doses of T4, the research findings with mentioned above methods application are inconsistent - the results of some studies signal deterioration of the health status, even if less significant than in patients after T4 discontinuation (Botella-Carretero et al., 2003, Tagay et al., 2005), other studies have not found disturbed health status (Eustatia-Rutten et al., 2006; Schroeder et al., 2006).

The first studies in general methods of quality of life have been carried out in China. Hou et al. (2001) have found out that the quality of life in patients with non-papillary carcinoma was worse in some aspects in comparison with other patients. Huang et al. (2004) have carried out measurement of patients' quality of life after removing the carcinoma surgically when the level of the result score was analogous to other chronically ill.

Recently, the research has especially focused on follow up of patients with differentiated thyroid cancer. Impaired health status and quality of life have been surveyed in them (Hoftijzer et al., 2008; Lee et al., 2010). Quality-of-life and health status parameters were inversely affected by duration of cure and consequently may be restored after prolonged follow-up (Giusti et al., 2011; Gómez et al., 2010; Hoftijzer et al., 2008; Malterling et al., 2010; Pelttari et al., 2009). Special attention should be paid in patients with more severe staging on diagnosis (Almeida et al., 2009; Giusti et al., 2011). An interesting qualitative study has been carried out in this topic (Sawka et al., 2009).

1.4.4 Researches in subclinical hypothyroidism and hyperthyroidism

In connection with laboratory diagnostics improvement the research of subclinical thyroid disorder moves forward. Some patients may suffer from clinical symptoms resembling hypothyroidism or hyperthyroidism, and others do not. There is not a consensus concerning the fact whether these diseases should be treated (Stárka, Zamrazil et al., 2005), therefore the research in health status and some aspects of quality of life are becoming more important.

A lot of studies observing patients with non-treated subclinical hypothyroidism proved deterioration in some aspects of the health status (Appolinario et al., 2005; Baldini et al., 1997, 2009; Monzani et al., 1993; Razvi et al., 2005). However, the results of works observing if the therapy with T4 hormone is beneficial are disputable. Some studies mention specific effects (Baldini et al., 1997, 2009; Bono et al., 2004; Jenšovský et al., 2000, 2002; Monzani et al., 1993;), other works do not prove positive changes (e.g. Parle et al., 2010). Recent study by Jorde et al. (2006) does not either demonstrate the profit of T4 treatment, but it does not find any differences among patients with subclinical hypothyroidism, concerning the health status, as well as by Vigário et al. (2009), Park et al. (2010).

Compared to the control group, the research results by Biondi et al. (2000) testify for deterioration of some health status aspects with non-treated patients with endogenous subclinical hyperthyroidism.

1.4.5 Researches in euthyroid goitre

Only little attention was paid to the patients with euthyroid goitre within the research of quality of life and health status. The results of the studies in non-treated and treated patients signal deteriorated health status in some aspects (Bianchi et al., 2004; Janečková, 2001, 2006; König et al., 2007).

It is supposed that just a regular monitoring of patient's euthyroid status with nodules in thyroid reduces the quality of his life; on the other hand, more significant deterioration of the quality of life would occur if the patient was not dispensarized within his course of life (Dietlein & Schicha, 2003; Vidal-Trécan et al., 2002).

2. Aims and background

The aim of our research was to map psychosocial aspects of thyroid disease (thyreopathy). We have especially focused on patients' quality of life, role of stress and coping with it, including protective factors (resilience and social support); at the same time we tried to compare the results with the healthy population. It dealt with comparing the patients in thyroid disease who have undergone an operation, including their follow up after surgery

We have looked into this topic from the viewpoint of two relatively young disciplines, namely health psychology and, at the same time, we are inspired by positive psychology. Health psychology represents one of the fastest developing spheres of present psychology; it is a relatively young discipline. Mostly there is a consensus that it is dealt with a discipline that applies psychological knowledge into the sphere of health, diseases and the healthcare system (comp. Kebza, 2005; Křivohlavý, 2009; Mohapl, 1992; Vašina, 1999). Many psychologists are aware of the necessity of a change, but not in a radical diversion from existing negative topics in psychology (basically given by the historic development), but rather in the sense of the whole picture completion with "positive" topics. It is due to the fact that absence of negative aspects is not the same as presence of the positive ones. Dissatisfaction with the existing state, newly oriented constituent psychological research, new attitudes to the representatives of different psychological disciplines have gradually flown into a bigger stream that has taken a shape and determined itself as the positive psychology (Kebza, 2005; Křivohlavý, 2010; Mareš, 2001; Seligman, 2000).

3. Design of the research

In correspondence with our research aim we have chosen non-experimental research plan (Hendl, 2006), where its core does not consist in an invasion or in a deliberate manipulation with the observed variables. Sometime such research plans are called as sample surveys. We understand our study as a descriptive research focused on exploration, description and orientation, or confirmation of carried out research, eventually prediction. We have used differentiation overview where we have compared patients in thyreopathy to health population, or patients with different types of thyreopathies among each other. We have presumed to compare health population with the ills in thyreopathy as a whole, because it is known from literature that within the course of this disease there can occur changes of hormonal status based on the disease or treatment character. We have used a development overview (a specific type of a differentiation overview) in the sense of longitudinal follow up of patients after 3 and 6 months since surgery where we try to capture a change of observed variables in time in patients with thyreopathy overall, or in the patients with different types of thyreopathies. We want to avoid frequent, quite easy process of measuring the status only before and after the change, what is rightly criticised (Břicháček, 2006), especially in measuring the quality of life (Mareš, 2005). We have also followed in our orientation research (Janečková, 2001, 2006), where we have especially focused on the thyroid disease as a mental strain (stress) and we have researched the consequences that this disease brings to the patients, its diagnostics and treatment. With respect to the research problem, the choice of a mixed research strategy has been considered as the most suitable one (quantitatively-qualitative).

The patients have almost always been asked by the doctor, who operated them on, to take part in this research. Then, the researcher conducted an interview with the patient. At first, he described him simply the aim and character of the research, then there was the dialogue itself and in the end, the patients were given questionnaires and instructions to them. The patient was informed to fill in the questionnaire 1 or 2 days before release from hospital (even due to the fact he will probably feel himself well), what was followed, with some exceptions. Being released from hospital, the researched person handed in the filled in questionnaire in a sealed envelope. Data collection after 3 and 6 months has also been realised in the hospital in a group form. The group was always formed by patients who were operated on within ± 14 days. At first, they filled in the questionnaires, then and individual semi-structured dialogue was carried out with them. The research has been approved by an ethics committee of the involved hospital.

4. Samples

The examined sample was created by the patients with thyroid operation carried out within the period from January 2006 to January 2007. The data were gained from 143 patients, 132 women (92.3 %) and 11 men (7.7 %). Average age of the patients was 51.9 ± 14.4 years. It was dealt with 45 patients with hyperthyroidism, 70 with nodular goitre, 17 with carcinoma (7 papillary carcinoma, 7 papillary microcarcinoma, 3 medullary carcinoma) and 11 with thyroiditis. Concerning the patients in nodular goitre, 36 of them underwent hemithyroidectomy and 34 of them total thyroidectomy. Patient's hormone level was adjusted within the hospitalisation in the way so that he would be euthyroid. Originally, according to thyroid function there were 45 patients hyperfunctional, 89 eufunctional and 9 hypofunctional. 68 patients did not take any specific medication, 39 took thyrostatics and 36 took synthetic thyroid hormones. An average length of thyreopathy from the diagnosis was 5.6 ± 8.7 years. Co-morbidity of diseases in patients with thyreopathy was also followed, when the doctor confirmed with all of them that, from an objective viewpoint, no one of them suffers from more serious disease than it corresponds to common population of the same age. We also inquired if the patient did not experience any important changes in his recent life. Persons from the control group were asked the same, because it could influence for example the results in the questionnaires.

Altogether 91.1% of addressed patients with thyreopathy took part in the research within their hospitalisation. After 3 months since surgery, 131 patients continued in the research and, after 6 months, 125 patients from the original sample (143 people). Altogether 87.4% of patients from the original sample finished the longitudinal follow up. "Wear and tear" of the sample occurred approximately in the same percentage with men and women. In general it can be said that we were successful in reaching quite a high percentage of filled in questionnaires and a small wear and tear of the sample (experimental mortality) during the longitudinal follow up. Probably due to this reason, that nearly all patients were enthusiastic about nice approach to them by the medical staff, especially by the doctor and they felt gratitude for that.

Selection of people into the control sample was given by respondents' availability and their willingness to participate in the research. In a maximum extent, we equalised this file with a group of patients according to criteria, such as sex, age and residence in the same region. We excluded people who were in the past, or who are currently treated with thyreopathy, or who are in medical dispensarization due to the mentioned above disease. Due to the fact that it was quite difficult to gather needed amount of healthy people, at the same time an avalanche selection, or the method of snowball, was applied (Ferjenčík,

2010; Miovský, 2006). Finally, the control sample was formed by 137 healthy people not suffering from thyreopathy, 127 women and 10 men. Average age of the respondents was 51.5 ± 14.8 years. Altogether, the questionnaires were filled in by 86.2 % of responded healthy people.

5. Methods

While choosing the method of data collection we endeavoured so that they were relevant to the aim of the research and observed variables based on the studied literature. We chose methods with good psychometric characteristics. All the persons were administrated with 7 tested methods and a semi-structured interview was carried out.

Antonovsky's Sense of Coherence Scale = SOC

SOC (sense of coherence) questionnaire contains 29 items, the extent of scores is 29 to 230. The method is based on Antonovsky's conception of SOC resilience and was translated by Křivohlavý. Except for the total coherence (integrity) of a personality, it measures 3 dimensions of SOC - comprehensibility (C), manageability (MA) and meaningfulness (ME). Křivohlavý (1990) mentions correlation of SOC, among others with Spielberger's STAI questionnaire.

Perceived Social Support Scale = PSSS

Perceived social support scale was surveyed by means of PSSS self-assessment method by Blumental et al. (1987). It consists of 12 basic and 4 additional items by means of which a person assesses availability of social support and satisfaction with it. The questionnaire items are assessed on a 7-point scale of Likert's type, where an individual expresses the extent of his agreement or disagreement with the given statement. A total score and 3 constituent scores are inquired - social support from an important, not specified person (PSSS_A), from family members (PSSS_B), and from friends (PSSS_C). Other 4 items (scales) that were added by Vašina (1999) allow to compare social support evaluation from the family, friends, co-workers and superiors.

COPE inventory

We used COPE questionnaire created by the team of Carver, Scheier and Weintraub (1989), in the Czech Republic translated by Vašina (2002), to find out coping strategies. Through 15 scales the method captures 15 groups, types of coping strategies. Each type is diagnosed with the help of 4 items on a 4-level scale from "I do not react like this" to "I react like this quite often". The authors of the method were thinking about a problem, whether the choise of specific types of reaction depends on a situation or on personal traits (similarly to Spielberger in STAI method), and with the help of a suitably chosen instruction they managed to capture dispositional and situational coping reactions (Vašina, 1999). In our study we have rather focused on general tendency of strategy selection. The questionnaire contains either, reactions that can be regarded as adaptive, effective, or maladaptive, ineffective. Each scale is unipolar, it means its missing does not mean that the present is the opposite. The method contains at least 2 pairs of opposite tendencies when it can be presupposed that a man can use wide repertoire of strategies in specific periods of life, including both opposite tendencies. Carver emphasizes that neither any total COPE score is counted from the method, nor the scales are divided into problem-focused and emotion-focused coping strategies. He rather pays attention to each scale separately and he observes what relation it is to other variables. He recommends so that each researcher would identify in their data own factors because different samples show different regularities of relations (dated 04/09/2011 available from http://www.psy.miami.edu/faculty/ccarver/sclCOPEF.html).

Schedule for the Evaluation of Individual Quality of Life = SEIQoL

SEIQoL is a method detecting individual quality of life, based on a interview. Altogether it requires a period of 10 to 20 minutes and it is suitable for research and clinical purposes (O'Boyle et al., 1994, as cited in Křivohlavý, 2009; O'Boyle et al., 1995). It has been used for different groups of patients even in healthy people (e.g. Buchtová, 2004; Koukola & Ondřejová, 2006; Rybářová et al., 2006; Řehulka & Řehulková, 2003). According to authors' conception, the quality of life of an individual, it depends on his own system of values that is fully respected within this method detection. The individual determines, considers and evaluates aspects of life that are essential for him in the specific situation and time (Křivohlavý, 2002). In the Czech Republic, this method was translated by Křivohlavý (2009). The result is calculation of a table (table - quality of life) and graphic presentation (line - life satisfaction). Analytic approach is necessary for the scale calculated from component areas, graphic scale requires holistic approach. Because most of the respondents wanted to fill in the form on their own, we especially built on written answers (similarly, e.g. Koukola & Ondřejová, 2006; Rybářová et al., 2006). We consider it as an advantage, because it is very difficult for a researcher not to influence a proband during the dialogue. Westerman et al. (2006) refer on the fact that it can easily happen the researcher (inadvertently) influences the interviewed and a big attention should be paid to this. Further on, they mention that, in different times, the patients indicate different key topics (reconceptualisation) and they can change the rate of importance in the same topics (recalibration), when both kinds of changes signal change of values (Schwartz & Sprangers, 1999, as cited in Westerman et al., 2006; comp. Mareš, 2005). Therefore, O'Boyle et al. (1995) recommend so that the respondents would always form new key areas in prospective studies, what we have kept. Křivohlavý (2002) also states that the areas can change within the course of life.

State-Trait Anxiety Inventory = STAI

To measure anxiety we have used STAI by Spielberger (1980) that we have translated from Slovak into Czech. This widely usable method enables to distinguish anxiety as a status and anxiety as a personality trait (anxiousness). This can be an advantage in usage with a longitudinal follow up. But it can be benefited from in patients even with first questionnaires administration after operation, because some patients can experience a high level of anxiety during hospitalisation, otherwise, they do not have the tendency to react in their lives like this. No less important advantage of this questionnaire compared to other ones is that it is more suitable for patients with thyreopathy. Anxiety is more likely deduced from feelings (feelings of tension, nervousness, fear, worries vs. feelings of calm, safety, satisfaction), than from physical symptoms, these could be more likely display of thyroid disorder that anxiety. State Anxiety Scale and Trait Anxiety Scale are always formed with 20 items that are assessed on the scale from 1 to 4.

Beck Depression Inventory = BDI

Beck's questionnaire BDI for detection of depression belongs among the most frequent self-assessment methods for detection of depressive symptoms. In order to burden the patient as little as possible, we have used shortened version in our study with 13 items that is also considered as valid and reliable enough (Reynold & Gould, 1981). A person evaluates each item on four-point assessment scale from 0 to 3.

Visual analogous scale Locus of Control = LOC

To detect Rotter's (1966, e.g. as cited in Kebza & Šolcová, 2008) LOC we have used visual analogue scale. The researched person was asked a question "To what extent do you suppose your life is in your hands (you can influence it, you control its course)?". As an answer he shall illustrate graphically his position between two extremes "not at all – completely" on a line segment of 100 mm long. LOC can reach the scores from 0 to 100. The more the score is closer to 100 (vs. closer to 0), the more it approaches internal locus of control (vs. external locus of control).

Semi-structured interviews

The interview was always carried out with approximately 80% of the patients, who filled in the questionnaires, in each administration of questionnaires (i.e. at the period of hospitalisation, 3 and 6 months since surgery). At least once a dialogue was carried out with each patient (except for 4), but usually three times. Altogether more than 300 dialogues of average length of approximately 20 minutes were realised. With respect to the research extensity, the interviews were recorded in a form of detailed notes. First three pilot depth interviews helped to map important topics and based on them a structure of semi-structured interview was created.

Statistical data processing was carried out with the help of statistical programme SPSS 14.0. To assess differences between averages of two groups, T-test was used (comp. Reiterová, 2007, 2009). To observe changes in patients in time, an analysis of variance was used for repeated measurements (general linear model). To detect level of the relation (dependence) tightness between two variables we used a correlation analysis. (Hendl, 2006). We assessed data of qualitative character through content analysis (Hendl, 2009; Silverman, 2005; Miovský, 2006). $\chi 2$ test of independence was used in SEIQoL method to detect whether frequency distribution in individual areas (life goals or cues) depends on (relates to) belonging to a group (the ills x the healthy). On the other hand, assessment of changes in frequency distribution in individual areas with 3 measurements in patients in time was detected with the help of Cochran's test. With respect to the low number of people, in some areas, it was not possible to carry out statistical test in all areas and to draw attention to all substantively significant differences.

6. Hypotheses and explorative questions

Based on the studies of these issues, we define the hypotheses as follows:

H1: We suppose the patient with thyreopathy will be less resilient (they will be with less sense of coherence and with a tendency to external locus of control) that the control group. It is described in the literature that people with a high level of resilience are physically healthier and there is a higher probability with them to stay healthy (e.g. Kebza, 2005; Kebza & Šolcová, 2008; Křivohlavý, 1990; Vašina, 1999). Moreover, a difficult life situation can result in lowering the feeling of control over the life (comp. Kebza, 2005; Křivohlavý, 2002).

H2: We suppose the ills with thyreopathy will use rather non-effective coping strategies compared to the control group. The problems of coping strategies with thyreopathies are not examined a lot, the attention was only paid to Graves' disease, and yet it is called for more research into modifying stress factors in this diagnose (e.g. Rosch, 1993). Kung's (1995) and Winsy et al.'s (1991) studies have not proved differences between the healthy and ills. On the other hand, Yoshiuchi et al. (1998b) has found out that the group of health women compared to the female patients scored higher in problem-focused coping strategy, the group of healthy men compared to the patients waited till the situation passes. Ma, Luo and Zeng (2002) have realised in ill people non-effective coping strategies, compared to the healthy ones.

H3: We suppose the patients with thyreopathy will show lower quality of life, less life satisfaction than the control group. Deteriorated health status and quality of life, limitations in usual activities, social and emotional troubles occur with not only untreated patients, but as well as with the half of treated patients, and with one third even anxiety and so on. (Razvi et al., 2005; Watt et al., 2006).

H4: We suppose the patients with thyreopathy will experience more negative emotions (depression and anxiety) that the control group. It is known that especially anxiety and depression occur in patients with different diagnoses (e.g. Kukleta, 2001; Vymětal, 2003).

H5: We suppose the patients with thyreopathy will perceive higher social support compared to the healhy ones. With regard to the fact it is dealt with a planned operation mobilisation of patient social network and providing increased social support can be presupposed, and even from the side of medical staff. Otherwise, social support has been researched only in patients with Graves' disease, and this areas also considers it as insufficient, e.g. Rosch (1993). Differences between the ills and healthy ones have not been proved (Winsa et al, 1991; Yoshiuschi et al., 1998b). Ma, Luo and Zeng's (2002; comp. Kukleta, 2001) research was an exception, were less support was shown in patients probably due to the reason the disease is developed with insufficient social support in an easier way.

H6: We suppose that increase of resilience occurs in time within a half-year follow up in patients (growth of the sense for coherence and tendency to internal locus of control). The researches show that even if the sense for coherence can show itself as a stable trait, difficult life situations can change man's view of the world (Schnyder, 2000). After experiencing surgery (situation with less control) patients can gradually perceived a growth of the control over their lives (comp. Kebza, 2005; Křivohlavý, 2002).

H7: We suppose that the patients with thyreopathy will begin to choose effective coping strategies in time within a half-year follow up. Even earlier experience plays a specific role in managing and choice of coping strategy (comp. Baumgartner, 2001). The patients could acquire more adaptive strategies of manageability with the help of coping with surgery and they could be stimulated to this by the contacts with doctors, and so on.

H8: We suppose there occur improvement in quality of life and life satisfaction in patients in time within a half-year follow up. Satisfaction and quality of life usually increases with decrease of health problems that we suppose after an operation (comp. Křivohlavý, 2002; Kebza, 2005; Křížová, 2005).

H9: We suppose that decrease of negative emotions (depression and anxiety) occur in patients with thyreopathy within a half-year follow up. There should be less negative emotions with presupposed improvement of the health status due to the surgery (comp. Vymětal, 2003).

H10: We suppose that decrease of perceived social support occur in patients with thyreopathy within a half-year follow up. After initial mobilisation of the social support (including medical staff) due to the surgery, there will be its decrease, when the surroundings begin to consider the patient as "healthy", "cured".

With respect to these unexplored issues we have also been interested in answers to the following explorative questions:

Q1: What are the differences in the observed variables among the patients with different thyreopathies? Insufficient defining the sample of patients (i.e. type of thyreopathy) is typical for contemporary studies dealing with patients with thyreopathy (Watt et al., 2006). We regard comparison of such type a very interesting and we have not been informed on any similar researches.

Q2: What is the composition of the key areas (life topics) in the framework of quality of life, what importance and satisfaction with individual areas patients with thyreopathy will mention within the follow up period and how it is going to be in the control group? It is necessary to await that disease, treatment effects the quality of life not only in its total height, but also concerning the composition and importance of individual areas (cues) and their satisfaction with them (Křivohlavý, 2002).

Q3: Which variable does the quality of life relate to? Connection of the quality of life with resilience and social support is described in the literature, on the contrary, stress and negative emotions should deteriorate it. (comp. Kebza, 2005; Křivohlavý, 2002, 2009).

7. Results and discussion

7.1 Results comparison of patients with thyreopathy to healthy population

1. A statistically significant difference between the patients and the control group has not been proved in average scores of the total sense of coherence. An significant difference of average scores have not been proved in scores between the patients and the control group, neither in comprehensibility, nor in manageability, or in meaningfulness. Significantly higher variance ($p < 0.05$) has been found out in comprehensibility with a healthy control group than in patients.
2. Statistically significant difference has not been proved in average scores of completely perceived social support between the experimental and control groups. Statistically significant difference has not been proved between the two groups in the social support from an important, not closely specified person, neither concerning the social support from friends. It shows that the patients perceive significantly higher ($p < 0.05$) social support from the family that in the control group.

3. Statistically significant difference of averages has not been found out in patients and healthy persons in any of the coping strategies. An exception is a strategy of "planning" where it has been showed on the edge of statistical significance, respectively closely behind it, that it is used more frequently by the healthy respondents than the ills with thyreopathy.
4. On the edge of statistical significance, respectively closely behind it, it is indicated that higher life satisfaction has been mentioned by the member of the control group that the patients. The patients have stated significantly higher quality of life ($p < 0.05$) than the persons not suffering from thyreopathy.
5. The ills have scored significantly higher ($p < 0.05$) in state anxiety and anxiousness than the healthy persons.
6. Statistically significant difference in average scores of depression has not been proved between the patients and the control group.
7. Significantly higher tendency ($p < 0.01$) to internality (internal locus of control) and, therefore, to the feeling they have the life in their hands, have had the healthy people compared to the ills. Higher variance in locus of control on the edge of statistical significance has been found out in the patients compared with controls.

Variables		**Patients compared to healthy ones**	
SOC	ME - meaningfulness		
	MA - manageability		
	C - comprehensibility		
	sense of coherence		
PSSS	A - significant others		
	B -family	↑	/p>0.05/
	C - friends		
	perceived social support		
COPE	planning	↓	close t. ed.
QoL	table - quality of life	↑	/p>0.05/
	line - life satisfaction	↓	close t. ed.
STAI	state anxiety	↑	/p>0.05/
	trait anxiety	↑	/p>0.05/
BDI	depression		
LOC	locus of control	↓	/p>0.01/

Caption: ↑ means that patients in the given variable scored higher than healthy population
↓ means that patients in the given variable scored lower than healthy population
„close t. ed." is an abbreviation for close to the edge of statistical significance

Table 1. Comparison of patients with thyreopathy to healthy population

Hypotheses H1 to H5 have been proved only partially (see Tab. 1). The patients with thyreopathy, compared to the healthy persons, significantly perceive higher social support from the family, they are more anxious and on the edge of significance they are less satisfied with the life. Even other literature resources state that the disease causes the need for help (e.g. Baštecká, 2003; Haškovcová, 1985). Razvi, McMillan, Weaver (2005) and Watt et al. (2006) summarize similar findings of some aspects sides concerning the quality of life. The healthy persons score significantly higher in locus of control and in coping strategy of "planning" on the edge of significance that is often regarded as an effective strategy. Differences between the patients and the healthy persons have not been found out in sense of coherence and depression. A paradox finding, that total higher quality of life is in patients compared to the healthy ones, has been explained in compliance with the quantitative data from the interviews. The patients have made an impression that they rather overestimated (idealised) the satisfaction evaluation in individual areas, especially within the period of hospitalisation, but also a little bit 3 months after it. As if due to the fact they have occurred in a difficult situation and they are to cope with it, they needed to see their life more positively and not to admit dissatisfaction with individual areas of life. Results graphically illustrated on the line segment of satisfaction level have been much more credible. Because the scale of life satisfaction requires holistic approach, but analytic assessment is necessary for the scale of total quality of life calculated from individual parts (comp. Rybářová et al., 2006), it is possible that real emotional status has been reflected on the line segment of satisfaction display, whereas the total calculated quality of life reflected their wish rather than the reality. On the other hand, for example Edelmann (1997, as cited in Baštecká et al., 2003), Moons et al. (2004) have stated that the quality of life does not have to unfold from the presence of a disease, so from the health status.

7.2 Follow up results of patients with thyreopathy since surgery during the period of six months

1. Statistically significant difference in average scores of the whole sense of coherence within the follow up period has not been proved. Statistically significant difference in average scores of manageability have not been proved, nor in the average scores of meaningfulness within the follow up period. The difference between the averages have been indicated on the edge of statistical significance and a significant linear growth ($p < 0.05$) of comprehensibility has been proved in the patients with thyroid disease during the follow up.
2. We have found out a statistically significant difference ($p < 0.05$) in average scores of total perceived social support within the follow up period and a significant quadratic trend has been proved ($p < 0.05$) – at first, more significant decrease of totally perceived social support occurs in the patients after 3 months and to its slight increase after 6 months. Statistically significant difference in averages of perceived social support from an important, not specified person has not been proved in patients within the follow up period. We have realised a statistically significant difference ($p < 0.05$) in average scores and a significant linear decrease ($p < 0.05$) of perceived social support from the family members in the patients within the follow up period. Also a statistically significant difference ($p < 0.05$) in averages of perceived social support from friends in patients within the follow up period a significant

quadratic trend ($p < 0.05$) has been found out - during the follow up period after the surgery, at first, the decrease of perceived social support from friends occurred after 3 months and, after 6 months, it increased.

3. A difference in averages, close to the edge of significance, appeared in patients during the follow up after the surgery, and on the edge of significance there was indicated a linear decrease in "use of emotional social support". Statistically significant difference ($p < 0.01$) has been found out in averages with scale of "focus on and venting of emotion" and it was dealt with a quadratic trend ($p < 0.05$) - within the follow up period after surgery, at first, decrease of average score in coping strategy of "focus on and venting of emotions" in patients after 3 months and, after 6 months, it increased. We have not found out any statistically significant differences in averages in other coping strategies within the follow up period.
4. Statistically significant difference in averages of the life satisfaction level in the patients has not been found out during the follow up. On the edge of statistical significance, respectively close to it there has been indicated a significant difference in averages and a significant linear decrease of quality of life ($p < 0.05$) has been proved in patients within the follow up period.
5. We have proved statistically significant difference ($p < 0.05$) in average scores and statistically significant linear decrease ($p < 0.05$) of state anxiety within the follow up period. Also a statistically significant difference ($p < 0.01$) in averages have been realised and a significant linear decrease ($p < 0.01$) of anxiousness during the follow up.
6. We have not proved a statistically significant difference of depression averages in patients during the follow up.
7. A difference in average scores on the edge of statistical significance has been indicated and a statistically significant linear trend ($p < 0.05$) to higher internality (internal locus of control) has been proved within the follow up period.

Hypothesis H10 has been confirmed, hypotheses H6 and H9 have been proved partially, hypotheses H7 and H8 have not been proved (see Tab. 2). During the half-year follow up period there occurred significant decrease of anxiety in patients, an increase in comprehensibility and in the feeling of the control over the situation has been indicated on the edge of significance (comp. Kebza, 2005; Kebza & Šolcová, 2008). Our finding is in compliance with the fact that in managing a difficult situation a man at first tries to understand it (comprehensibility) (comp. Mareš, 2007, 2008, 2009; Mareš et al., 2007). A linear decrease in coping strategy of "use of emotional social support" was indicated in patients within the follow up, and a significant decrease was indicated in perceived social support from the family, apparently due to the fact the stress situation of operation passed. Total social support, support from friends and coping strategy of "focus on and venting of emotions" changed in a quadratic way - at first, there was a significant decrease after 3 months, and a slight increase after 6 months after hospitalisation. Apparently it relates to the fact, the patient can feel himself isolated during the first 3 months after the surgery. Close to the edge of statistical significance a decrease in total quality of life was indicated in patients within the follow up, that relates to original overvaluation of life satisfaction with individual areas, but at the same time it can relate to the fact what was apparent in first interviews with them- inappropriate expectations in relation to the medical intervention (they expected complete cure). It is similarly reflected by Vavrda (2005), comp. Calman (1984, as cited in Křivohlavý, 2002).

Variables		Follow up of patients during 6 months (trend)	
SOC	ME - meaningfulness		
	MA - manageability		
	C - comprehensibility	linear ↑	ed.
	sense of coherence		
PSSS	A - significant others		
	B -family	linear ↓	/p>0.05/
	C - friends	quadratic	/p>0.05/
	perceived social support	quadratic	/p>0.05/
COPE	use of emotional social support	linear ↓	close t. ed.
	focus on & venting of emotions	quadratic	/p>0.01/
QoL	table - quality of life	linear ↓	close t. ed.
	line - life satisfaction		
STAI	state anxiety	linear ↓	/p>0.05/
	trait anxiety	linear ↓	/p>0.01/
BDI	depression		
LOC	locus of control	linear ↑	ed.

Caption: ↑ means that the given variable was dealt with a linear increase
↓ means that the given variable was dealt with a linear decrease
depicted curve illustrates course of a quadratic trend
„ed." is an abbreviation for edge of statistical significance
„close t. ed. " is an abbreviation for close to the edge of statistical significance

Table 2. Follow up of patients with thyreopathy since surgery during the period of six months

7.3 Comparison of results in patients with different types of thyreopathies

1. There were not found out statistically significant differences of averages among the patients with different types of thyreopathies, nor in the total sense of coherence, or in manageability or meaningfulness within any of the 3 measurements. Comparing the average scores of comprehensibility there were not found any significant differences during 1st measurement, bur with 2nd and 3rd measurements, there were indicated lower average scores of comprehensibility on the edge of statistical significance in patients with carcinoma compared to other types of thyreopathies.
2. Statistically significant differences of averages were not proved in patients with different types of thyreopathies, neither in total perceived social support, nor in the social support from significant others, in social support from family members and from friends. Concerning the variances there was not found any statistically significant difference in the sphere of social support from friends within 1st measurement, but they

showed higher variance in social support from friends in 2nd measurement ($p < 0.05$) and, the patients with carcinoma especially in 3rd measurement, compared to other ills.

3. We did not prove any statistically significant differences of average scores in different coping strategies, except for 2, in 1st measurement among the patients with different types of thyreopathies. The results on the edge of statistical significance indicate that the patients with carcinoma probably coped stress more often through "positive reinterpretation and growth" within 1st measurement, and, conversely, they used less coping strategy of "humour", compared to the patients with other types of thyreopathies.
4. During 2nd measurement, the patients with thyroid carcinoma use coping strategy of "humour" significantly less frequently ($p < 0.05$) and more frequent "use of instrumental social support" was indicated on the edge of significance than in patients with nodular goitre. The patients with hyperthyroidism used significantly more often ($p < 0.05$) "planning" strategy during 2nd measurement and more frequent coping through "suppression of competing activities", through "restraint coping" and through "focusing on and venting of emotions" was indicated on the edge of statistical significance, compared to other patients. During 2nd measurement there were not proved any statistically significant differences of averages in other coping strategies among the patients with different types of thyreopathies.
5. We did not find statistically significant differences of averages in any of the coping strategies in patients with different types of thyreopathies within 3rd measurement.
6. Higher variance in coping strategy of "religious coping" was indicated in patients with carcinoma, compared to other patients, on the edge of significance, within 2nd measurement, and especially within 3rd measurement ($p < 0.05$).
7. Results on the edge of statistical significance ($p = 0.05$) within 1st measurement indicate higher life satisfaction in patients with nodular goitre compared to other patients. During 2nd and 3rd measurements, any statistically significant differences in averages of satisfaction were not found out. Statistically significant difference in averages with quality of live among the patients with different types of thyreopathies was not proved in any of the measurements.
8. Statistically significant difference in averages of anxiousness among the patients with different types of thyreopathies was not proved in any of the measurements. Higher average scores of state anxiety in patients with carcinoma were indicated on the edge of significance during 2nd and 3rd measurements compared to other ills. During 2nd measurement there was indicated difference in variances on the edge of significance, where the highest variance was in the results of patients with carcinoma.
9. Statistically significant difference in depression among patients with different types of thyreopathies was not proved within any measurement.
10. Comparing the average scores of locus of control there were not found any statistically significant differences in 1st and 3rd measurements. A higher tendency to externality (external locus of control) and the feeling they cannot influence their lives were indicated in patients with carcinoma on the edge of statistical significance during 2nd measuring compared to other patients.

Comparison of patients with different types of thyreopathies brought interesting results (see Tab. 3.). The patients with nodular goitre were significantly more satisfied with life at the time of surgery than other patients. The most significant difference from other types of

Variables		Carcinomas		
		Sugery	3 months	6 months
SOC	C - comprehensibility		↓ ed.	↓ ed
PSSS	C - friends		↑s^2 /p>0.05/	↑s^2 /p>0.01/
COPE	suppression of competing activities		↓ ed.	
	use of instrumental social support		↑ ed.	
	positive reinterpretation & growth	↑ ed.		
	focus on & venting of emotions		↓ ed.	
	religious coping		↑s^2 ed.	↑s^2 /p>0.05/
	humor	↓ ed.	↓ /p>0.05/	
STAI	state anxiety		↑ ed.	↑ ed.
LOC	locus of control		↓ ed.	
Variables		**Nodular goitres at the time of surgery**		
QoL	line - life satisfaction	↑ ed.		
Variables		**Hyperthyroidism after 3 months since surgery**		
COPE	planning	↑ /p>0.05/		
	suppression of competing activities	↑ ed.		
	restraint coping	↑ ed.		
	focus on & venting of emotions	↑ ed.		

Caption: ↑ means that patients with this diagnose scored higher in the given variable that other patients
↓ means that patients with this diagnose scored lower in the given variable that other patients
„ ed." is an abbreviation for edge of statistical significance

Table 3. Comparison of results in patients with different types of thyreopathies

thyreopathies is in patients with thyroid carcinoma. Only a small amount of these was in our researched file, but we will try to indicate statistically significant and marginally significant differences and trends. The biggest differences appear after 3 months since surgery when patients with carcinoma score lower in coping strategies as "humour", "suppression of competing activities" and "focus on and venting emotions", as well as in locus of control. In the period after 3 and 6 months since surgery the patients with carcinoma are more anxious compared to the others and score lower in comprehensibility. Bigger interindividual differences can be captured in carcinomas compared to the others after 3 and 6 months since surgery in coping strategy in "religious coping" and in social support from friends. Support from friends is probably related to what the patients referred to during the interviews; some of them hid till the end of observation from their family and friends that thyroid cancer had been found out with them. Tschuschke (2004) also refers on similar findings, for example a tendency to apply mechanisms of suppression and increased level of anxiety in patients with carcinoma.

7.4 Follow up results of patients with different types of thyreopathies since surgery during the period of six months in selected variables

1. Statistically significant difference in average scores of life satisfaction was not proved, neither in total quality of life within the observed period, nor in patients with hyperthyroidism, or in patients with carcinoma. We found out a statistically significant difference in average scores in patients with nodular goitre and a significant linear decrease of life satisfaction was proved (always for $p < 0.05$) and in total quality of life (always to $p < 0.01$). Patients with nodular goitre, who underwent total thyroidectomy, had lower level of life satisfaction in 3rd measuring on the edge of significance compared to those who underwent hemithyroidectomy. We attribute this finding to the fact that nodular goitre recently undergoing total intervention experienced more changes in life than those with hemithyroidectomy.
2. Statistically significant difference in averages of locus of control was not proved during the follow up period in patients with nodular goitre. The patients with nodular goitre, who had already undergone hemithyroidectomy, had higher tendency to internality (internal locus of control) with 3rd measurement on the edge of significance compared to those who had undergone total thyroidectomy. We attribute this finding to the fact that nodular goitre recently undergoing total intervention experienced more changes in life than those with hemithyroidectomy. Differences on the edge of significance in average scores of locus of control were indicated in patients with hyperthyroidism and carcinoma within the observed period. During operation follow up, the linear trend to higher internality (internal locus of control) was indicated on the edge of significance in patients with hyperthyroidism. During operation follow up, the quadratic trend was indicated on the edge of significance in patients with carcinoma - at first, after 3 months, there was a tendency to higher externality (external locus of control) and after 6 month, conversely, to higher internality (internal locus of control) than the original level was.

The results indicate (see Tab. 4, Fig. 1-3), that it is probable, the observed changes in time in life satisfaction rate, in total quality of life and in locus of control are effected by type of thyreopathy. Concerning nodular goitres, there occur a significant reduction in the level of life satisfaction and total quality of life during the half-year follow up; in other types of thyreopathies, significant changes of these variables do not occur in any direction. This corresponds with our finding resulting from interviews that people who had some difficulties before intervention adapt better and express higher satisfaction with their status than people who did not have any problems (most often nodular goitres). In patients with hyperthyroidism there occurs increase of internality on the edge of significance during follow up, but in the patients with carcinoma, at first a significant decrease occurs after 3 months and, after 6 months, there occurs increase to higher level that it was at the time of hospitalisation. Last-mentioned disease can be considered as the most serious from the viewpoint of control loss over the situation development (comp. Kebza, 2005; Kebza & Šolcová, 2008).

Variables		Nodular goitre follow up during 6 months (trend)	
QoL	table - quality of life	linear ↓	/p>0.01/
	line - life satisfaction	linear ↓	/p>0.05/
Variables		**Carcinomas follow up during 6 months (trend)**	
LOC	locus of control	quadratic ◡	ed.
Variables		**Hyperthyroidism follow up during 6 months (trend)**	
LOC	locus of control	linear ↑	ed.

Caption: ↑ means that the given variable was dealt with a linear increase
↓ means that the given variable was dealt with a linear decrease
depicted curve illustrates course of a quadratic trend
„ ed.“ is an abbreviation for edge of statistical significance

Table 4. Follow up results of patients with different types of thyreopathies since sugery during the period of six months in selected variables

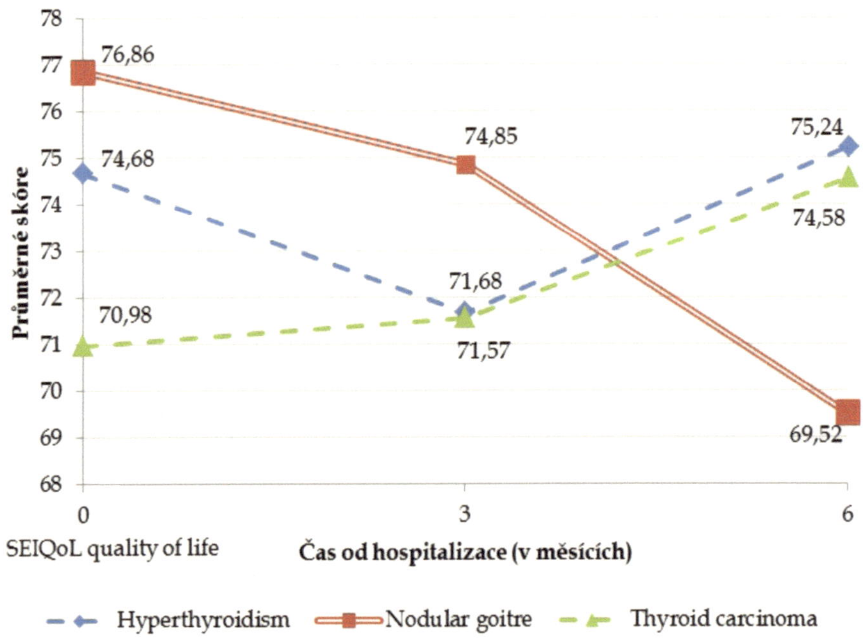

Caption: __________ (double line) statistically significant trend in time
_ _ _ _ _ _ _ (dashed line) statistically insignificant trend in time

Fig. 1. Monitoring of average scores of total quality of life in SEIQoL (table) during the six-month period in patients with different types of thyreopathies

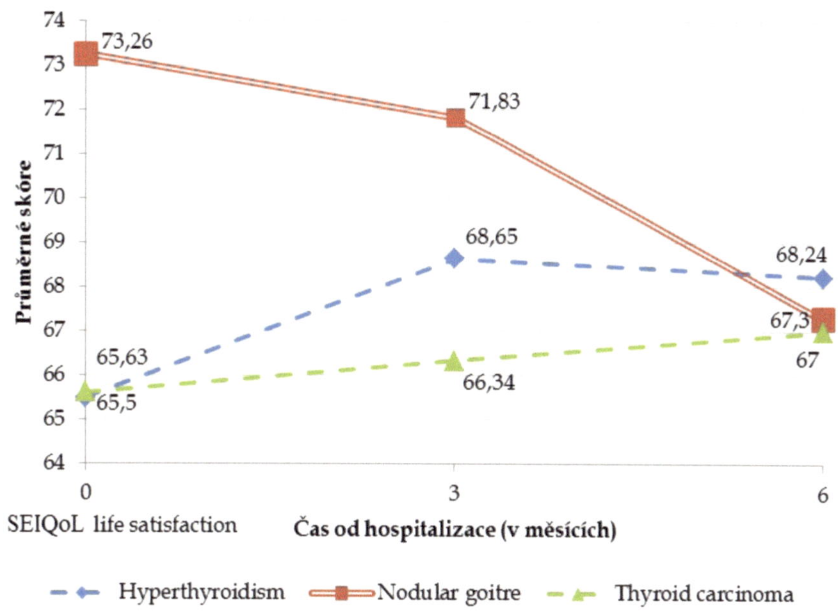

Caption: __________ (double line) statistically significant trend in time
_ _ _ _ _ _ _ (dashed line) statistically insignificant trend in time

Fig. 2. Monitoring of average scores of life satisfaction in SEIQoL (line) during the six-month period in patients with different types of thyreopathies

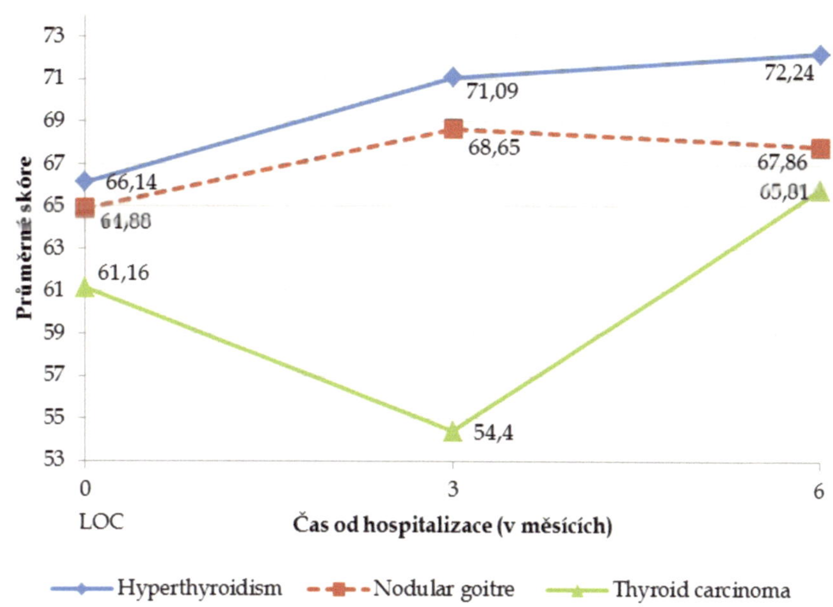

Caption: __________ (single line) trend in time on the edge of statistical significance
_ _ _ _ _ _ _ (dashed line) statistically insignificant trend in time

Fig. 3. Monitoring of average scores of LOC (locus of control) during the six-month period in patients with different types of thyreopathies

7.5 Results for quality life assessment measured by SEIQoL method acquired from individual areas (life goals or cues)

1. Respondents' answers regarding quality of life were divided into 11 categories (excluding a collective category: other): family, health, work, interpersonal relationships, leisure, material security, mental well-being, spiritual dimension, education, living conditions and good old age. All above mentioned categories appeared in the group of patients and in the control group. Patients with thyroid gland, when compared to healthy people, mentioned life and social security within more categories (work, mental well-being, living conditions). In category family, they reported close people, mainly those that are somehow depended on them (children, old parents). Patients, more than the controls, had more answers connected with health of close people. During follow up, patients didn´t change their understanding of content of individual categories.
2. Respondents of all groups most often mentioned cues: 1. family, 2. health and 3. work. Patients frequently reported life goals as good old age, or mental well-being, while the control group reported more leisure and education. During the follow up of patients with thyreopathy changes occurred in the distribution of frequencies (significant and the significance edge) for more than half the categories.
3. The most important cues for all respondent groups were 1. family, 2. health, 3. spiritual dimension, rarely good old age, which otherwise closely followed the spiritual dimension. It seems that during follow up of patients there was, on the edge of significance, a sign of decline for family and increase for health. Apparently there is also a change in the spiritual dimension category; its importance (with probands who recorded it) is highly evaluated within 3 months after surgery.
4. We have a reason to believe that the patients rather overevaluated (idealized) a situation while evaluating satisfaction for individual categories, sometimes slightly also after 3 months; therefore we cannot objectively assess the shift over time or differences between patients and control group. All observed groups assessed life conditions and material security as the least satisfactory, patients at the time of surgery recorded little satisfaction with mental well-being and after 3 to 6 month showed little satisfaction with category work.

The answers of respondents in the quality of life were categorized into 11 (or 12) areas that occurred both in patients and controls. Patients put more emphasis on life securities and care for close people dependent on them. In connection with their own illness they were apparently aware of what would happen to their children or parents dependent on them if something happened to them. Respondents of all groups mentioned as the most frequent and the most important goals family and health. Findings of Buchtová (2004) and Rybářová et al. (2006) correspond. Spiritual dimension category was little recorded but the people that recorded it saw its importance right after family and health (comp. Rybářová et al., 2006). Patients frequently reported categories of good old age and mental well-being because these areas can be threaten by the disease. Also, at the time of surgery, they were least satisfied with mental well-being. Their dissatisfaction with the work within 3 and 6 months after surgery is probably due to return to work, which can be difficult. The spiritual dimension is gaining importance within 3 months after surgery which is likely due to demands for coping with surgery. Experiencing difficult situations can lead to awareness of the importance of faith (comp. Hodačová, 2007). In our findings there were changes in patients´ reconceptualisation (change of key topics), and recalibration (change of importance) (e.g. Schwartz & Sprangers, 1999, as cited in Westerman et al., 2006; comp. Mareš, 2005). During interviews we noted that one of our patients with carcinoma, 6 months after surgery, had so called posttraumatic growth. Higher levels of satisfaction of patients are explained by their overvaluation (idealization) of a life situation (see also chap. 7.1 and 7.9).

7.5.1 Content analysis of categories (life goals or cues) reported by respondents in the SEIQoL method

Category family

It included mentions of family members - mostly mentioned children, mainly by patients, desire for having children, then a partner, siblings, and only patients recorded in their answers parents. Patients seem to be more aware of what would happen to their children or parents dependent on them if something happened to them. Healthy and ill people associated this category with concepts such as family relationships and satisfaction, happiness in family. They perceived the family as a place that should provide support and help with governance of love, peace, cohesiveness, harmony and understanding. They recorded also a topic of raising children.

Category health

It contained mainly answers specifying the person or persons who should be healthy - the most frequent goal was to be healthy and health of close people, a lot of responses concerned the health of loved ones (most frequently with patients), only little less his/her own health. Healthy people rather than patients stated a healthy lifestyle. Sometimes formulation in terms of: health is the most important value, appeared.

Category mental well-being

Answers related to feelings of satisfaction, peace and happiness. Patients are featured responses expressing a desire for life securities.

Category work

It included themes of work, employment, profession - his/her own work was most mentioned, and then the same number of responses focused on career and caring for family members to have a job and succeed in it. A number of formulations expressed a goal to have a job. The patients had a topic of having secured job.

Patients and healthy persons expected peace, satisfaction and financial security at work they also show the importance of interpersonal relationships in the workplace, the work to be interesting, allowing self-realization.

Category living conditions

It contained topics related to awareness of society, nature - respondents mostly wished for world peace, the same number of responses went to topics about environment and events in society, politics. Patients recorded answers about social security.

Category interpersonal relationships

It contained mainly friendly relations and relationships with people in general - in connection with this, the respondents mentioned love, understanding and harmony between people. Some of them were also aware of their own share in relationships and reported character behaviour to others (willingness to help, be polite, etc.). Several responses were related to relations with neighbours.

Category education

The answers were mainly related to respondents' own education and training, but also to education of their children.

Category good old age

It included the pursuit of contented old age, some people mentioned self-sufficiency. This category was recorded by both groups of respondents in their elderly age.

Category leisure

It contained a variety of leisure activities, rest was mentioned only exceptionally. As for activities, respondents most frequently reported sport, followed by gardening, culture, travel, household chores, but also reading, nature (including walks in the countryside) and others.

Category material security

In both groups it related to material and financial security, provisions. About 2/3 of answers were formed by subcategory finance, 1/3 was associated with housing.

Category spiritual dimension

It included topics related to faith or spiritual life. There were not only traditional religious answers (God, prayer, etc.), but also answers expressing some sort of overlap (spiritual growth, to understand the meaning of life, respect for life, look for better side of matters, etc.)

7.6 Determination of proximity of relations (correlation) between the monitored variables particularly in regards to results of SEIQoL method

1. Patients more satisfied with life, healthy people more satisfied with life and healthy people reporting about higher quality of life were more resilient (rather with internal locus of control, with a higher sense of coherence), perceived higher social support and were less anxious and depressed. Results of all questionnaires and scales in patients were more dependent of level of life satisfaction than total quality of life consisting of different areas.
2. The results of all methods used for patients do not depend on the length of diagnosis, nor the age or marital status as in the control group, they usually only moderately correlate with recent in/experienced life changes. Educated patients and educated healthy people have a higher sense of coherence and are less anxious.

Our findings regarding the relationship of other variables to measure satisfaction and overall quality of life correspond with the findings reported in several studies (e.g. Matuz, 2006) as well as in literature about health psychology (e.g. Kebza, 2005; Křivohlavý, 2009).

7.7 Factor analysis of a questionnaire for coping strategies COPE

1. We identified four types of general coping strategies based on preference or rejection of some partial methods of coping, as measured using the COPE method. They were strategies that we called strategy of active, constructive coping, a passive strategy, a emotion-focused strategy and strategy for obtaining a distance.

In many respects, our results correspond with Vašina's (2002) findings.

7.8 Comparison of results of people depending on their economic activity

For completeness, we mapped the psychosocial factors of patients with thyroid gland, depending on their economic activity. Patients with thyroid gland didn´t show any statistically significant differences in any of the examined characteristics between economically active people and pensioners. In this case an intervening variable is obviously important- most likely it is the thyroid gland disease.

Whereas in old-age pensioners not suffering from thyroid disease we found significantly higher levels of anxiousness ($p < 0,01$) compared with healthy economically active people. Compared to old-age pensioners not suffering from thyroid disease, healthy economically active people scored significantly in sense of coherence ($p < 0,05$) and had more internal locus of control ($p = 0,055$). Higher levels of anxiousness in old-age pensioners is probably related to their age and situation, as well as feeling that their life is determined by external circumstances, which they cannot affect. Křivohlavý (2009) indicates higher anxiety associated with a lower level of sense of coherence.

7.9 Results from semi-structured interviews

1. Many patients did not felt subjectively well, long before the correct diagnosis was established. Thyroid disease in the early days was often mistaken for mental illness - by both healthcare professionals and patients who then feared to search the doctors.
2. Patients in the time before surgery reported diverse and varying physical and mental symptoms - especially tiredness, anxiety, irritability, sadness.
3. The patients considered a psychological stress as the most common reason for a disease breakout (roughly half of patients). All expected a full recovery after the surgery, which is not possible.
4. At the time of surgery, patients felt social support from their families, but not at work. They rather feared situations at work, and thought they might lose their jobs.
5. The patients gave the impression of overestimating (idealizing) the situation when evaluating satisfaction for each category, especially at the time of surgery, and a little after 3 months.
6. Patients would need more information about the recovery, especially in the first 3 months, (primarily about the state of scars) and further prognosis for thyreopathy.
7. Satisfaction or dissatisfaction, which they expressed with their health status, related to whether and to what extent they experienced difficulties resulting from illness prior to surgery, and whether and with what effect they have been previously treated. The patients, who experienced difficulties resulting from their disease and hadn´t been cured, were more satisfied with their health status after the surgery.

8. If patients had no difficulties after the surgery, they believed that they will feel as good in future. If they had difficulties, they hoped to feel better.
9. Patients with cancer experienced disease differently than others. There were significant interindividual differences in coping with illness. 3 months after surgery, when they often responded with denial, were more dissatisfied with their condition than other patients. It was difficult for them to tell their close ones diagnosis. Compared to other patients, the topic of disease was topical even after 6 month after the surgery. In this time, one patient with cancer showed so called posttraumatic growth.
10. During follow up, patients reported more positive than negative consequences of surgery. As the most positive they considered improvement of health, further re-evaluation of values, which could indicate the direction to posttraumatic growth (comp. Costa & Pakenham, 2011). As the most negative consequences of the surgery they reported a scar and use of medication.

Overall, we observed three types of attitudes to an interview. The first type of patients was willing to share their illness and their life experiences. The second type of patients was particularly willing to share their experience with thyroid disease, physical condition, the diagnosis and treatment, in other areas they were less willing to share (seems consistent with the classical biomedical model). The third type consisted of patients who were generally more reserved, and answered any type of questions briefly.

8. Conclusion

Comparisons of people with thyroid gland disease and healthy people, and longitudinal follow up of patients were carried out. In some psychosocial aspects the patients with thyreopathy differ from the general population, which does not suffer from this disease, independently of the thyreopathy type. Statistically, the patients were significantly more anxious and perceived higher social support from family when compared with the control group. The control group scored significantly higher in locus of control and on the edge of significance they felt more satisfied with life than the patients. During the six-month follow up after the surgery, some indicators of quality of life were improved. We found a statistically significant decrease in anxiety and social support. Comprehensibility and the feeling of having my life firmly in my hands increased on the edge of significance. One patient with cancer we even saw so called posttraumatic growth. Results of total quality of life calculated from individual categories cannot be evaluated fully psychometrically, since the situation was most likely overvalued (idealized) by patients mainly during hospitalization and a bit after 3 month after the surgery. Results recorded in graphics on segment line of life satisfaction were more plausible. Life satisfaction and quality of life significantly positively correlated with sense of coherence, with the locus of control and perceived social support, and significantly negatively correlated with anxiety and depression.

Division of patients by type of thyreopathy to nodular goitre (including thyroiditis), hyperthyroidism, and cancer was critical for the research. Patients with eufunctional nodular goitre in some respects also differ from healthy population. These have been studied very rarely; they are even assigned to the control group as healthy people during research on other types of thyreopathies. Patients who benefited from surgery the most were those who had some difficulties before the surgery (usually with hyperthyroidism) they better adapted to the surgery and expressed satisfaction with their condition.

Dissatisfaction or worse quality of life was recorded by patients who had an impression of being without difficulties before the surgery, and suddenly they experience some and must use hormone replacement (usually nodular goitre, rarely carcinomas). The biggest relief is experienced by patients, who had some symptoms and were not treated by other means than surgical, as manifestations of their disease didn´t last long. Patients with thyroid carcinoma differ from other types of thyreopathies the most.

Patients in our country do not have comparable information in terms of quantity and quality when compared to patients in traditionally democratic countries, and they do not have background of patient organizations.

We are aware of the limitations of our work. In particular, it would be necessary to increase the number of surveyed people. It would be necessary to include a larger number of men into the set of surveyed people (but there is low incidence of this disease with men). Members of the control group in our survey honestly declared that they are not, and were not, treated or monitored for thyroid disease. When choosing members of the control group, it would be most suitable to have each member screened for thyreopathy, which would be, on the other hand, costly. When comparing patients with healthy population it would be better to set a paired control group and adjust it according to status and demographic features. In regards to the specificity of the sample, results cannot be generalized or only with some reservations. On the other hand, it is a six-month follow up of almost the entire population of patients who underwent thyroid surgery in one of the hospitals in the Czech Republic, which is very valuable for better exploration of this issue. It would be useful to verify our results in another, similar department or collect data from more departments focusing on thyroid surgeries, in the same time. In future, it would be good to keep only the most informative methods in a battery of tests, in order not to bother the patients unnecessarily. It should be strictly monitored whether patients fill out a questionnaire at the time of hospitalization under the same conditions. As for the longitudinal follow up, it would be necessary to make more than 3 measurements in time to be able to better predict events. It would also be valuable if follow up could last longer than 6 months. Research of patients treated by means other than surgical could be very useful. We believe that it would be very desirable to continue in the research of these issues, because the current findings give us more questions and directions of interest than „finished " and clear answers.

We are not aware of any similar research in the Czech Republic on this topic. The performed research is in such a stage and complexity unique even for the English literature. We believe that this issue deserves a greater attention of researchers and psychotherapists because many of the untreated and treated patients may suffer from a variety of symptoms, experience worse health status and quality of life. It would be useful to concentrate on preoperative preparation of a patient and work with his expectations while doing it.

9. References

Abraham-Nordling et al. (2005). Graves' disease: A long term quality of life follow-up of patients randomized to treatment with antithyroid drugs, radioiodine or surgery. *Thyroid*, Vol.15 (Suppl.1), pp. S27-S28, ISSN 1050-7256

Air et al. (2006). Outdated and missing: A review of the quality of thyroid cancer information on the internet. *Thyroid*, Vol.16, p. 865, ISSN 1050-7256

Air et al. (2007). Thyroid net outdated and incomplete: A review of thyroid cancer on the world wide web. *Thyroid*, Vol.17, pp. 259-265, ISSN 1050-7256

Almeida, J., Vartanian, J. G. & Kowalski L. P. (2009). Clinical predictors of quality of life in patients with initial differentiated thyroid cancers. *Archives of Otolaryngology-Head and Neck Surgery*, Vol.35, pp. 342-346, ISSN 0886-4470

Appelhof, B. C. et al. (2005). Combined therapy with levothyroxine and liothyronine in two ratios, compared with levothyroxine monotherapy in primary hypothyroidism. *Journal of Clinical Endocrinology and Metabolism*, Vol.90, pp. 2666-2674, ISSN 0021-972X

Appolinario, J. C., Fontenelle, L. F., Rodrigues, A. L. C., Segenreich, D. & Fontes, R. (2005). Symptoms of depression and anxiety among patients with subclinical hypothyroidism. *Jornal Brasileiro de Psiquiatria*, Vol.54, pp. 94-97, ISSN 0047-2085

Baldini, M. et al. (1997). Psychopathological and cognitive features in subclinical hypothyroidism. *Progress in Neuro-Psychopharmacology & Biological Psychiatry*, Vol.21, pp. 925-935, ISSN 0278-5846

Baldini, M. et al. (2009). Neuropsychological functions and metabolic aspects in subclinical hypothyroidism: The effects of L-thyroxine. *Progress in Neuro-Psychopharmacology & Biological Psychiatry*, Vol.33, pp. 854-859, ISSN 0278-5846

Baštecká, B. et al. (2003). *Klinická psychologie v praxi*. Portál, ISBN 80-7178-735-3, Prague, Czech Republic

Baštecký, J., Šavlík, J. & Šimek, J. (1993). *Psychosomatická medicína*. Grada Avicenum, ISBN 80-7169-031-7, Prague, Czech Republic

Baumgartner, F. (2001). Zvládanie stresu - coping. In: *Aplikovaná sociální psychologie II.*, J. Výrost, I. Slaměník, (Eds.), 113-128. Grada Publishing, ISBN 80-247-0042-5, Prague, Czech Republic

Bianchi, G. P. et al. (2004). Health-related quality of life in patients with thyroid disorders. *Quality of Life Research*, Vol.13, pp. 45-54, ISSN 0962-9343

Biondi, B. et al. (2000). Endogenous subclinical hyperthyroidism affects quality of life and cardiac morphology and function in young and middle-aged patients. *Journal of Clinical Endocrinology and Metabolism*, Vol.85, pp. 4701-4705, ISSN 0021-972X

Blumenthal, J. A. et al. (1987). Social support, type A behavior, and coronary artery disease. *Psychosomatic Medicine*, Vol.49, pp. 331-340, ISSN 0033-3174

Bono, G., Fancellu, R., Blandini, F., Santoro, G. & Mauri, M. (2004). Cognitive and affective status in mild hypothyroidism and interactions with L-thyroxine treatment. *Acta Neurologica Scandinavica*, Vol.110, pp. 59-66, ISSN 0001-6314

Botella-Carretero, J. I., Galán, J. M., Caballero, C., Sancho, J. & Escobar-Morreale, H. F. (2003). Quality of life and psychometric functionality in patients with differentiated thyroid carcinoma. *Endocrine-Related Cancer*, Vol.10, pp. 601–610, ISSN 1351-0088

Brown, B. T., Bonello, R., Pollard, H. & Graham, P. (2010). The influence of a biopsychosocial-based treatment approach to primary overt hypothyroidism: a protocol for a pilot study. *Trials*, Vol.11, No.106, ISSN 1745-6215

Břicháček, V. (2006). Dlouhodobé výzkumné projekty v psychologii zdraví. In: *Psychologie zdraví a kvalita života*, B. Koukola, J. Mareš, (Eds.), 116-117, MSD, ISBN 80-86633-66-7, Brno, Czech Republic

Buchtová, B. (2004). Kvalita života dlouhodobě nezaměstnaných. *Československá psychologie*, Vol.48, pp. 121- 135, ISSN 0009-062X

Bunevičius, R., Kažanavičius, G., Žalinkevičius, R. & Prange, A. J. Jr (1999). Effects of thyroxine as compared with thyroxine plus triiodothyronine in patients with hypothyroidism. *New England Journal of Medicine*, Vol.340, pp. 424-429, ISSN 0028-4793

Bunevičius, R. & Prange, A. J. Jr (2000). Mental improvement after replacement therapy with thyroxine plus triiodothyronine: Relationship to cause of hypothyroidism. *International Journal of Neuropsychopharmacology*, Vol.3, pp. 167-174, ISSN 1461-1457

Bunevičius, R. et al. (2002). Thyroxine vs thyroxine plus triiodothyronine in treatment of hypothyroidism after thyroidectomy for Graves' disease. *Endocrine*, Vol.18, pp. 129-133, ISSN 1355-008X

Caparevic, Z. V., Diligenski, V. M., Stojanovic, D. M. & Bojkovic, G. D. (2005). Psychological evaluation of patients with a nodular goiter before and after surgical treatment. *Advances in psychology research*, Vol.37, pp. 47-61), ISSN 1532-723X

Carver, Ch. S., Scheier, M. F. & Weintraub, J. K. (1989). Assesing coping strategies: A theoretically based approach. *Journal of Personality and Social Psychology*, Vol.56, pp. 267-283, ISSN 0022-3514

Clyde, P. W et al. (2003). Combined levothyroxine plus liothyronine compared with levothyroxine alone in primary hypothyroidism. *JAMA*, Vol.290, pp. 2952-2958, ISSN 0098-7484

Costa, R. V. & Pakenham, K. I. (2011). Associations between benefit finding and adjustment outcomes in thyroid cancer. *Psychooncology*, Mar 17. doi: 10.1002/pon.1960, ISSN 1057-9249

Dietlein, M. & Schicha, H. (2003). Lifetime follow-up care is necessary for all patients with treated thyroid nodules. *European Journal of Endocrinology*, Vol.148, pp. 377-379, ISSN 0804-4643

Dow, K. H., Ferrell, B. R. & Anello, C. (1997). Quality- of-life changes in patients with thyroid cancer after withdrawal of thyroid hormone therapy. *Thyroid*, Vol.7, pp. 613-619, ISSN 1050-7256

Duntas, L. H. & Biondi, B. (2007). Short-term hypothyroidism after levothyroxine-withdrawal in patients with differentiated thyroid cancer: clinical and quality of life consequences. *European Journal of Endocrinology*, Vol.156, pp. 13-19, ISSN 0804-4643

Egle, U. T. et al. (1999). The relevance of physical and psychosocial factors for the quality of life in patients with thyroid-associated orbitopathy (TAO). *Experimental and Clinical Endocrinology and Diabetes*, Vol.107 (Suppl.5), pp. S168 - S171, ISSN 0947-7349

Elberling, T. V. et al. (2004). Impaired health-related quality of life in Graves' disease. A prospective study. *European Journal of Endocrinology*, Vol.151, pp. 549-555, ISSN 0804-4643

Estcourt, S., Vaidya, B., Quinn, A. & Shepherd, M. (2008). The impact of thyroid eye disease upon patients' wellbeing: a qualitative analysis.*Clinical Endocrinology*, Vol.68, No.4, pp.635-639, ISSN 0300-0664

Eustatia-Rutten, C. F. A. et al. (2006). Quality of life in longterm exogenous subclinical hyperthyroidism and the effects of restoration of euthyroidism, a randomized controlled trial. *Clinical Endocrinology*, Vol.64, pp. 284-291, ISSN 0300-0664

Fahrenfort, J. J., Wilterdink, A. M. & van der Veen, E. A. (2000). Long-term residual complaints and psychological sequelae after remission, of hyperthyroidism. *Psychoneuroendocrinology*, Vol.25, pp. 201-211, ISSN 0306-4530

Ferjenčík, J. (2010). *Úvod do metodologie psychologického výzkumu* (2nd ed.), Portál, ISBN 978-80-7367-815-9, Prague, Czech Republic

Filická, K., Hadačová, M. (2006). Úloha sestry v terapeutickom procese endokrinných ochorení - špecifiká a význam informovanosti pacienta. *Diabetologie, metabolismus, endokrinologie, výživa*, No.3, p. 145, ISSN 1211-9326

Fukao, A. et al. (2003). The relationship of psychological factors to the prognosis of hyperthyroidism in antithyroid drug-treated patients with Graves' disease. *Clinical Endocrinology*, Vol.58, pp. 550-551, ISSN 0300-0664

Gerding, M. N. et al. (1997). Quality of life in patients with Graves' ophthalmopathy is markedly decreased: Measurement by the medical outcomes study instrument. *Thyroid*, Vol.6, pp. 885-889, ISSN 1050-7256

Giusti, M. et al. (2011). Five-year longitudinal evaluation of quality of life in a cohort of patients with differentiated thyroid carcinoma. *Journal of Zhejiang University. Science. B.*, Vol.12, No.3, pp. 163-173, ISSN 1673-1581

Gómez, M. M. N., Gutiérrez, R. M. V., Castellanos, S. A. O., Vergara, M. P. & Pradilla, Y. K. R. (2010). Psychological well-being and quality of life in patients treated for thyroid cancer after surgery. *Terapia Psicológica*, Vol.28, No.1, pp. 69-84, ISSN 0716-6184

Grozinsky-Glasberg, S., Fraser, A., Nahshoni, E., Weizman, A. & Leibovici, L. (2006). Thyroxine-triiodthyronine combination therapy versus thyroxine monotherapy for clinical hypothyroidism: Meta-analysis of randomized controlled trials. *Journal of Clinical Endocrinology and Metabolism*, Vol.91, pp. 2592-2599, ISSN 0021-972X

Harineková, M. (1976). Struma v školskom veku a jej odraz v psychickej oblasti. *Československá psychologie*, Vol.20, pp. 257-258, ISSN 0009-062X

Harris, T., Creed, F. & Brugha, T. S. (1992). Stressful life events and Graves' disease. *British Journal of Psychiatry*, Vol.161, pp. 535-541, ISSN 0007-1250

Haškovcová, H. (1985). *Spoutaný život*, Panorama, Prague, Czech Republic

Hendl, J. (2006). *Přehled statistických metod zpracování dat: analýza metaanalýza dat* (2nd ed.), Portál, ISBN 80-7178-820-1, Prague, Czech Republic

Hendl, J. (2009). *Kvalitativní výzkum* (2nd ed.), Portál, ISBN 978-80-7367-485-4, Prague, Czech Republic

Hirsch, D. et al. (2009). Illness perception in patients with differentiated epithelial cell thyroid cancer. *Thyroid*, Vol.19, No.5, pp. 459-65, ISSN 1050-7256

Hobbs, J. R. (1992). Stress and Graves' disease. *Lancet*, Vol.339, pp. 427-428, ISSN 0140-6736

Hodačová, L. (2007). Posttraumatický rozvoj a změna v prožívání spirituality. In: *Kvalita života u dětí a dospívajících II.*, J. Mareš et al., (Eds.), 35-47, MSD, ISBN 987-80-7392-009-8, Brno, Czech Republic

Hoftijzer, H. C. et al. (2008). Quality of life in cured patients with differentiated thyroid carcinoma. *Journal of Clinical Endocrinology and Metabolism*, Vol.93, No.1, pp. 200-203, ISSN 0021-972X

Hou, T. et al. (2001). Quality of life of patients operated on for thyroid tumor. *Chinese Mental Health Journal*, Vol.15, pp. 312-314, ISSN 1000-6729

Huang, S. M., Lee, CH. H, Chien, L. Y., Liu H. E. & Tai, Ch. J. (2004). Postoperative quality of life among patients with thyroid cancer. *Journal of Advanced Nursing*, Vol.47, pp. 492-499, ISSN 0309-2402

Janečková, P. (2001). *Problematika psychické zátěže u tyreopatie* (Dissertation), FF UP, Olomouc, Czech Republic

Janečková, P. (2006). Psychological distress in patients with thyroid gland disease. *Homeostasis in Health and Diseases*, Vol.44, No.1-2, pp. 83-87, ISSN 0960-7560

Janečková, P. (2007a). Psychosocial aspects of thyroid disease. Proceedings of *10th European Congress of Psychology* (Mapping of Psychological Knowledge), ISBN 978-80-7064-017-2, ČMPS, Prague, Czech Republic, July

Janečková, P. (2007b). Současné výzkumy psychosociálních aspektů tyreopatie. *Československá psychologie*, Vol.51, No.6, pp. 635-654, ISSN 0009-062X

Janečková, P. (2007c). Výzkum psychosociálních aspektů tyreopatie. In: *Psychologie zdraví a kvalita života II.*, B. Koukola, J. Mareš, (Eds.), 36-41, MSD, ISBN 987-80-7392-009-8, Brno, Czech Republic

Janečková, P. (2008a). Onemocnění štítné žlázy z psychosociálního hlediska/Zjištění o kvalitě života/. In: *Psychologie zdraví a kvalita života 2008*, B. Koukola, J. Mareš, (Eds.), 45-53, MSD, ISBN 978-80-7392-074-6, Brno, Czech Republic

Janečková, P. (2008b). *Psychosociální aspekty tyreopatie* (Dissertation), FSS MU, Brno, Czech Republic

Janečková, P. (2008c). Základní poznatky z výzkumů psychosociálních aspektů onemocnění štítné žlázy. Proceedings of *Dokbat*, ISBN 978-80-7318-664-7, UTB, Zlín, Czech Republic, April

Jenšovský, J., Špačková, N., Hejduková, B. & Růžička, E. (2000). Vliv normalizace izolovaně zvýšeného TSH na neuropsychologický profil pacientů. *Časopis lékařů českých*, Vol.139, No.10, pp. 313-316, ISSN 0008-7335

Jenšovský, J., Růžička, E., Špačková, N. & Hejduková, B. (2002). Changes of event related potential and cognitive processes in patients with subclinical hypothyroidism after thyroxine treatment. *Endocrine regulations*, Vol.36, pp. 115-122, ISSN 1210-0668

Joffe, R. T. et al. (2004). Does substitution of T4 with T3 plus T4 for T4 replacement improve depressive symptoms in patients with hypothyroidism? *Annals of the New York Academy of Sciences*, Vol.1032, pp. 287-88, ISSN 0077-8923

Jorde, R. et al. (2006). Neuropsychological function and symptoms in subjects with subclinical hypothyroidism and the effect of thyroxine treatment. *Journal of Clinical Endocrinology and Metabolism*, Vol.91, pp. 145-153, ISSN 0021-972X

Kahaly, G. J., Hardt, J., Petrak, F. & Egle, U. T. (2002). Psychosocial factors in subjects with thyroid - associated ophthalmopathy. *Thyroid*, Vol.12, s. 237-239, ISSN 1050-7256

Kahaly, G. J., Petrak, F., Hardt, J., Pitz, S. & Egle, U. T. (2005). Psychosocial morbidity of Graves' orbitopathy. *Clinical Endocrinology*, Vol.63, pp. 395-402, ISSN 0300-0664

Kaplan, H. I., Sadock & B. J., Grebb, J. A. (1994). *Synopsis of Psychiatry: Behavioral Sciences, Clinical Psychiatry* (7th ed.). Williams & Wilkins, Baltimore, USA

Kaplan, M. M., Sarne, D. H. & Schneider, A. B. (2003). In search of the impossible dream? Thyroid hormone replacement therapy that treats all symptoms in all hypothyroid patients. *Journal of Clinical Endocrinology and Metabolism*, Vol.88, pp. 4540-4542, ISSN 0021-972X

Kebza, V. (2005). *Psychosociální determinanty zdraví*, Academia, ISBN 80-200-1307-5, Prague, Czech Republic

Kebza, V. & Šolcová, I. (2008). Hlavní koncepce psychické odolnosti. *Československá psychologie*, Vol.52, pp. 1-19, ISSN 0009-062X

König, D., Jagsch, R., Beirer, A., Kryspin-Exner, I. & Koriska, K. (2007). Patient reported outcomes in treatment for thyroid diseases. Proceedings of *10th European Congress of Psychology* (Mapping of Psychological Knowledge), ISBN 978-80-7064-017-2, ČMPS, Prague, Czech Republic, July

Koukola, B. & Ondřejová, E. (2006). Kvalita života vysokoškoláků zjišťovaná metodou SEIQoL. In: *Psychologie zdraví a kvalita života*, B. Koukola, J. Mareš, (Eds.), 149-151, MSD, ISBN 80-86633-66-7, Brno, Czech Republic

Křivohlavý, J. (1990). Nezdolnost v pojetí SOC. *Československá psychologie*, Vol.34, pp. 511 - 517, ISSN 0009-062X

Křivohlavý, J. (2002). *Psychologie nemoci*, Grada Publishing, ISBN 80-247-0179-0, Prague, Czech Republic

Křivohlavý, J. (2009). *Psychologie zdraví* (2nd ed.), Portál, ISBN 978-80-7367-568-4, Prague, Czech Republic

Křivohlavý, J. (2010). *Pozitivní psychologie* (2nd ed.), Portál, ISBN 978-80-7367-726-8, Prague, Czech Republic

Křížová, E. (2005). Sociologické podmínky kvality života. In: *Kvalita života a zdraví*, J. Payne et al., (Eds.), 351-364, Triton, ISBN 80-7254-657-0, Prague, Czech Republic

Kukleta, M. (2001). Psychosocial stress and health. *Homeostasis in Health and Diseases*, Vol.41, No.1-2, pp.35-40, ISSN 0960-7560

Kung, A. W. C. (1995). Life events, daily stresses and coping in patients with Graves' disease. *Clinical Endocrinology*, Vol.42, pp. 303-308, ISSN 0300-0664

Lamberts, S. W. J., Romijn, J. A. & Wiersinga, W. M. (2003). The future endocrine patient. Reflections on the future of clinical endocrinology. *European Journal of Endocrinology*, Vol.149, pp. 169-175, ISSN 0804-4643

Lee, I. T. et al. (2003). Relationship of stressful life events, anxiety and depression to hyperthyroidism in an asian population. *Hormone Research*, Vol.60, pp. 247-251, ISSN 0301-0163

Lee, J. I. et al. (2010). Decreased health-related quality of life in disease-free survivors of differentiated thyroid cancer in Korea. *Health and Quality of Life Outcomes*, Vol.8, No.101, ISSN 1477-7525

Lincoln, N. B. et al. (2000). Patient education in thyrotoxicosis. *Patient Education and Counseling*, Vol.40, pp. 143-149, ISSN 0738-3991

Ma, L., Luo, G. & Zeng Z. (2002). Psychological factors in patients with Graves' Disease. *Chinese Mental Health Journal*, Vol.16, p. 616, ISSN 1000-6729

Ma, C. et al. (2009). Thyroxine alone or thyroxine plus triiodothyronine replacement therapy for hypothyroidism. *Nuclear Medicine Communications*, Vol.30, No.8, pp. 586-593, ISSN 0143-3636

Malterling, R. R. et al. (2010). Differentiated thyroid cancer in a Swedish county - long-term results and quality of life. *Acta Oncologica*, Vol.49, pp. 454–459, ISSN 0284-186X

Mandincová, P. (2008a). Česká studie psychosociálních aspektů onemocnění štítné žlázy. Proceedings of *XXVI. Psychologické dny*, ISBN 978-80-210-4938-3, FSS MU & ČMPS, Brno, Czech Republic, September

Mandincová, P. (2008b). Primární a sekundární prevence tyreopatie–pohled psychologa. Proceedings of *Integrující přístupy k prevenci a péči o zdraví*, ISBN 978-80-7318-778-1, UTB, Zlín, Czech Republic, November

Mandincová, P. (2009a). Některé psychosociální ukazatele kvality života a ekonomická aktivita. Proceedings of *Dokbat*, ISBN 978-80-7318-811-5, UTB, Zlín, Czech Republic, April

Mandincová, P. (2009b). Klíčové oblasti kvality života u pacientů operovaných pro onemocnění štítné žlázy. Proceedings of *Konference psychologie zdraví*, ČMPS, Vernířovice, Czech Republic, May

Mandincová, P. (2010). Psychosociální pomoc pacientům s onemocněním štítné žlázy. Proceedings of *Konference psychologie zdraví*, ČMPS, Vernířovice, Czech Republic, May

Mandincová, P. (2011a). Pohled pacientů na onemocnění štítné žlázy. Proceedings of *Konference psychologie zdraví*, ČMPS, Vernířovice, Czech Republic, May

Mandincová, P. (2011b) *Psychosociální aspekty péče o nemocného: Onemocnění štítné žlázy*, Grada Publishing, ISBN 978-80-247-3811-6, Prague, Czech Republic

Markalous, B. & Gregorová, M. (2007). *Nemoci štítné žlázy – otázky a odpovědi pro pacienty a jejich rodiny* (3rd ed.), Triton, ISBN 80-7254-961-8, Prague, Czech Republic

Mareš, J. (2001). Pozitivní psychologie: důvod k zamyšlení i výzva. *Československá psychologie*, Vol.45, pp. 97-117, ISSN 0009-062X

Mareš, J. (2005). Kvalita života a její proměny v čase u téhož jedince. *Československá psychologie*, Vol.49, pp. 19-33, ISSN 0009-062X

Mareš, J. (2007). Posttraumatický rozvoj u dětí a dospívajících. In: *Kvalita života u dětí a dospívajících II.*, J. Mareš et al., (Eds.), 9-33, MSD, ISBN 978-80-7392-008-1, Brno, Czech Republic

Mareš, J. (2008). Posttraumatický rozvoj: nové pohledy, nové teorie a modely. *Československá psychologie*, Vol.52, No.6, pp. 567-583, ISSN 0009-062X

Mareš, J. (2009). Posttraumatický rozvoj: výzkum, diagnostika, intervence. *Československá psychologie*, Vol.53, No.3, pp. 271-290, ISSN 0009-062X

Mareš, J., Rybářová, M. & Tůmová, Š. (2007). Posttraumatický rozvoj mediků. In: *Kvalita života u dětí u dospívajících II.*, J. Mareš et al., (Eds.), 225-234, MSD, ISBN 978-80-7392-008-1, Brno, Czech Republic

Matos-Santos, A. et al. (2001). Relationship between the number of impact of stressful life events and the onset of Graves' disease and toxic nodular goitre. *Clinical Endocrinology*, Vol.55, pp. 15-19, ISSN 0300-0664

Matuz, T. (2006). End of life decisions and psychological aspects in amyotrophic lateral sclerosis - empirical ethics and neuropsychological approaches. Proceedings of *17th International Symposium on ALS/MND*, Yokohama, Japan, November

McMillan et al. (2004). Design of new questionnaires to measure quality of life and treatment satisfaction in hypothyroidism. *Thyroid*, Vol.14, pp. 916-925, ISSN 1050-7256

McMillan, C. V., Bradley, C., Razvi, S. & Weaver, J. U. (2005). Psychometric validation of new measures of hypothyroid-dependent quality of life (QoL) and symptoms. *Endocrine Abstracts*, Vol.9, P151, ISSN 1470-3947

McMillan, C. V., Bradley, C., Razvi, S. & Weaver, J. U. (2008). Evaluation of new Measures of the impact of hypothyroidism on quality of life and symptoms: The ThyDQoL and ThySRQ. *Value in Health*, Vol.11, No.2, pp. 285-294, ISSN 1098-3015

Meng,W. et al. (2004). Replacement therapy with thyroxine plus triiodothyronine (14 : 1) is not superior to thyroxine alone with respect to the psychical and physical wellbeing of patients with hypothyroidism. *Experimental and Clinical Endocrinology and Diabetes*, Vol.112, p. S26, ISSN 0947-7349

Miovský, M. (2006). *Kvalitativní výzkum a metody v psychologickém výzkumu*, Grada Publishing, ISBN 80-247-1362-4, Prague, Czech Republic

Mizokami, T., Wu Li, A., El-Kaissi, S. & Wall, J. R. (2004). Stresss and thyroid autoimmunity. *Thyroid*, Vol.14, pp. 1047-1055, ISSN 1050-7256

Mohapl, P. (1992). *Úvod do psychologie nemoci a zdraví*, UP, Olomouc, Czech Republic

Monzani, F. et al. (1993). Subclinical hypothyroidism: Neurobehavioral features and beneficial effect of L-thyroxine treatment. *Journal of Clinical Investigation*, Vol.71, pp. 367-371, ISSN 0021-9738

Moons, P., Marquet, K., Budts, W. & De Geest, S. (2004). Validity, reliability and responsiveness of the „Schedule for the Evaluation of Individual Quality of Life – Direct Weighting" (SEIQoL-DW) in congenital heart disease. *Health and Quality of Life Outcomes*, Vol.2, No.27, ISSN 1477-7525

Nygaard, B., Jensen, E. W., Kvetny, J., Jarløv, A. & Faber, J. (2009). Effect of combination therapy with thyroxine (T4) and 3,5,30-triiodothyronine versus T4 monotherapy in patients with hypothyroidism, a double-blind, randomised cross-over study. *European Journal of Endocrinology*, Vol.161, pp. 895–902, ISSN 0804-4643

O'Boyle, C. A., Browne, J., Hickey, A., McGee, H. & Joyce, C. R. B. (1995). *Schedule for the Evaluation of Individual Quality of Life (SEIQoL): a Direct Weighting procedure for Quality of Life Domains (SEIQoL-DW)* (Administration Manual), Royal College of Surgeons Dublin, Ireland

Olosová, Ľ., Filická, A. (2006). Úloha sestry v diagnotickom procese endokrinných ochorení – špecifiká a význam informovanosti pacienta. *Diabetologie, metabolismus, endokrinologie, výživa*, No.3, p. 147, ISSN 1211-9326

Pacini, F. et al. (2006). Radioiodine ablation of thyroid remnants after preparation with recombinant human thyrotropin in differentiated thyroid carcinoma: Results of an international, randomized, controlled study. *Journal of Clinical Endocrinology and Metabolism*, Vol.91, pp. 926-932, ISSN 0021-972X

Park, Y. J. et al. (2010). Subclinical hypothyroidism (SCH) is not associated with metabolic derangement, cognitive impairment, depression or poor quality of life (QoL) in elderly subjects. *Archives of Gerontology and Geriatrics*, Vol.50, pp. e68–e73, ISSN 0167-4943

Parle, J. et al. (2010). A randomized controlled trial of the effect of thyroxine replacement on cognitive function in community-living elderly subjects with subclinical hypothyroidism: The Birmingham elderly thyroid study. *Journal of Clinical Endocrinology and Metabolism*, Vol.95, No.8, pp. 3623–3632, ISSN 0021-972X

Pelttari, H., Sintonen, H., Schalin-Jäntti, C. & Välimäki, M. J. (2009). Health-related quality of life in long-term follow-up of patients with cured TNM Stage I or II differentiated thyroid carcinoma. *Clinical Endocrinology*, Vol.70, No.3, pp. 493-7, ISSN 0300-0664

Ponto, K. A. & Kahaly, G. J. (2010). Quality of life in patients suffering from thyroid orbitopathy. *Pediatric endocrinology reviews*, Vol.7 (Suppl.2), pp. 245-249, ISSN 1565-4753

Radosavljević, V. R., Janković, S. M. & Marinković, J. M. (1996). Stressful life events in the pathogenesis of Graves' disease. *European Journal of Endocrinology*, Vol.134, pp. 699-701, ISSN 0804-4643

Razvi, S., Ingoe, L. E., McMillan, C. V. & Weaver, J. U. (2005). Health status in patients with sub-clinical hypothyroidism. *European Journal of Endocrinology*, Vol.152, pp. 713-717, ISSN 0804-4643

Razvi, S., McMillan, C. V. & Weaver, J. U. (2005). Instruments used in measuring symptoms, health status and quality of life in hypothyroidism: a systematic qualitative review. *Clinical Endocrinology*, Vol.63, pp. 617-624, ISSN 0300-0664

Regalbuto, C. et al. (2007). Effects of either LT4 monotherapy or LT4/LT3 combined therapy in patients totally thyroidectomized for thyroid cancer. *Thyroid*, Vol.17, pp. 323-331, ISSN 1050-7256

Reiterová, E. (2007). *Statistické metody v psychologickém výzkumu*, FF UP, ISBN 978-80-244-1678-6, Olomouc, Czech Republic

Reiterová, E. (2009). *Základy statistiky pro studenty psychologie* (3rd ed.), FF UP, ISBN 978-80-244-2316-6, Olomouc, Czech Republic

Reynolds, W. M. & Gould, J. W. (1981). A Psychometric Investigation of the Standard and Short Form Beck Depression Inventory. *Journal of Consulting and Clinical Psychology*, Vol.49, pp. 306-307, ISSN 0022-006X

Robbins, L. R. & Vinson, D. B. (1960). Objective psychologic assessment of the thyrotoxic patient and the response to treatment: preliminary report. *Journal of Clinical Endocrinology*, Vol.20, pp. 120-129, ISSN 0368-1610

Roberts, K. J., Lepore, S. J. & Urken, M. L. (2008). Quality of life after thyroid cancer: An assessment of patient needs and preferences for information and support. *Journal of Cancer Education*, Vol.23, No.3, pp. 186-191, ISSN 0885-8195

Rodewig, K. (1993). Psychosomatische Aspekte der Hyperthyreose unter besonderer Berücksichtigung des Morbus Basedow. Ein Überblick. *Psychotherapie, Psychosomatik, medizinische Psychologie*, Vol.43, pp. 271-277, ISSN 0937-2032

Romijn, J. A., Smit, J. W. A. & Lamberts, S. W. J. (2003). Intrinsic imperfections of endocrine replacement therapy. *European Journal of Endocrinology*, Vol.149, pp. 91-97, ISSN 0804-4643

Rosch, P. J. (1993). Stressful life events and Graves' disease. *Lancet*, Vol.342, pp. 566-567, ISSN 0140-6736

Rybářová, M., Mareš, J., Ježek, S. & Tůmová, Š. (2006). Kvalita života vysokoškoláků zjišťována zjednodušenou metodou SEIQoL. In: *Kvalita života u dětí a dospívajících I.*, J. Mareš et al., (Eds.), 189-198, MSD, ISBN 80-86633-65-9, Brno, Czech Republic

Řehulka, E., Řehulková, O. (2003). Teachers and quality of life. In: *Teachers and health 5*, E. Řehulka, (Ed.), 177-197, Nakladatelství Pavel Křepela, ISBN 80-8669-02-5, Brno, Czech Republic

Saravanan, P. et al. (2002). Psychological well-being in patients on 'adequate' doses of L-thyroxine: results of a large, controlled community-based questionnaire study. *Clinical Endocrinology*, Vol.57, pp. 577-585, ISSN 0300-0664

Saravanan, P. et al. (2005). Partial substitution of thyroxine (T4) with tri-iodothyronine in patients on T4 replacement therapy. *Journal of Clinical Endocrinology and Metabolism*, Vol.90, pp. 805-812, ISSN 0021-972X

Sawka, A. M. et al. (2003). Does a combination regimen of thyroxine (T4) and 3,5,3' - triiodothyronine improve depressive symptoms better than T4 alone in patients with hypothyroidism? *Journal of Clinical Endocrinology and Metabolism*, Vol.88, pp. 4551-4555, ISSN 0021-972X

Sawka, A. M. et al. (2009). The impact of thyroid cancer and post-surgical radioactive iodine treatment on the lives of thyroid cancer survivors: A qualitative study. *PLoS One*, Vol.4, No.1, e4191, ISSN 1932-6203

Sawka, A. M. et al. (2011). How can we meet the information needs of patients with early stage papillary thyroid cancer considering radioactive iodine remnant ablation? *Clinical Endocrinology*, Vol.74, No.4, pp. 419-23, ISSN 0300-0664

Seligman, M. (2000). Positive psychology. In: *The Science of Optimism and Hope (Research Essays in Honor of Martin E. P. Seligman)*, J. E. Gillham, (Ed.), 415-429, Templeton Foundation Press, ISBN 978-1-890151-26-3, Philadelphia, USA

Schnyder, N. et al. (2000). Antonovsky's sense of coherence: Trait or state? *Psychotherapy and Psychosomatics*, Vol.69, pp. 296-302, ISSN 0033-3190

Schreiber, V. (1985). *Stres: Patofyziologie, endokrinologie, klinika*, Avicenum, Prague, Czech Republic

Schroeder, P. R. et al. (2006). A comparison of short-term changes in health-related quality of life in thyroid carcinoma patients undergoing diagnostic evaluation with recombinant human thyrotropin compared with thyroid hormone withdrawal. *Journal of Clinical Endocrinology and Metabolism*, Vol.91, pp. 878-884, ISSN 0021-972X

Siegmund, W. et al. (2004). Replacement therapy with levothyroxine plus triiodothyronine (bioavailable molar ratio 14 : 1) is not superior to thyroxine alone to improve well-being and cognitive performance in hypothyroidism. *Clinical Endocrinology*, Vol.60, pp. 750-757, ISSN 0300-0664

Sinclair, D. L. (2006). The interface of psychology and thyroid disorders. *Dissertation Abstracts International. Section B: Physical Sciences and Engineering*, Vol.66, 12-B, p. 6936, ISSN 0419-4217

Silverman, D. (2005). *Ako robiť kvalitatívny výskum: praktická příručka*, Ikar, ISBN 80-551-0904-4, Bratislava, Slovakia

Sonino, N. & Fava, G. A. (1998). Psychological aspects of endocrine disease. *Clinical Endocrinology*, Vol.49, pp. 1-7, ISSN 0300-0664

Sonino, N. et al. (1993). Life events in the pathogenesis of Graves' disease. A controlled study. *Acta Endocrinologica*, Vol.128, pp. 293-296, ISSN 0001-5598

Spielberger, C. D. (1980). *Dotazník na meranie úzkosti a úzkostlivosti STAI*. Psychodiagnostika, Bratislava, Slovakia

Stárka, L. & Zamrazil, V. et al. (2005). *Základy klinické endokrinologie* (2nd ed.). Maxdorf, ISBN 80-7345-066-6, Prague, Czech Republic

Tagay, S. et al. (2005). Health-related quality of life, anxiety and depression in thyroid cancer patients under short-term hypothyroidism and TSH-suppressive levothyroxine treatment. *European Journal of Endocrinology*, Vol.153, pp. 755-763, ISSN 0804-4643

Terwee, C. B., Gerding, M. N., Dekker, F. W., Prummel, M. F. & Wiersinga, W. M. (1998). Development of a disease specific quality od life questionnaire for patients with Graves' ophtalmopathy: the GO-QOL. *British Journal of Ophthalmology*, Vol.82, pp. 773-779, ISSN 0007-1161

Terwee, C. B. et al. (1999). Test-retest reliability of the GO-QOL: a disease-specific quality of life questionnaire for patients with Graves' ophthalmopathy. *Journal of Clinical Epidemiology*, Vol.52, pp. 875-84, ISSN 0895-4356

Terwee, C. B. et al. (2001). Interpretation and validity of changes in scores on the Graves' ophthalmopathy quality of life questionnaire (GO-QOL) after different treatments. *Clinical Endocrinology*, Vol.54, pp. 391-398, ISSN 0300-0664

Terwee, C. B. et al. (2002). Long-term effects of Graves' ophthalmopathy on health-related quality of life. *European Journal of Endocrinology*, Vol.146, pp. 751-757, ISSN 0804-4643

Tschuschke, V. (2004). *Psychoonkologie: psychologické aspekty vzniku a zvládnutí rakoviny*, Portál, ISBN 80-7178-826-0, Prague, Czech Republic

Vašina, B. (1999). *Psychologie zdraví*, FF OV, Ostrava, Czech Republic

Vašina, B. (2002). Osobnostní vlastnosti a copingové strategie. In: *Učitelé a zdraví 4*, E. Řehulka, (Ed.), 39-52, Nakladatelství Pavel Křepela, ISBN 80-902653-9-4, Brno, Czech Republic

Valizadeh, M. et al. (2009). Efficacy of combined levothyroxine and liothyronine as compared with levothyroxine monotherapy in primary hypothyroidism: a randomized controlled trial. *Endocrine Research*, Vol.34, No.3, pp.80-89, ISSN 0743-5800

Vavrda, V. (2005). Změna kvality života: očekávání a realita. In: *Kvalita života a zdraví*, J. Payne et al., (Eds.), 176-180, Triton, ISBN 80-7254-657-0, Prague, Czech Republic

Vidal-Trécan, G. M., Stahl, J. E. & Durand-Zaleski, I. (2002). Managing toxic thyroid adenoma: a cost-effectivness analysis. *European Journal of Endocrinology*, Vol.146, pp. 283-294, ISSN 0804-4643

Vigário, P. et al. (2009). Perceived health status of women with overt and subclinical hypothyroidism. *Medical Principles and Practise*, Vol.18, pp. 317-322, ISSN 1011-7571

Vymětal, J. (2003). *Lékařská psychologie* (3rd ed.). Portál, ISBN 80-7178-740-X, Prague, Czech Republic

Walsh, J. P. et al. (2003). Combined thyroxine/liothyronine treatment does not improve well-being, quality of life, or cognitive function compared to thyroxine alone. *Journal of Clinical Endocrinology and Metabolism*, Vol.88, pp. 4543-4550, ISSN 0021-972X

Watt, T. et al. (2005). Which aspects of quality of life are relevant to patients with Graves' disease? *Thyroid*, Vol.15 (Suppl.1), p. S209, ISSN 1050-7256

Watt, T. et al. (2006). Quality of life in patients with benign thyroid disorders. A review. *European Journal of Endocrinology*, Vol.154, pp. 501-510, ISSN 0804-4643

Watt, T. et al. (2009). Establishing construct validity for the thyroid-specific patient reported outcome measure (ThyPRO): an initial examination. *Quality of Life Research*, Vol.18, pp. 483-496, ISSN 0962-9343

Wekking et al. (2005). Cognitive functioning and well-being in euthyroid patients on thyroxine replacement therapy for primary hypothyroidism. *European Journal of Endocrinology*, Vol.153, pp. 747-753, ISSN 0804-4643

Westerman M., Hak T., The, A. M., Groen, H. & van der Wal, G. (2006). Problems Eliciting Cues in SEIQoL-DW: Quality of Life Areas in Small-Cell Lung Cancer Patients. *Quality of Life Research*, Vol.15, pp. 441-449, ISSN 0962-9343

Whybrow, P. C. (1991). Behavioral and psychiatric aspects of thyrotoxicosis. In: *Werner and Ingbar's the Thyroid: a Fundamental and Clinical Text*, L. E. Braverman, R. D. Utiger, (Eds.), 863-870, J. B. Lippincott Company, Philadelphia, USA

Wiersinga, W. M., Prummel, M. F. & Terwee, C. B. (2004). Effects of Graves' ophthalmopathy on quality of life. *Journal of Endocrinological Investigation*, Vol.27, pp. 259-264, ISSN 0391-4097

Winsa, B. et al. (1991). Stressful life events and Graves' disease. *Lancet*, Vol.338, pp. 1475-1479, ISSN 0140-6736

Yang, H. & Zang, D. (2001). Coping style and personality of patients with Graves disease. *Chinese Mental Health Journal*, Vol.15, pp. 156-157, ISSN 1000-6729

Yoshiuchi, K. et al. (1998a). Psychosocial factors influencing the short-term outcome of antithyroid drug therapy in Graves' disease. *Psychosomatic Medicine*, Vol.60, pp. 592-596, ISSN 0033-3174

Yoshiuchi, K. et al. (1998b). Stressful life events and smoking were associated with Graves' disease in women, but not in man. *Psychosomatic Medicine*, Vol.60, pp. 182-185, ISSN 0033-3174

Zeng, Z., Ma, L., Luo, G. & Zhou, H. (2003). Clinical study of combined psychological treatments on hyperthyroidism. *Chinese Mental Health Journal*, Vol.17, pp. 382-384, ISSN 1000-6729